Current Topics In Inflammation and Infection

INTERNATIONAL ACADEMY OF PATHOLOGY

MONOGRAPHS IN PATHOLOGY

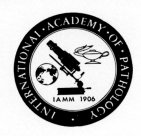

SERIES EDITOR, Nathan Kaufman, M.D.

Secretary-Treasurer
US-Canadian Division
International Academy of Pathology

INTERNATIONAL ACADEMY OF PATHOLOGY MONOGRAPH

Current Topics in Inflammation and Infection

EDITED BY **GUIDO MAJNO, M.D.**

Professor and Chairman
Department of Pathology
University of Massachusetts Medical School
Worchester, Massachusetts

RAMZI S. COTRAN, M.D.

F. B. Mallory Professor of Pathology
Harvard Medical School
and
Chairman
Department of Pathology
Brigham and Women's Hospital
Boston, Massachusetts

AND **NATHAN KAUFMAN, M.D.**

Secretary-Treasurer
United States-Canadian Division
International Academy of Pathology
Augusta, Georgia

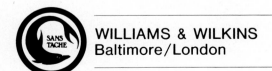

WILLIAMS & WILKINS
Baltimore/London

Made in the United States of America

Library of Congress Cataloging in Publication Data

Main entry under title:

Current topics in inflammation and infection.

   (Monographs in pathology; no. 23)
   Includes index.
1. Inflammation. 2. Infection. I. Majno, Guido. II. Cotran, Ramzi S. III. Kaufman, Nathan, 1915- IV. Series
RB131.C88   616'.047   81-16311
ISBN 0-683-05401-5   AACR2

Composed and Printed at
Waverly Press, Inc.
Mt. Royal and Guilford Aves.
Baltimore, MD 21202, U.S.A.

Foreword

This is the 23rd Monograph in the series of Monographs in Pathology initiated by the International Academy of Pathology in 1953. The various chapters are based on presentations for the Long Course entitled "The Inflammatory Process and Infectious Diseases" given on March 4, 1981, at the time of the 70th Annual Meeting of the United States-Canadian Division.

The Monograph allows for a more extensive treatment of each subject than was possible at the time of presentation and has the additional advantage of including a wide list of references which can serve as a convenient access to the recent literature.

Dr. Guido Majno, Professor and Chairman, Department of Pathology, University of Massachusetts Medical School, and Dr. Ramzi S. Cotran, F. B. Mallory Professor of Pathology, Harvard Medical School and Chairman, Department of Pathology, Brigham and Women's Hospital, were the Directors of the course and are the editors of this monograph. They have gathered an impressive group of scientists and clinicians as faculty for the course and as authors for the various chapters of the monograph.

The monograph deals briefly with a historical review, but the main thrust is the emphasis on recent developments in the basic understanding of the inflammatory process and the application of recent knowledge.

The Academy wishes to express its appreciation to Dr. Guido Majno, Dr. Ramzi Cotran, to the other distinguished contributors to this monograph, and to the publisher, The Williams & Wilkins Company, for their valuable support and cooperation.

NATHAN KAUFMAN, M.D.
Series Editor

Preface

Dangerous as it may be to use the word *never*, we have good reasons to suspect that there has never been a book entitled "Inflammation and Infection."

Why this one?

It is only too obvious that the two processes form a natural pair. We do teach our students that infection and inflammation can occur separately, but on the whole they do tend to occur together—and when they do there is a certain yin and yang quality to the association. Indeed, if we take the long view of evolution, it seems most likely that infection was a key stimulus for the development of the inflammatory reaction. The very neutrophils seem to have been created as antibacterial machines; when they appear on the scene in situations in which their favorite prey is absent (as in many allergic reactions), they perform their act anyway and do more harm than good.

There is no need to further justify the association of inflammation and infection, but we would like to point out that the two processes have acquired a novel order of unity within the framework of cell biology. Bacteria are cells (even if pathologists tend to frown at the notion) no less than basophils or endothelial cells. They use the language of receptors, as all cells do; they have devised all manner of cellular tricks for frustrating the defenses of tissue cells; they even take part in the inflammatory reaction by secreting, of all things, some of the inflammatory mediators: an absurd, suicidal effort, so great a mistake (on the part of the bacteria) that it leads one to wonder whether there may not be a broader picture that we do not see. In any event, here are the aggressors siding with the defenses. There is yin and yang, we are told.

An exhaustive coverage of both fields would have produced another series of volumes, which few would have cared to read. A more condensed format was suggested by the very mechanism that gave birth to the book: the content was originally planned as a program for a one-day course on "The Inflammatory Process and Infectious Diseases," under the aegis of the United States-Canadian Division of the International Academy of Pathology. We therefore attempted to select, for half-hour lectures, those aspects of inflammation and infection that seemed to be more novel, more exciting, more inspiring, and, in some cases, more unusual. The choice was arbitrary, and we apologize for all that was left out; we do believe, however, that what is here should provide enrichment to many colleagues, as it did to us.

GUIDO MAJNO
RAMZI S. COTRAN
Monograph Editors

Contributors

HARVEY CARP, PH.D.
Fellow in Pathology, University of New York at Stony Brook, Stony Brook, New York

DANIEL H. CONNOR, M.D.
The Director, Department of Infectious Disease, Armed Forces Institute of Pathology, Washington, D.C.

RAMZI S. COTRAN, M.D.
F. B. Mallory Professor of Pathology, Harvard Medical School and Chairman, Department of Pathology, Brigham and Women's Hospital, Boston, Massachusetts

JOHN E. CRAIGHEAD, M.D.
Professor and Chairman, Department of Pathology, University of Vermont School of Medicine, Burlington, Vermont

DEAN W. GIBSON, PH.D.
Research Scientist, Armed Forces Institute of Pathology, Washington, D.C.

AARON JANOFF, PH.D.
Professor of Pathology, University of New York at Stony Brook, Stony Brook, New York

GERALD T. KEUSCH, M.D.
Professor of Medicine, Chief, Division of Geographic Medicine, Tufts-New England Medical Center, Boston, Massachusetts

HELEN M. KORCHAK, PH.D.
Fellow in Medicine, Division of Rheumatology, New York University School of Medicine, New York, New York

GUIDO MAJNO, M.D.
Professor and Chairman, Department of Pathology, University of Massachusetts Medical School, Worchester, Massachusetts

RICHARD L. MYEROWITZ, M.D.
Director of Laboratories, Forbes Health System, and Clinical Associate Professor of Pathology, University of Pittsburgh, Pittsburgh, Pennsylvania

R. NEAL PINCKARD, PH.D.
Professor of Pathology and Medicine, University of Texas Health Sciences Center, San Antonio, Texas

EMANUEL RUBIN, M.D.
Professor and Chairman, Department of Pathology and Laboratory Medicine, Hahnemann Medical College and Hospital, Philadelphia, Pennsylvania

CHARLES N. SERHAN, B.S.
    Predoctoral Fellow in Pathology, New York University School of Medicine, New York, New York

FRANCIS A. WALDVOGEL, M.D.
    Professor of Medicine, Infectious Disease Division, Department of Medicine, University Hospital, Geneva, Switzerland

DAVID H. WALKER, M.D.
    Associate Professor of Pathology, University of North Carolina School of Medicine, Chapel Hill, North Carolina

PETER A. WARD, M.D.
    Professor and Chairman, Department of Pathology, The University of Michigan School of Medicine, Ann Arbor, Michigan

GERALD WEISSMANN, M.D.
    Professor of Medicine, New York University School of Medicine, New York, New York

EVGENYA ZHKARINSKY, M.D.
    Research Associate, Department of Pathology and Laboratory Medicine, Hahnemann Medical College and Hospital, Philadelphia, Pennsylvania

ANNEMARIE ZIEFER, M.D.
    Visiting Scientist, Armed Forces Institute of Pathology, Washington, D.C.

Contents

Chapter 1

Inflammation and Infection: Historic Highlights

GUIDO MAJNO

Before we plunge into the intricacies of prostaglandins and slow viruses, it will be appropriate to acknowledge that we are not the first to explore the depths of inflammation and infection. The roots of both concepts can be traced back almost as far as the earliest written records.

Medical terms for a clinical entity identifiable as "inflammation" can be found in the clay tablets of Mesopotamia as well as in the earliest Egyptian medical papyri (19). Clay tablets referring to inflammation are not rare in King Assurban-ipal's great library, which was buried with the destruction of Nineveh in 612 B.C.; three are reproduced in Figure 1.1. Notice that in each one of these the word meaning "inflamed" is written differently; this is due to the complexities of cuneiform spelling: the word as represented derives in each case from the verb *napāḫu*, which means *to blow*. In the mind of an Akkadian, blowing and heat were closely linked; like the American Indians and many other ancient people, the Akkadians started their fires with a drill, a procedure which requires a great deal of puffing. To qualify a reddened skin as "blown skin" made very good sense in that setting.

Another term used in medical texts to mean "the hot thing" is *ummu*, which can be—depending on the context—either fever or inflammation. The ideogram for *ummu* (Fig. 1.2) means nothing to most of us today. With the aid of the late Professor Labat of the Collège de France, I was able to trace its derivation, and to convince myself that the symbol for the word *ummu* as we find it in 700 B.C. is actually the last stage of a slow transformation: a Sumerian pictogram (Fig. 1.3, *bottom*) was simplified, then rotated counterclockwise by 90° for convenience in writing, then reproduced with many separate cuneiform signs printed (rather than drawn) into the clay, and then again simplified. When this sequence is traced backward to the source, we find that *ummu* derives from an ancient Sumerian pictogram representing a flaming brazier, perhaps 2000 years older than *ummu* as spelled at the time of Assurbanipal.

You may wonder whether this bit of information could be applied in any way in your daily life. I can think of one possible application. There is another Akkadian word (again from the time of Assurbanipal) in which *ummu* is inscribed inside a kind of frame (Fig. 1.4, *top*). Now trace that complicated sign back to the origin, as we did for *ummu*; rotate it back by 90° clockwise; and find the

1

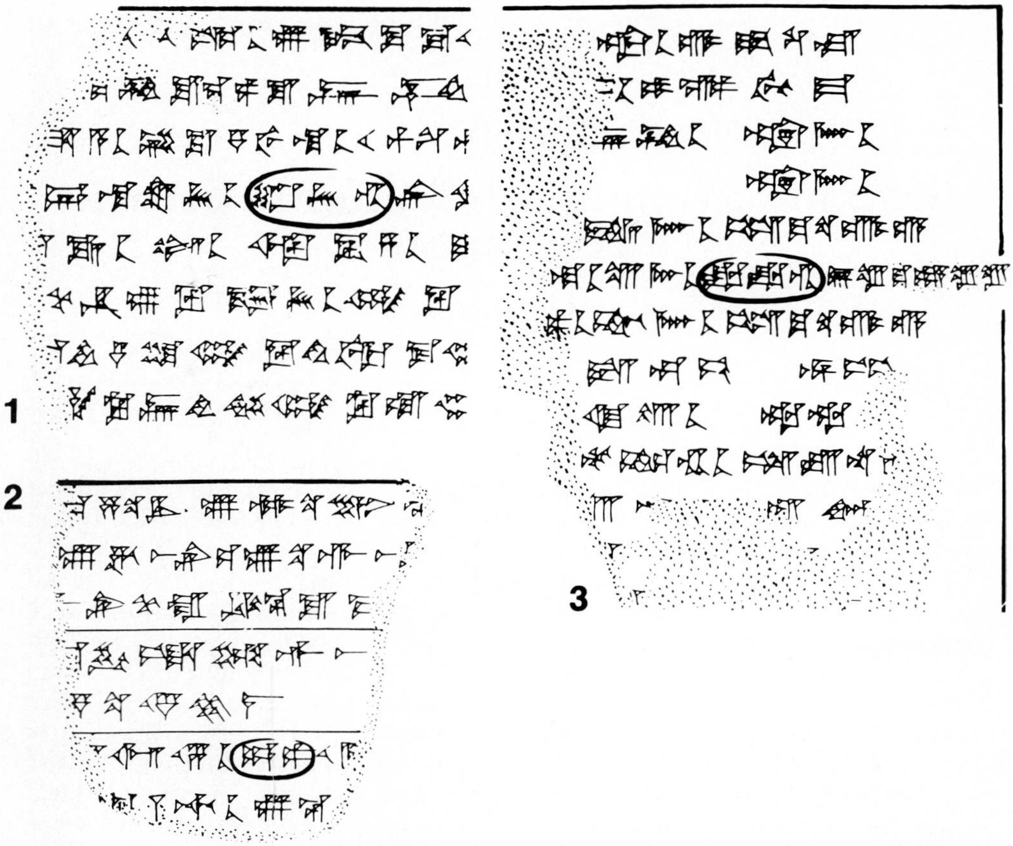

FIG. 1.1. Fragments of three cuneiform tablets found in the archives of King Assurbanipal (7th century B.C.). The words encircled mean *inflamed*: (1) "If a man, his right eye is inflamed ... " (2 *and 3*) ... his guts are inflamed ... " (Reproduced with permission from G. Majno (19).)

corresponding Sumerian pictogram: this is again a flaming brazier inside something that looks like a bottle. Actually, this frame is the outline of a human chest. So we have obtained *inflammation inside the chest*: your professional background may lead you to suspect that we are dealing with the most ancient record of pericarditis. In fact, the condition—heat inside the chest—is far more benign: this was the Sumerian sign for *love* (19).

The ancient Egyptians, too, had words to denote inflammation; they recur, among others, in the famous Smith Papyrus, also referred to as the "Surgical Papyrus," which dates from about 1650 B.C. but represents the copy of a much older text, perhaps from 2500 B.C. (19).

In hieroglyphic writing the words are represented by consonants only; we must guess the vowels, for which we have very few clues. To make these awkward clusters of consonants readable, it is customary to fill the vowel spaces with as many e's as necessary; thus *nfr*, good, will be read *nefer*.

One of the terms used for *inflammation* or *inflamed* is s-r-f (*seref*) (Fig. 1.5). Note that after the word there is a peculiar oblong sign. This is not pronounced;

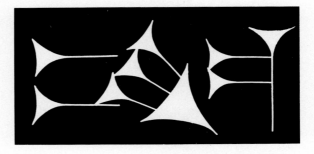

FIG. 1.2. This word, written in cuneiform script, reads *ummu*; it can mean either *fever* or *inflammation*. Its origin is explained in the next figure (Reproduced with permission from G. Majno (19).)

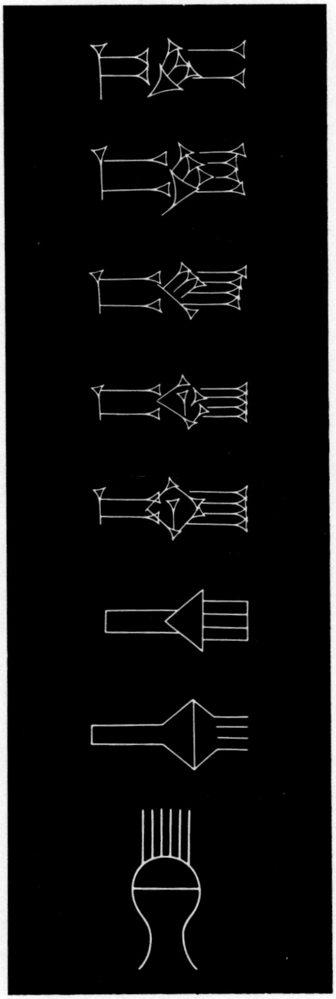

FIG. 1.3. The cuneiform rendition of the word *ummu* (*top*) derives from the stepwise transformation of a much older Sumerian pictogram (*bottom*) representing a flaming brazier.

it is one of about 100 such signs called *determinatives* (Fig. 1.6) that were used to give the general concept of the preceding word. The determinative was a handy device for distinguishing two unrelated words that had the same consonants and were therefore written the same way (consider the problem of distinguishing

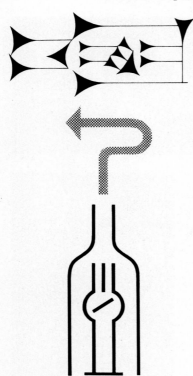

FIG. 1.4. The Akkadian word for *love* (*top*) is written with the word *ummu* (fever or inflammation) inside a frame. This seemingly obscure set of signs derives from a much older Summerian pictogram (*below*) which clearly explains the significance of the composition: *a flaming brazier inside a human chest.*

FIG. 1.5. One of the ancient Egyptian words for *inflammation* is spelled s-r-f (today's guess at the pronounciation is *seref*). It also stood for "warmth, passion" (9). It is written with three signs (a folded cloth, a mouth, a horned viper) that correspond to s,r,f, as indicated below each symbol. The last sign at the right—the key to the whole word—is explained in the following figure.

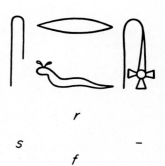

between *cat* and *act*, if both were spelled *ct*) (10). In this particular case, *seref* means something hot; hence, the little sign used as determinative is a flaming brazier. When it is fully painted in color, *e.g.*, in the illustration of a papyrus scroll, the details clearly show a pot with two handles, filled with burning oil, and surmounted by a plume of smoke curling downward.

So, at the origin of both the Mesopotamian and the Egyptian words for inflammation, we find a flaming brazier. There is no doubt that those ancient medical texts were dealing with *the hot thing*.

All this may sound very remote, but it is closer than you may suspect. The

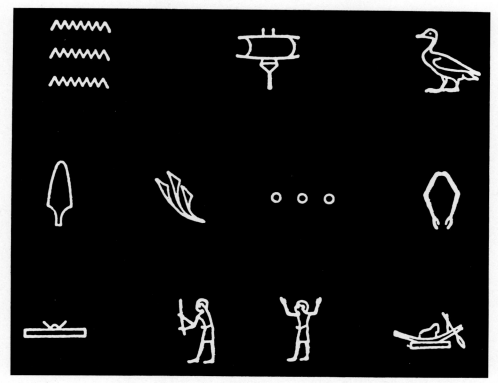

FIG. 1.6. To avoid the ambiguity due to spelling without vowels, many Egyptian words were followed by a sign called *determinative*, which explained the general idea of the word; here are some determinatives (from *top left* to *bottom right*): "watery thing," "windy thing," "bird," "tree," "bush," "mineral" (grains), "embracing," "theoretical concept [a papyrus scroll tied with a knot], "done with effort," "high, joyful" "boat" (10).

word *seref* has the typical structure of semitic words, which are built around three consonants (s + r + f). A Hebrew word still used today, *saraf*, means *to burn, to destroy by fire* (Fig. 1.7); *sarefet* means "boil, phlegmon" and *saraf* means *angel* (seraphim): guardian angel (1), surely the ultimate transformation of *inflammation*.

As regards the history of infection, I will certainly not attempt an overview; interested readers may find good sources (4, 15, 28, 30, 32, 33). Since most of us tend to correlate the discovery of infection with the works of Pasteur and Lister, I will limit my "highlights" to a few key episodes in the history of infection before Pasteur and Lister, episodes that are much less known but deserve greater recognition.

The notion that live agents can invade the body, make their home within it, and cause disease has been very difficult to accept for the medical profession. It meant that a new, impalpable threat was lurking in the outside world, whereas traditional medicine had taught for two millennia that disease came from inside, from an imbalance of the humors. This may explain why the concept of infection has such an unlikely history.

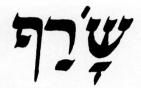

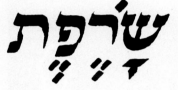

FIG. 1.7. The semitic root *srf* which gave rise to the ancient Egyptian word for *inflammation* survives in many words of modern Hebrew: here are some examples (from *top* to *bottom*): *saraf*, to burn, to destroy by fire; *sarefet*, boil, phlegmon, contusion; *saraf*, angel (seraphim).

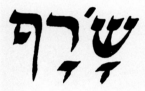

It did not burst into blossom with the discovery of bacteria; in fact this discovery had very little impact on medicine for almost 200 years. Bacteria, as well as man, were drawn into the act relatively late, after the basic principles of parasitism had been worked out thanks to maggots, itch mites, gallnuts, silk-worms, and fungi. Human infectious diseases were actually studied as applied science after infectious diseases of milk, beer, and wine had been conquered as industrial problems, a curious reversal of applied science as currently understood.

The key words related to infection show that we are dealing with a very ancient concept. *Sepsis* was a well established notion for Aristotle (2); it referred to fermentation and especially putrefaction, and was opposed to *pepsis*, digestion without putrefaction (18). The term *antisepsis*, instead, did not appear until 1712 (29). *Infectio* is a Latin noun corresponding to the verb *inficere*, which means literally to *put in*, hence, to dip, to dye, to stain, to darken, to taint, to spoil (17).

The transmission of disease from one human being to another is recorded—once again—in the clay tablets of Mesopotamia: "If his testicles are inflamed, if his penis is covered with sores, he has gone to the High Priestess of his god" (19) (a reference to the custom of ritual prostitution). This may have been a double infection: chancroid plus gonorrhea, which often caused bilateral epididymo-orchitis before the era of penicillin. However, we can only say that the contagion was *recorded*; it may not have been *perceived* as such. In the context of Mesopotamian thinking, the High Priestess might well have punished her male devotee for having previously committed a sin.

Oddly enough, we have nothing to learn about contagion from the Hippocratic books; infection, contagion, and even venereal disease are simply not discussed among the 70 works that constitute the Hippocratic collection, apart from a single remark to the effect that epidemic diseases must be caused "by the air that we breathe" (12). Surely, this cannot mean that physicians at the time of Hippocrates (~460–380 B.C.) did not recognize the existence of infection and contagion; we can only surmise that some pertinent book was lost. Consider, for instance, that there is not a single reference to snake bite in the Hippocratic collection; it is inconceivable that Greek physicians should not have been trained to deal with snake bite, which is to this day a concern in all the Mediterranean world.

For once, where the Greek texts are silent, we must credit the Romans with a bit of insight that may be original with them. Marcus Terentius Varro, a contemporary of Julius Caesar, wrote that swamps breed tiny animals that cannot be seen with the eye, but when they penetrate into the body through the nose and mouth, they cause severe diseases (31).

A few specific infectious diseases can be identified in the texts of antiquity. Mumps is clearly described in a Hippocratic book (11); the Persian physician Rhazes (~850–923 A.D.) described smallpox (24). Today it seems obvious that such diseases are transmissible; it was not so obvious to medieval physicians trained in the tradition of Greek, Arabic, or Indian medicine, all of which believed in the doctrine of faulty humors. When the medical profession was faced with epidemics of catastrophic proportions—such as the Black Death—this endogenous mechanism was difficult to defend; yet, it was essential to find an acceptable explanation, so that a rational prevention could be worked out. During the Middle Ages the public at large tended to believe in *contagion, i.e.,* in the transmission of some mysterious agent by contact with the sick person or with a contaminated object; whereas the medical profession, impressed by the fact that many individuals were "contacted" but never caught the disease, felt that there had to be some other explanation, and leaned toward the concept of *miasma* (32). By this was meant a mysterious atmospheric change that hung over towns and villages like a cloud, arising perhaps from swamps or from corpses rotting in the open. Preventive measures varied accordingly. Those who believed in contagion practiced cleanliness and avoided human contacts; by contrast, the notion of miasma implied running away, or creating suitable smokes to purify the air, and breathing as little as possible (this is actually recommended in that single Hippocratic passage on epidemic disease (12)). Consider what might happen to a ship landing in Palermo, Sicily, in the early 1500s and suspected of carrying the plague (32). All men were sent ashore to a secluded place, where there garments were removed (some were burned, some washed and perfumed for 50 days); the men were then exposed to fumes of boiling pitch and washed down with vinegar. Each type of cargo was treated in a specific manner: barrels were washed with sea water and then with vinegar; salt was considered not infectable and was not treated. Other merchandise was aired and perfumed ashore for 50 days; the sails and ropes of the ship were taken down, sunk in the sea for a week, then hung from the masts until the end of the quarantine; last, the inside of the ship was fumigated with cauldrons of boiling pitch for 50 days. How did *Yersinia pestis* fare throughout all these travails? If it was carried by the ships' rats and their fleas (as textbooks say), it probably survived the ordeal; if it was carried primarily by human fleas (as was recently proposed (8)) the public health officers had not worked in vain.

THE THEORY OF CONTAGION: GIROLAMO FRACASTORO
(1484–1553)

The most dreaded diseases of the Middle Ages and early Renaissance were the black plague and leprosy, to which syphilis was added at the close of the 15th century. Somehow, the first two had no outstanding champion (although books about the plague sprang up everywhere). Syphilis, instead, became a source of inspiration to an Italian physician of Verona, Girolamo Fracastoro, who was also a poet, latinist, physicist, astronomer, pathologist, and geologist as well; he was the first to refer to the magnetic poles of the earth and shared with Leonardo the first true interpretation of fossils. However, his major claim to fame rests on two books: one on syphilis (which he thus named) and one on contagion, which appeared in 1546 (9). This book is extraordinarily important in the history of infection, because it shows how far one can go by simple observation and by studying what we now call the *natural history* of diseases. Here is a summary (32) of Fracastoro's concept of the mechanism of infection drawn from his clinical experience: (a) many diseases are caused by transmissible, self-propagating entities, which he conceives as chemical substances; (b) each disease has its own specific agent; (c) the agent propagates itself in the tissue of the host, and causes disease by setting up chemical, putrefactive changes; (d) the agents vary in their capacity to survive in the environment; (e) the agents may originate in the body or outside; (f) the agents are spread by contact, at a distance, or by the intermediary of "fomites" (infected objects); (g) to produce disease, each agent must find an analogy in the tissues of the host; and (h) the treatment must destroy the agent, check the putrefactive processes set up by them, and neutralize the action by "antipathetic" substances.

This is perhaps the most brilliant piece of insight between Hippocrates and Pasteur. Consider that *it was achieved without the benefit of a single experiment*. This was, in fact, its very weakness: lacking proof, and being 300 years ahead of its time, it left its followers with little firm ground to stand upon.

THE "LIVING CONTAGION" (CONTAGIUM ANIMATUM):
ATHANASIUS KIRCHER (1602–1680)

About 70 years after Fracastoro's death, simple microscopes became available. A Jesuit working in Rome, Athanasius Kircher, became an ardent microscopist; he was also a physician, mathematician, physicist, optician, musician, egyptologist, and genius or quack, depending on the sources. He studied the blood of "feverish" people and saw "thousands of little worms" (14). It is pointless to speculate what species of protozoa he might have been able to see with his microscope, because he also reports an experiment with putrid water in which these little worms developed wings and flew out. Whatever he actually saw or imagined, he became enthused with the notion that contagion can be caused by living creatures: *contagium animatum*. So, *as Fracastoro had proposed a correct microscopic theory of infection without a microscope, Kircher improved upon the theory by misinterpreting his microscopic experiments*.

Kircher was right for the wrong reasons, but he still persisted in believing that his little worms were generated within the body. With characteristic exuberance he submitted his works to a celebrated Italian physician, Francesco Redi; the response was extremely courteous but skeptical (22): Redi himself had already dealt the first blow to the theory of spontaneous generation.

MAGGOTS, MITES AND GENIUS: FRANCESCO REDI (1626–1697)

Redi practiced in Florence (Fig. 1.8); he lived the leisurely life of a *gentiluomo*, but was also a born student of natural phenomena, a skillful user of the microscope, and a member of the prestigious Florentine Academy of Science (the Accademia della Crusca). He corresponded with top scientists of his time (including Kircher, the gentle Malpighi, and Steno (25) and was a poet of some repute, especially for his verses in praise of good wine. The Grand Duke of Tuscany used

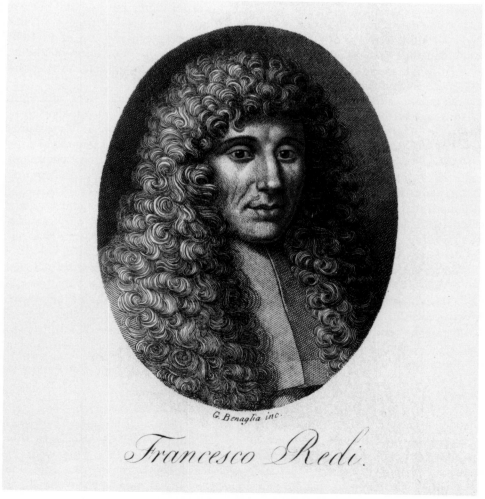

G. Benaglia inc.

Francesco Redi.

FIG. 1.8. Francesco Redi (1626–1697).

to send him all the unusual objects of nature that came to his attention (a huge sea turtle, a bottle of French "hemostatic water") so that Redi might work out their mysteries, which he did very objectively. In 1684 Redi published—with appropriate inserts of poetry—his study of spontaneous generation. This theory had been generally accepted ever since Aristotle; a scientist of great fame, van Helmont (1577–1644), to whom we owe the word *gas* and pioneer studies on digestion, had recently offered this formula for making mice: take a jar, put into it a dirty shirt and some grain, store it away in a warm place, and after a time the mice will appear (32)!

One of the "proofs" of spontaneous generation was the appearance of hordes of insects, including maggots, in and around rotting bodies. Redi began experimenting with maggots, for which he did not even need his microscope. He put pieces of fresh meat or fish into a jar, and left it open; after several days the flesh was teeming with maggots. Then he repeated the experiment, but covered the jar with a fine gauze: no maggots ever developed inside this jar, but frustrated flies could be seen flying above the cover and depositing eggs on top of it. Redi concluded that "rotten stuff has no other function in the generation of insects than to provide a suitable place for laying eggs at the proper time, so that the offspring will find therein a convenient pasture" (23).

This simple experiment opened a wide crack in the foundations of classic Aristotelian biology. Having established that the maggots in rotten food were really the offspring of flies, Redi went on to study the little wormy creatures found in live cherries, peaches, and pears, and proposed that the same held true.

His friend Malpighi was quick to grasp the message: in the second volume of his little known *Anatomy of Plants*, the gallnut is properly explained as a reaction to a parasite (4, 20).

Thus, at this point, it was established that *rotten food, as well as plants, could be parasitized by an insect*. Notice that this first step in the study of parasitism was performed with creatures visible to the naked eye; the microscope was not yet necessary.

We owe the next step to a young pupil of Redi, Giovancosimo Bonomo (1666–1696) and to his friend Giacinto Cestoni, a pharmacist, who owned a microscope (4). They chose to study scabies, which plagued the inmates of their home town, Livorno (also in Tuscany). The minuscule itch mite that causes scabies, *Acarus scabiei*, had already been seen; it was even known to Shakespeare (27). In Romeo and Juliet—what unlikely company for itch mites—Mercutio fantasizes about a tiny fairy wagon, driven by

> A small grey-coated gnat
> Not half as big as a round little worm
> Prick'd from the lazy finger of a maid
> .... (27)

Worm may not be accurate, but *round* certainly is, and we also learn that laziness was supposed to breed these creatures in the fingers (27). They were the smallest animals visible with the naked eye: in fact the words *acarus, mite*, and *atom* convey the same meaning of *indivisible* (28). It was then believed that black bile reached the skin and caused it to produce mites; thus the therapy was strictly internal: purging and bleeding to remove the bile. Now Bonomo and Cestoni discovered that the mites were insects like all others: they even laid eggs! This decisive event actually happened, just once, under their microscope: it was witnessed by their artist while he was portraying the mite (Fig. 1.9). If the mites developed from eggs, and not from humors of the patient's body, it was most likely that they came from outside to infect the skin, like Redi's flies had flown into the jar to parasitize the meat.

Thus, just 8 years after Redi's experiment, we have an application to man (1687): it had important therapeutic significance, because if the itch mites came from outside, proper therapy had nothing to do with bleeding and purging: the best hope was in the *local* application of an ointment to kill the mites. Bonomo and Testoni tried it, and it worked.

THE DISCOVERY OF BACTERIA: ANTONI VAN LEEUWENHOEK (1632–1723)

At the same time that Redi was working with his maggots, a janitor of the City Hall in Delft, Holland—a draper by trade—was busy making microscopes of his own design; throughout his long life he built some 247 of those, and wrote up his observations in 375 papers. The story of van Leeuwenhoek is too well known to be retold here; the only point that I wish to make is that he first observed bacteria in 1676 (16): thus the bicentennial of the United States was also the tricentennial of a great discovery (which, as far as I know, was never celebrated). Van Leeuwenhoek discovered his bacteria ("animalcula") accidentally, in water in which he had suspended some pepper, hoping to discover why it tasted so hot. He found more animalcula in the whitish material collected between his own teeth. It never occurred to him that such creatures might cause disease. During the 1700s, this idea did surface here and there; in Italy, for instance, Bartolomeo Cogrossi, a Milanese physician, had read about the itch mite and about Leeuwenhoek and proposed that some such creature could explain the epidemic disease that was destroying the cattle in his time (4, 6). In London, in 1720, Benjamin Marten thought that invisible creatures could also be the cause of tuberculosis (21). There was even a charlatan, one Dr. Boyle, who operated in Paris between 1726 and 1727 and attempted to make a fortune by demonstrating to patients the "animalculae" which he collected from their blood; he sold appropriate "anti-animalculae" specific for each disease (4). His trick was discovered, and he vanished. In essence, during the 1700s, no significant progress was made in the understanding of infection.

Yet it should have been possible to formulate the germ theory of disease (32): Fracastoro had postulated the rules of contagion; Kircher had proposed the notion of *contagium animatum*; Redi and his group had demonstrated the exogenous origin of parasites; Leeuwenhoek had discovered bacteria. *Why did all these discoveries lie dormant for a whole century?* It has been said that the responsibility may rest upon the shoulders of Thomas Sydenham (1624–1689), the "British Hippocrates," who had a near total disregard for the concept of contagion. For Sydenham, diseases followed a vaguely metaphysical, unchangeable course of 30 or 40 years; epidemics were linked to a particular "constitution"

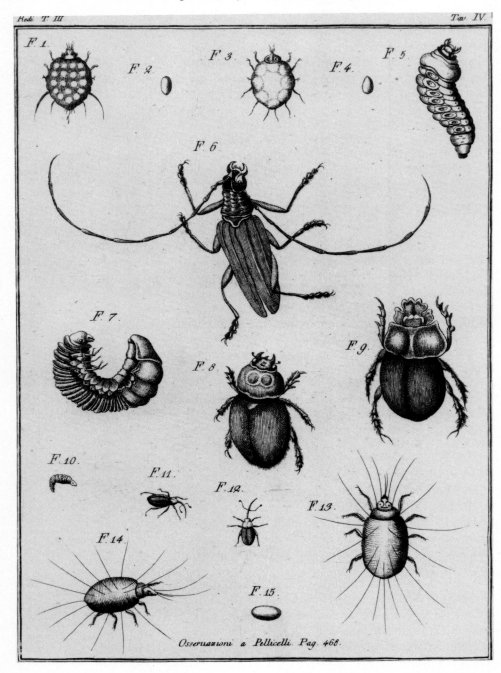

FIG. 1.9. A plate from the complete works of Francesco Redi. *Top left, Acarus scabiei (F. 1),* which two of Redi's associates recognized as the cause of scabies. Next to it is the egg that it had laid under the microscope. (The other insects were thrown in for good measure.)

of a given year, and this constitution was "dependent upon a certain secret and inexplicable alteration of the bowels of the earth, such as the air becomes impregnated with effluvia as subject human bodies to particular distempers" (32).

It may be too much to say that Sydenham held back epidemiological progress for 2 centuries (32), but his influence must have played a role in this stagnation.

FUNGI AS A CAUSE OF DISEASE: AGOSTINO BASSI (1773–1856)

At the very end of the 1700s (1798), there graduated in Pavia, near Milan, a young man called Agostino Bassi. To please his parents he took his degree in the law, but he had managed to sneak in some courses in mathematics, physics, chemistry, and natural history, so as to "follow his own inclinations" (4). Among his teachers was Spallanzani, whose experiments against spontaneous generation are today better known than those of Redi. A mysterious eye disease forced Bassi to abandon the law and to work as an administrator of estates; thus he became acquainted with a peculiar disease of silkworms (*moscardino*) which was threatening to destroy the silk industry of northern Italy. In a series of very simple experiments, Bassi demonstrated that the disease was caused by a contagious agent, which he identified as a fungus (3) (how his eye disease could prevent him from studying the law, while allowing him to use the microscope, was never explained). The general astonishment at this discovery was so great that the fungus, which belonged to the species *Botrytis*, was named *Botrytis paradoxa* (it is now called *Botrytis bassiana*). Botrytis, incidentally, is not always a wicked fungus: it is also the agent of the "noble rot" which gives sweet wines their taste (19).

The news spread like wildfire; Bassi's dead, dried-up little silkworms were requested all over Europe. Some landed in Zurich, in the hands of Johann-Lucas Schoenlein, a famed clinician (1793–1864). Schoenlein had already been wondering as to the possible "botanical" nature of certain human diseases of the skin; excited by the discovery of Agostino Bassi, he looked up some patients suffering from what he called *Porrigo lupinosa*, scraped their skin, and found in it the fungus that became *Achorion schoenleinii*. He published this discovery in a single page, in *Virchows Archiv*, in 1839 (26). Five years after the discovery of Agostino Bassi it was realized that *fungi could infect human beings.* The concept of infection was now well established. At this time, Louis Pasteur was about 17 years old.

PHYSICIANS AS A CAUSE OF INFECTION: OLIVER WENDELL HOLMES (1809–1894)

Shortly after Schoenlein's communication, another paper that could have saved thousands of lives appeared in an obscure medical journal on the far side of the Atlantic Ocean: the *New England Quarterly Journal of Medicine and Surgery* of April 1843 (13). The journal ceased to be published a year later, and the paper—by Oliver Wendell Holmes—was largely forgotten.

Holmes was another poet-physician, as well as Professor of Anatomy at Harvard Medical School. He was 34 at the time and had no experiments to report; his impassionate message consisted of clinical observations and literature on

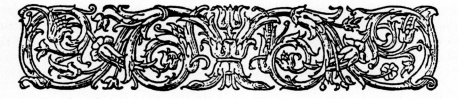

Puerperal Fever as a Private Pestilence

BY

OLIVER WENDELL HOLMES, M.D.

Parkman Professor of Anatomy and Physiology in Harvard University

INTRODUCTION

IT HAPPENED, some years ago, that a discussion arose in a Medical Society, of which I was a member, involving the subject of a certain supposed cause of disease, about which something was known, a good deal suspected, and not a little feared. The discussion was suggested by a case, reported at the preceding meeting, of a physician who made an examination of the body of a patient who had died with puerperal fever, and who himself died in less than a week, apparently in consequence of a wound received at the examination, having attended several women in confinement in the mean time, all of whom, as alleged, were attacked with puerperal fever.

FIG. 1.10. The historic paper by Oliver Wendell Holmes (13). Opening page.

puerperal fever. For instance (Fig. 1.10) it had been reported "locally" (note the merciful expression) that "a physician who made an examination of the body of a patient who had died with puerperal fever . . . himself died in less than a week, apparently in consequence of a wound received at the examination"; in the meantime he had "attended several women in confinement . . . all of whom were attacked with puerperal fever." Dr. Holmes had become almost obsessed with the notion that puerperal fever was due to a "poison" carried by the physician and listed a horrifying series of examples proving that "within the walls of lying-in hospitals there is often generated a miasma, palpable as the chlorine used to destroy it, tenacious . . . and deadly in some institutions as the plague." He felt that this morbid poison was "generated in the course of the disease," correctly related it to erysipelas, and concluded that some physicians carried it on them-

selves as a *private pestilence*; hence, the title of his second paper on this subject
12 years later. (Because his first publication had made no impact, except for
arousing detractors, he republished it word for word in 1855 under the title
Puerperal Fever as a Private Pestilence (13).) In this reprint Holmes adds
statistics to his arguments and concludes that puerperal fever is "professional
homicide . . . taught from the chairs [*of his detractors in Philadelphia*]. The
pestilence carrier in the lying-in chamber must look to God for pardon, for man
will never forgive him." This paper, written in the most florid, emphatic, colorful
but highly accurate style, should be required reading for every medical student.
It was reprinted as a "Medical Classic" in 1936 and stands as an everlasting
example of crystal-clear reasoning based on clinical observation.

The credit for the discovery of puerperal fever as an infectious disease usually
goes to Ignaz Semmelweis (1818–1865), who had not yet graduated from medical
school when Holme's paper appeared; however, in the 1855 reprint, among the
new references there appears a communication from France, reporting observations of a Monsieur "Semmeliveis."

I mention Oliver Wendell Holmes in this context because his first paper saw
the light two decades before Pasteur's fundamental works and represents another
step toward establishing that human disease can be caused by a transmissible
"miasma" capable of propagating itself.

INFECTION OF WOUNDS: HOSPITAL GANGRENE

The lying-in hospitals of the 18th and 19th century provided Holmes and
Semmelweis with a tragic mass experiment on women, leading to the discovery
that puerperal fever was an infection carried by physicians; at the same time
another mass experiment led to a similar conclusion for wounded men—in the
military hospitals.

This chapter is less well known, and I can only summarize it here. "Hospital
gangrene" (called in French *pourriture d'hôpital*, "hospital rot") was a dreaded
disease, primarily in military hospitals. Today, it is easy to explain it as the result
of massive acute infection of wounds, in the days preceding asepsis and antisepsis.
English and French medical texts of the early 1800s are filled with studies of
hospital gangrene; there was much debate as to its nature, and whether it was
contagious or not.

In 1815, a little-known *mémoire* was published in France by a surgeon, J.
Delpech (7); it was a report on hospital gangrene among thousands of wounded
soldiers, victims of Napoleon's campaigns, when they were crowded into the
hospitals of Montpellier. The conclusions of Dr. Delpech are startling because
they state in unmistakable terms some of the principles of Lord Lister. The cause
of hospital gangrene, said Dr. Delpech, is always external; the disease is "essentially contagious"; the nature of the contagion "seems to be animal"; the miasma
"is not just derived from the material that brought the contagion: *it seems that
the infected surface has the property of reproducing a material quite similar to
that which caused the infection.*" The contagion was definitely caused by contact
with unclean materials, such as lint and surgical instruments; *when the instruments were washed in vinegar or flamed, the gangrene became far less common!*

This *mémoire* was written in 1815; ironically, it was lost from memory—

although it had come from a highly authoritative source. Why was it buried? Perhaps (and this was suggested to me by a medical student) because it was military medicine of the losing side.

It is not enough to be right: one has to be right at the right time, in the right place.

The purpose of this short essay was to outline some of the incidents, accidents, and discoveries that paved the way to Pasteur and Lister. If any lessons may be drawn from it, they are self evident. I will simply point out, in closing, that among the seven or eight main figures in our story, one was a draper, one was a lawyer, and three were poets.

ACKNOWLEDGMENTS

This work was supported in part by a grant from the Commonwealth Fund. I am also indebted to Professor Luigi Belloni of Milan for constant help and advice; his excellent papers on the theory of *contagium vivum* were a key to this chapter. It is a pleasure to thank Daniel Z. Silverstone, who pointed out to me the link between the Egyptian and the Hebrew srf; Dr. David Neiman of the Department of Theology, Boston College, for the Hebrew calligraphy; and Dr. Harold M. Constantian, who suggested a diagnosis for the devotee of the High Priestess.

REFERENCES

1. Alcalay, R. *Complete Hebrew-English Dictionary.* Tel Aviv, Masada Press, 1965.
2. Aristotle. *Historia animalium*, VI, 569a 28, London, Loeb Classics Library, W. Heinemann; Cambridge, Mass., Harvard University Press, Tranlated by A. L. Peck, Vol. II. pp. 282–283, 1970.
3. Bassi, A. Del Mal del Segno Calcinaccio o Moscardino. Torino, 1837.
4. Belloni, L. I secoli Italiani della dottrina del contagio vivo. In: *Per la Storia della Medicina*, edited by L. Belloni, pp. 111–126. Milan, A. Forni, 1980.
5. Bonomo, G. Osservazioni intorno a' pellicelli del corpor umano, altre volte pubblicato sott 'l nome del Signor Dottor Giovancosimo Bonomo. (Reprinted in: Redi, F., *Opere*, Milano, Vol. III, pp. 439–468, 1809–1811.)
6. Cogrossi, C. F. *Nuova idea del male contagioso de' buoi.* Milan, 1714. (Reprinted and translated by L. Belloni and D. M. Schullian (eds.), c/o Sez. Lombarda Soc. Ital. Microbiol., VI Internatl. Congr. Microbiol., Rome, Nov. 2–6, 1953.)
7. Delpech, J. Mémoire sur la complication des plaies et des ulceres, connue sous le nom de pourriture d' hôpital. Paris, 1815.
8. Ell, S. R. Interhuman transmission of medieval plague. *Bull. Hist. Med. 54:* 497–510, 1980.
9. Fracastoro, G. *Hieronymi Fracastorii, Liber i De Sympathia et Antipathia Rerum. Liber i de Contagione, et Contagiosis Morbis et Eorum Curatione* . . . Lugduni, 1550.
10. Gardiner, A. *Egyptian Grammar.* London, Oxford University Press, 1966.
11. Hippocrates. *Epidemics I,* i (Loeb Classics Library, Cambridge, Mass., Harvard University Press; London, W. Heinemann, translated by W. H. S. Jones, Vol. I, pp. 146–149).
12. Hippocrates. *Nature of Man*, XI (Loeb Classics Library, London, W. Heinemann, and Cambridge, Mass., Harvard University Press, translated by W. H. S. Jones, pp. 26–29, 1959).
13. Holmes, O. W. *The Contagiousness of Puerperal Fever (1843)* and *Puerperal Fever as a Private Pestilence (1855).* (Reprinted in: *Medical Classics*, E. C. Kelly (ed.), pp. 194–268. Baltimore, Williams & Wilkins, 1936.
14. Kircher, A. Athanasii Kircheri e Societate Iesu Scrutinium Physico-Medicum Contagiosae Luis, quae Pestis dicitur . . . Romae, Typis Mascardi, 1658.
15. Klebs, A. C. The history of infection. *Ann. Med. Hist.,* x. I, 169–173, 1917.
16. Van Leeuwenhoek, A. *The Collected Letters of Antoni van Leeuwenhoek,* edited and annotated by a committee of Dutch scientists, Vol. II. Amsterdam, Swets and Zeitlinger, 1941.

17. Lewis, C. T., and Short, C. *A Latin Dictionary*, p. 945, Oxford, Clarendon Press, 1962.
18. Liddell, G. L., and Scott, R. *A Greek-English Lexicon*, p. 1398. Oxford, Clarendon Press, 1968.
19. Majno, G. *The Healing Hand*. Cambridge, Mass. Harvard University Press, 1975.
20. Malpighi, M. Anatomes plantarum. In: *Malpighi, Opera Omnia*, Lugduni Batavorum, P. Vander, 1687, Vol. II, *De Gallis*, pp. 112–132.
21. Marten, B. *A New Theory of Consumptions*. London, 1720.
22. Redi, F. *Opere*. Milan, 1809–1811.
23. Redi, F. *Opere*, Vol. III, pp. 1–201, Milan, 1803–1811.
24. Rhazes (al-Razi) Muhammad ibn Zakariyya: *A Treatise on Smallpox and Measles*, English translation by W. A. Greenhill. London, Sydenham Society, 1848.
25. Scherz, G. *Steno. Geological papers*. Odense University Press, 1969.
26. Schoenlein, J. L. Zur Pathogenie der Impetigines. Arch. Anat. Physiol. Wiss. Med. 82, 1839.
27. Shakespeare, W. *The Tragedy of Romeo and Juliet*, R. Holsey (ed.), Act I, Sc. 4. New Haven, Yale University Press, 1954.
28. Singer, C. and Singer, D. The development of the doctrine of *contagium vivum*, 1500–1750. XVII Internatl. Congr. Med., Sect. Hist. Med., pp. 187–207, 1913.
29. Skinner, A. *The Origin of Medical Terms*, p. 34. Baltimore, Williams & Wilkins, 1961.
30. Temkin, O. An historical analysis of the concept of infection. In *Studies in Intellectual History*, Boas *et al.* (eds.) pp. 123–147. Baltimore, The Johns Hopkins Press, 1953.
31. Varro, Marcus Terentius *On Agriculture*, I xii (Loeb Class. Lib., London, W. Heinemann, and Cambridge, Mass., Harvard University Press, Translated by W. D. Hooper, pp. 208–209, 1967).
32. Winslow, C-E. A. *The Conquest of Epidemic Disease*. Princeton University Press, 1943.
33. Wood, W. B. *From Miasmas to Molecules*. New York, Columbia University Press, 1961.

Chapter 2

The Endothelium and Inflammation:
New Insights

RAMZI S. COTRAN

The role played by vascular endothelium in inflammation has been recognized since the days of Cohnheim, who witnessed the exudation of fluid and cells across the lining of blood vessels in the frog's tongue. Until the past decade, however, the endothelial cell was regarded as a relatively passive cellular membrane, forming the interface between blood and tissues. This notion was based on two considerations: first, the simple structure of endothelial cells which are hardly visible with the light microscope and poorly endowed with the usual cell organelles; and, second, the conclusion of physiological studies that transfer of water and solutes across capillary endothelium was determined largely by physical factors, such as blood flow and pressure gradients, and not by cell activity. Even in inflammation, the role of endothelium was thought to be a *reactive* one. Chemical mediators derived from other cells or plasma separated the endothelial junctions, causing vascular leakage, and neutrophils and monocytes—responding to some stimulus outside the vessel wall—squeezed between endothelial cells into the interstitial space. The endothelial cell "just sat there."

Historically, the first suggestion that endothelium was a more active participant in acute inflammation was the observation by my coeditor, Guido Majno *et al.*[99] that gaps between endothelial cells induced by histamine, formed not because this mediator loosened some tight intercellular junction but because endothelial cells actively contracted in response to a specific stimulus.

Today, our concept of endothelium has totally changed, and it has become clear that the endothelial cell is a functionally active component of the vessel wall, is capable of a variety of metabolic, synthetic, and regenerative activities, and is involved in the regulation of such phenomena as blood flow, coagulation, growth of vascular wall cells, immunological reactivity, and also in the organism's response to pathological stimuli.

The major advances in endothelial research began with the development by Jaffe *et al.*[82] and Gimbrone *et al.*[59] of reproducible methods for endothelial culture. These investigators first used human umbilical vein endothelium as a culture source, but it has since become possible to culture endothelia from a variety of species and from veins, arteries, and even capillaries (see review by Gimbrone).[56] The most recent advance in the culture field is the long-term culture of capillary endothelial cells, and the elegant demonstration by Folkman and his associates[43, 44] of the formation of entire capillary networks *in vitro* from single clusters of capillary endothelial cells.

Much of the impetus for current endothelial research comes from formulation of two concepts seemingly unrelated to inflammation: the first is the "response to injury" hypothesis of atherosclerosis, which considers endothelial injury as the initial event in atherogenesis,[119] and the second is the concept that new blood vessel formation, so-called neovascularization, is an important control point in the growth of tumors (tumor angiogenesis).[42] However, the contributions from the numerous studies concerned with these two areas of research are also relevant to the role of endothelium in classical inflammatory responses, since atherosclerosis appears—in large part—to be the arterial reaction to injury and exhibits many features of classical inflammation.[86] Furthermore, neovascularization is a prominent component of wound healing and chronic inflammatory responses.[42]

This chapter will briefly review only selected aspects of recent endothelial research. For more comprehensive coverage of the subject, the reader is referred to recent reviews and books.[1, 4, 27, 42, 54–56, 78, 97, 121, 126, 145, 150, 152]

ENDOTHELIAL PERMEABILITY AND ENDOCYTOSIS

The well-known function of endothelium as a selective permeability barrier between blood and tissues continues to be the subject of considerable investigation. However, the long-standing uncertainty as to the ultrastructural basis of endothelial permeability to small molecular weight lipid-insoluble substances is still unresolved. While there is general agreement that the pinocytotic vesicles in continuous capillary endothelium[110] represent the large-pore system postulated by physiologists (~500 Å),[150] the issue of whether the "small pores" are represented by the pinocytotic vesicles or the intercellular junctions is still controversial. Earlier studies using horseradish peroxidase (MW 40,000) as tracer suggested that this protein traversed the endothelium across intercellular junctions, at least in the myocardium and diaphragm.[88] More recently, however, Simionescu *et al.*, using smaller hemepeptides (MW 1,900), provided evidence for transport across vesicles, particularly in the true capillaries of the diaphragm.[129-133] These authors showed that such vesicular transport occurs either because a single vesicle fuses with the luminal and abluminal membranes, giving rise to a short channel, or chains of fused micropinocytotic vesicles give rise to a longer transendothelial channel. Such channels are thought to be transient and are focally narrowed by strictures related to the points of fusion; the strictures are presumed to be the equivalent of the restrictive "small pore."[131] In addition, diaphragms similar to those seen in fenestrated endothelium sometimes bridge the openings of vesicles, and these are interpreted as another mechanism for size restriction. While the photographic evidence provided in these studies is impressive, the distribution and frequency of transendothelial channels has not been established. Several authors have failed to confirm their presence with sufficient frequency to account for macromolecular transfer.[18, 150, 156] What has become clear from the studies of the past few years is that endothelia vary considerably as to structural and permeability characteristics not only from tissue to tissue, but also even within different segments of the microcirculation in the same organ. Thus, in the diaphragm, the intercellular junctions of the arterioles, and the entire length of the capillary, are impermeable to the hemeundecapeptide (20 Å), while in the small venules, about one quarter of the junctions are sufficiently open to allow passage of this tracer.[131, 132] Such differences in junctional permeability are also reflected by ultrastructural differences, as seen by freeze etch techniques.[132]

Beyond the issue of pores, pore sizes, and intercellular junctions, recent data suggest an interesting influence of the surface properties or the metabolic state of endothelium upon the process of pinocytosis or transfer by these cells.

The luminal surface of vascular endothelia is covered by a cell coat (glycocalyx) containing abundant anionic sites, which can be stained by such cationic substances as ruthenium red and cationized ferritin.[94, 114, 140] In certain endothelia, there is preferential concentration of such anionic sites in certain microdomains of the luminal plasma membrane, e.g., the fenestral diaphragms of fenestrated pancreatic and intestinal capillaries.[134, 135] Biochemical and enzyme digestion studies indicate that these anionic sites contain sialoglycoproteins and proteoglycans, the most important of the latter being heparin sulfate.[5, 19, 50, 125] The sialoproteins and proteoglycans probably play diverse roles in endothelial function (some of these will be discussed later in this chapter), but recent evidence suggests strongly that these anionic sites influence the process of pinocytosis, and possibly also transendothelial permeability. Almost a decade ago, Garby and Areekul[51] showed increased permeability to neutral dextran, as compared to the negatively charged dextran sulfate in rabbit ear vessels.[51] More recently, Davies *et al.*[32] studied the effects of endothelial surface charge on endocytosis and degradation by bovine aortic endothelium in culture. Figure 2.1 shows the quantitative uptake of three different preparations of horseradish peroxidase, one negatively charged (pI < 3.6), one slightly catonic (pI 8), and one cationic (pI 9.5–10.5); although the molecules were of equal size, the uptake of the anionic molecule was significantly lower than that of native peroxidase, and the latter in turn was lower than that of cationic peroxidase. The difference in uptake was not due to an effect of the charged molecules themselves on the rate of pinocytosis, since uptake of labeled sucrose measured simultaneously was the same under the three conditions. Of

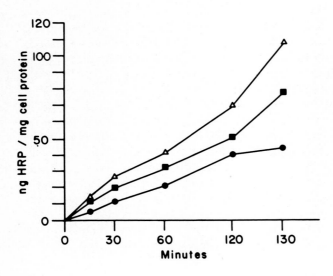

Fig. 2.1. Uptake of anionic (●), native (■), and cationic (△) HRPases in confluent cultured arterial cells at 37°C. Cells were incubated with 1 mg HRPase/ml medium. Intracellular HRPase activity was determined in duplicate cultures following washing, dispersal of cells with trypsin, and solution in Triton X-100. (Reproduced with permission from P. F. Davies, H. G. Rennke, and R. S. Cotran (34).)

equal interest is that altering the charge of the molecule affected not only the pinocytosis, but also degradation. Thus, the half-life for anionic horseradish peroxidase was 95 hours, that for neutral peroxidase 18 hours, and that for cationic peroxidase 8.2 hours. It was further shown that the speed of degradation of one molecule could be altered by previous exposure to another charged molecule.

The precise influence of charge-dependent pinocytosis on transendothelial permeability *in vivo* is unclear, as is the potential significance of changes in endothelial anionic sites under pathological conditions. However, the importance of anionic sites to the permeability of renal glomeruli is now well established,[16, 117, 148] and it may well be that the reported differences in distribution of anionic sites in fenestrated endothelium may be involved in the control of endothelial permeability in such vessels.[134] Studies of experimental atherosclerosis suggest that one of the early events in experimental hypercholesterolemia may be a decrease in anionic sites of endothelium in atherosclerosis-susceptible areas of the arterial system.[53]

Another potentially important influence on pinocytosis is the cell cycle state of endothelium. Davies *et al.* found that the rate of fluid pinocytosis increased in actively growing cells as compared to quiescent cells.[33, 34] Vlodavsky *et al.*[149] showed increased uptake of low density lipoprotein (LDL) by replicating endothelium, and Davies presented evidence that increased LDL binding is closely related to the cell cycle, though apparently uncoupled from actual cell growth. These well cycle-dependent changes may well affect the uptake of lipoproteins into the endothelium in atherogenesis.

One word of caution: these studies on pinocytosis in culture measure uptake and interiorization, not transfer. The former processes may be relevant to diverse other functions of endothelium, rather than to transendothelial permeability.

ANTIPLATELET AND ANTITHROMBOTIC PROPERTIES OF ENDOTHELIUM

One of the fundamental properties of normal endothelium is that it does not promote the adherence of platelets or activation of the blood coagulation system.[152] Indeed, it remains as true today as first suggested by Virchow that endothelial injury is the major stimulus for the initiation of local thrombus formation. *In vivo* and culture studies of the past decade have shown that this property is due not only to the presence of endothelium as a physical barrier between blood and thrombogenic subendothelial connective tissue, but also to active antithrombotic functions of endothelium, serving to limit thrombus formation in the vicinity of foci of endothelial injury. Some of these antithrombotic activities are listed in Table 2.1.

PROSTACYCLIN (PGI₂)

In 1975, Gimbrone and Alexander[58] demonstrated that cultured human umbilical vein endothelial cells were stimulated to produce prostaglandin E by certain vasoactive agents, and suggested that such prostaglandins might be important in modulating platelet function in hemostasis. In 1976, Moncada *et al.*[105, 106] reported the presence of prostacyclin (PGI-2) in microsomal factions of aorta and showed that prostacyclin is one of the most potent inhibitors of platelet aggregation.[105, 106]

Prostacyclin (PGI₂)
Plasminogen activator
Thrombin-binding sites
    Antithrombin III cofactor
      Protein C activation cofactor
Heparin/heparan sulfate
Alpha-2-macroglobulin
Ecto-ADPase

Subsequently, Weksler and her associates[154] confirmed the synthesis of PGI-2 by human umbilical vein and bovine aortic endothelial cell cultures, and it now appears that the most important antithrombotic activity of endothelium is PGI-2 production.[9, 10, 62, 154] While normal endothelial cells in culture show little PGI-2 production, marked stimulation of PGI-2 synthesis occurs after addition of arachidonic acid,[62, 154] or in the presence of *thrombin*.[154] One scenario postulated for the role of PGI-2 in thrombus formation is as follows: a focus of injury to endothelium results in loss of PGI-2 production which tends to promote thrombosis. Thrombin is then formed at the site of injury, and this stimulates PGI-2 synthesis by endothelial cells in adjacent *noninjured* areas, tending to limit the number of platelets involved in the primary response and helping to localize thrombus formation. Under such circumstances, therefore, endothelial cells contribute both to thrombus formation and to the localization of the thrombus. PGI₂, however, does not appear to be the factor preventing *adhesion* (rather than aggregation) of platelets to normal endothelium.[31]

PLASMINOGEN ACTIVATOR

It has long been known from studies with the fibrin gel technique that endothelium is associated with fibrinolytic activity and thus may contribute to clot dissolution. Studies by Loskutoff and his associates[90, 92, 93] have recently shown that this fibrinolytic activity is due to the presence of a membrane-associated plasminogen activator (PA) which converts plasminogen to plasmin. Of interest is that in some endothelia, such as rabbit venous endothelium, this fibrinolytic activity is obscured by the presence of an inhibitor of plasminogen activator in the cytosol of endothelial cells. Inhibition occurs at the level of plasmin formation, not plasmin activity, and the inhibitor appears to be distinct from the inhibitory antifibrinolytic activity observed in plasma, platelets, and other cell types.[93] These findings suggest that fibrinolytic activity in endothelium represents a balance between activator and inhibitor properties and that certain stimuli might well affect one or the other of these two activities and thus influence fibrin deposition in areas of local injury. Thus, the tumor-promoting molecule phorbol-myristate acetate (PMA) markedly stimulates plasminogen activator activity, but thrombin results in marked *inhibition* of PA activity.[93a]

THROMBIN BINDING

Awbrey *et al.*[7] have recently shown that thrombin binds to cultured human umbilical vein endothelium rapidly, irreversibly, and with high affinity. Such thrombin binding is potentially antithrombotic in two ways: (a) Lollar and Owen[91] provided evidence that inactivation of thrombin by antithrombin III may be catalyzed by thrombin binding to endothelium *in vivo*, and (b) Esmon and Owen[38] also showed the presence of a cofactor in endothelial cultures which enhances the rate of activation of vitamin K-dependent protein-C. The latter exerts a potent anticoagulant effect by inactivating factors V A, VIII A, and the platelet receptor for factor X A. Both of these activities are potentially antithrombotic. How they relate to each other is still unclear, as is the relationship of such thrombin binding to the presence of heparin or heparan sulfate on the endothelial surface. It is at least theoretically possible that deficiencies in these binding sites, or in the cofactor, or potential inhibitors of these activities may play a role in the induction of thrombotic disorders.

Of interest to the issue of thrombin binding is the recent report by Savion *et al.*[123] that subsequent to internalization and degradation of thrombin by corneal endothelial cells in culture, there was a curious *up regulation* of thrombin binding sites, as contrasted to the usual down regulation which occurs after binding; these authors suggested that this up regulation may represent a mechanism for maintaining relatively low levels of extracellular thrombin.

OTHER ANTITHROMBOTIC PROPERTIES

(a) *Heparan Sulfate.* As stated earlier, the endothelial surface contains several glycosoaminoglycans, including heparan sulfate. Heparan sulfate is among the small family of sulfated glycans known to catalyze the thrombin-antithrombin III reaction. One possibility is that this heparin-like substance on the endothelial surface is responsible for the binding of thrombin and catalysis of the thrombin-antithrombin III reaction described earlier[91]; (b) *Alpha 2 macroglobulin* appears to be an integral component of the endothelial lining.[13] Alpha 2 macroglobulin is known to have broad antiprotease activity, and it may well influence enzyme reactions of the coagulation and fibrinolytic process; (c) Finally, the endothelial surface has an ecto-ADPase activity which serves to convert adenosine diphosphate released from platelets to adenosine, which is a platelet inhibitor of great potency. Pearson *et al.*[111-113] also suggested that this ectoenzyme may act in injured endothelial cells which release with ATP and ADP.

ENDOTHELIUM AND THE METABOLISM OF VASOACTIVE MEDIATORS

Vascular endothelium participates in the metabolism of or appears to secrete a number of vasoactive mediators which play a role in the regulation of vascular tone and in the vascular response in inflammation (Table 2.2). Endothelium contains kininase-2 activity, which serves to degrade the vasoconstrictive agent bradykinin[72]; this seems to be similar to angiotensin-converting enzyme, which converts angiotensin I to the powerful vasoconstrictive agent angiotensin-2.[23, 72, 85, 120, 155] Several metabolites of arachidonic acid metabolism, including PGE-2, PGF-2α, and prostacyclin (PGI-2) are synthesized by endothelium, and their synthesis is stimulated by a variety of physiological and pathological stimuli.[9, 10, 58, 62, 154] The majority of these activities are vasodilatory, but recently thromboxane, a vasoconstricting agent, has been added to the list,[79] and it is possible that

TABLE 2.2. ENDOTHELIAL METABOLISM AND VASOACTIVE MEDIATORS

Bradykinin degradation (kininase II)
Angiotensin-converting enzyme activity
Arachidonic acid (AA) metabolism
    Production of PGI_2, PGE_2, and $PGF_{2\alpha}$
    ? Other AA metabolites
Uptake and degradation of amines (serotonin, catecholamines)
Histamine formation?

other byproducts of the lipo-oxygenase catalytic system may also be elaborated by endothelium (see Chapter 3). Endothelium, particularly pulmonary endothelium, also appears to degrade vasoactive amines, including serotonin and catecholamines, and substance P, a vasoactive peptide, is also inactivated by human endothelial cells in culture.[83, 87, 109, 118, 127, 128, 141] In addition, endothelial cells are said to have histamine-forming capacity, through the presence of the enzyme histidine decarboxylase.[35]

At present, the precise interactions among all of these activities—some causing vasoconstriction and others vasodilatation—is unclear. However, the scenario that emerges is that there must be an important relationship between the endothelium and the underlying smooth muscle which reacts to cause vasoconstriction or vasodilation. Such a relationship has been shown in recent experiments in which bradykinin and acetylcholine caused relaxation of pulmonary arteries only when the endothelium was left intact.[26]

ENDOTHELIAL RECEPTORS AND BINDING SITES

In concert with what is known for other cell types, it might well turn out that many of the activities of endothelium are due to the presence of receptors to the various vasoactive mediators, coagulation proteins, hormones, lipoproteins and, as we shall see later, growth factors[20] (Table 2.3). The demonstration of high affinity binding sites for thrombin has been discussed earlier.[7] The endothelium has also been shown to have receptors for insulin, and Schafer *et al.*[124] demonstrated the presence of beta-adrenergic adenyl cyclase-driven receptors, suggesting that some endothelial functions may be regulated by circulating vasoactive hormones that raise cellular cyclic nucleotide content. Friedman *et al* showed that whereas normal endothelium does not possess Fc or C3 receptors, such receptors can be induced by viral infection *in vitro*. These receptors may serve to bind immune reactants to virally infected cells.[46, 47]

TABLE 2.3. SOME ENDOTHELIAL RECEPTORS AND BINDING SITES

Thrombin
Insulin
Beta-adrenergic
Fc or C3 (inducible)
Chemotactic peptides
Plasmodium-infected erythrocytes

One receptor system that I find particularly appealing is that recently suggested by experiments of Hoover and his associates,[76, 77] namely that endothelial cells possess receptors for *chemotactic peptides*.[76, 77] These authors quantitated the adhesion of neutrophils to cultured endothelium using scanning microscopy and ^{51}Cr-labeled neutrophils. Their most interesting finding is that pretreatment of either polymorphonuclear leukocytes or endothelial cells with chemotactic agents, including synthetic chemopeptides (*e.g.*, formyl-methionyl-leucyl-phenyl-alanine) caused increased adherence of neutrophils. Scatchard plot analyses of the binding of the radioactive peptide fMet-Leu-Phe suggested a small population of high affinity specific binding sites for this chemopeptide.Whether these receptors for chemotactic agents are present *in vivo* is, of course, unknown. However, if true, these findings may be critical to the process of leukocytic margination in inflammation. By binding to endothelium, the chemotactic agents may render it more adhesive, thus directing the neutrophils to the site of injury. Here again, the endothelium serves to actively direct the traffic of leukocytes into the inflammatory focus, rather than react passively to these events.

More recently, Udeinya *et al.*[146] found that erythrocytes infected with the late stages of the human malarial parasite *Plasomodium falciparum* adhere to cultured human endothelial cells by knob-like protrusions. The authors suggested that there is a specific receptor-like interaction between endothelial cells and a component in the knob of infected erythrocytes. Such interactions also may be important in the adhesion and penetration of other infection agents across the vessel wall.

ANTIGENS ON THE ENDOTHELIAL SURFACE

In spite of highly sophisticated techniques for tissue typing, rejection remains a major cause of graft failure. Curiously, the difference in graft survival for patients with HLA identical renal transplants is no more than 30% better than for patients transplanted with fully mismatched kidneys.[11, 12] In addition, 30–40% of totally mismatched kidneys appeared to function over 5 years. Recently, it has been suggested that these discrepancies may be due, in some part, to the fact that vascular endothelial cells, which are the primary interface between vascularized organs and tissues, possess HLA-DR and endothelial specific antigens and might be more important in graft rejection than the traditional HLA A and B histocompatibility antigens. Indeed, the Leiden group has shown that typing for the more recently defined HLA-DR antigens may have a greater impact on graft survival.[11, 12]

Table 2.4 lists some of the antigens shown to be present on endothelium. In addition to the HLA-AB and HLA-DR systems, endothelial cells possess specific antigens which are shared only with monocytes (E-M antigens)[107]; the latter are found in highest concentrations in the kidney on peritubular capillaries. Baldwin *et al.*[12] further showed that DR antigens appear to be present in larger quantities

TABLE 2.4. IMMUNOLOGICALLY IMPORTANT ENDOTHELIAL CELL ANTIGENS

ABD blood group antigens
HLA-A,B,C antigens
HLA-D antigen*
HLA-DR antigens
Endothelial-monocyte alloantigens (E antigens)

[a] Detected by proliferation of allogeneic lymphocytes.

in endothelium than in tubules. This may explain the frequent occurrence of vasculitis in renal rejection. Although it is too early to assess the significance of these new findings, a detailed study of the antigenic profile of endothelium may be of critical importance to the understanding of graft survival.

Of equal interest is the demonstration that endothelial cells may function as *accessory cells* for T cell activation,[89] in a manner similar to the accepted accessory role of monocytes and dendritic cells in these reactions. The evidence for this is as follows: (a) Freshly isolated endothelial cells and endothelium *in situ* express Ia antigens as judged by immunofluorescence microscopy.[71] (b) endothelial cells in culture stimulate a mixed lymphocyte reaction.[74, 75, 104] (c) human umbilical vein endothelial cells in culture display antigen presenting properties in an *in vitro* system, replacing monocytes in this reaction.[21, 73] Human umbilical vein endothelial cells can also replace monocytes in mitogen-induced human T cell activation *in vitro*.[2] Despite this evidence, however, it must be cautioned that the most minimal contamination with monocytes or dendritic cells or their products may negate these findings. Thus, the role of endothelium as an antigen-presenting cell in immunobiology must await further investigations.

ENDOTHELIAL INJURY

The ultrastructural studies of the 1960s established two fundamental types of endothelial injury in inflammation.[28, 29, 98, 121] The first, termed *"histamine type"* vascular injury consists of the formation of intercellular gaps in the endothelium and accounts for much of the characteristic vascular leakage in inflammation. These gaps occur almost exclusively in small- and medium-sized venules. Majno *et al*[99] presented persuasive evidence that the gaps form as a result of contraction of endothelial cells mediated by vasoactive agents. This sort of injury is relatively short-lived (at least after single injections of vasoactive agents) and seems to be common to the vast majority of permeability-increasing chemical mediators studied, such as histamine, serotonin, bradykinin, and C3 and C5a. Similar studies have not been performed with the new class of chemical mediators, such as the prostaglandins, the leukotrienes, and acetyl glyceryl ether phosphoryl choline (AgePC) (Chapter 3). The second type of endothelial injury, known as *"direct vascular injury,"* is characterized by outright endothelial necrosis, resulting in increased vascular permeability and frequently in local thrombus formation.[30] This type of injury is thought to result from the direct effects of the injurious agent (*e.g.*, a burn or chemical), but there is no *a priori* reason that endothelial necrosis and denudation could not also be caused by a chemical mediator. Indeed, recent evidence suggests that endothelial injury sufficient to cause Cr51 release in endothelial cultures[122] (and marked edema in the lung) may be caused by oxygen-derived free radicals released from leukocytes adherent to endothelium. It is also possible that some of the new mediators of inflammation, particularly the potent lipid molecules, may result in severe injury resembling the so-called direct type (see also Chapters 3 and 6).

In addition to these two types of injury, which affect mainly endothelial barrier function, there is increasing evidence that endothelial injury may be reflected by alterations in any one of the many functions of endothelium described earlier *without necessarily causing endothelial denudation* or *endothelial gaps*. This concept of *"endothelial dysfunction,"* well-developed by Gimbrone[55] in context of the "response to injury" hypothesis of atherosclerosis, may also well hold true in the classical inflammatory response. Thus, while overt endothelial desquamation is rarely seen early in the development of atherosclerosis in hypercholesterolemic animals, such animals exhibit foci of increased endothelial replication,[41] increased permeability to horseradish peroxidase (without denudation),[143] diminution in surface anionic sites,[53] and increased monocyte adhesion.[52, 53] Another example of such endothelial dysfunction is the altered pinocytosis caused either by changes in surface charge or in the cell cycle, as detailed earlier (p. 21). Finally, it has been shown that virally or chemically transformed endothelial cells,[31, 158] unlike normal endothelial cells, are highly adhesive to platelets in culture. Gimbrone postulates that transient interactions of circulating platelets with such altered endothelial cells could result in platelet adhesion and release of products which contribute to the acute inflammatory response in the absence of overt desquamation, at least initially.[56] Table 2.5 lists the several documented or postulated types of endothelial injury.

TABLE 2.5. TYPES OF ENDOTHELIAL INJURY

Interendothelial gaps
    Histamine-type chemical mediators (lesions restricted to venules)
    ? Direct-delayed injury (lesions in capillaries and venules) (48)
Endothelial necrosis and desquamation
    Direct injury (lesions in all segments of microcirculation)
    ? "New" chemical mediators
    ? Oxygen-derived radicals
Endothelial "dysfunction" (injury without desquamation)
    altered pinocytosis
    widening of intercellular junctions
    altered cell replication
    increased leukocyte adhesion
    increased platelet adhesion
    others

ENDOTHELIAL REPAIR, NEOVASCULARIZATION, AND THE ROLE OF MACROPHAGES

One of the main components of wound healing and of chronic inflammatory responses is the formation of new blood vessels, so-called neovascularization. This process has been the subject of intensive study because of the demonstration by Folkman and his associates[42, 45] that neovascularization induced by tumors (tumor angiogenesis) is of great importance in the growth of solid tumors *in vivo*. These studies have shown that tumor-induced and inflammatory neovascularization are fundamentally similar responses, although they are more sustained in the case of tumors, and are governed by different stimuli. Four processes appear to underlie the formation of new blood vessels, induced either by tumors or by inflammatory stimuli[4, 6] (Fig. 2.2): (a) migration; (b) proliferation; (c) maturation of endothelial cells; and (d) alterations in the extracellular matrix, including basement membrane, allowing for the extension of vascular sprouts. Although these four processes may be under separate control mechanisms, the vast majority of studies in the past few years have dealt with the identification of factors that

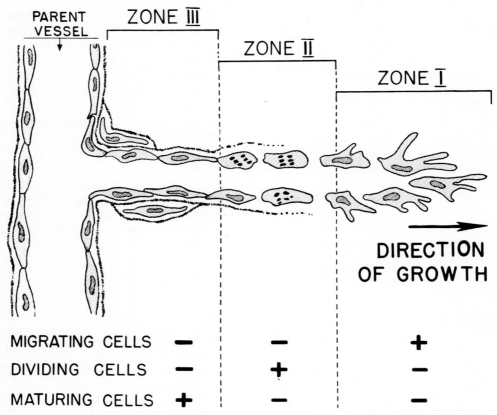

Fig. 2.2. Diagram of various processes in formation of a new capillary sprout—migration, proliferation, and maturation of endothelial cells. The fourth process involves alterations in the extracellular matrix and basement membranes (see text). (Reproduced with permission from D. H. Ausprunk (4).)

TABLE 2.6. FACTORS REPORTED TO CAUSE NEOVASCULARIZATION *IN VIVO* OR STIMULATION OF ENDOTHELIAL GROWTH *IN VITRO*

	Neovascularization *in Vivo*	Stimulation of Cell Growth or DNA-synthesis *in Vivo*
Tumor-derived factors (TAF)	+ (45)	+ (3, 15, 39, 43)
Macrophage-derived growth factor	+ (115, 144)	+ (69, 102, 151)
Epidermal growth factor	+ (64, 66, 67)	+ (64, 66, 67)
Fibroblast growth factor	+ (64, 66, 67)	+ (64, 66, 67)
Endothelial conditioned medium	+ (49, 70)	+ (49, 70)
Submaxillary gland extract	+ (84)	+ (84)
Hypothalamic extract	ND	+ (96)
3T3 adipocytes	ND	+ (25)
Corpus luteum	+ (68)	ND
Plasminogen activator	+ (14)	ND
Retinal growth factor	+ (61)	+ (61)

[a] References are in parentheses ( ) and are not all-inclusive. A more comprehensive list appears in ref. 126.

induce endothelial cell proliferation.[126] Table 2.6 lists some of the factors reported to cause endothelial cell growth *in vitro*, or angiogenesis *in vivo*. It can be seen that they represent a heterogeneous group of substances derived from plasma, inflammatory cells, mesenchymal cells, or tumors. Here I would like to briefly review evidence from our own laboratory implicating a macrophage-derived factor in inflammatory neovascularization and in the growth of endothelial cells, fibroblasts, and smooth muscle.[57, 60, 100–103, 115, 116, 136–139]

A role for macrophages in neovascularization is suggested by a number of *in vivo* observations. First, there is the well-known histological association of macrophages with proliferating capillaries in granulation tissue. Secondly, Polverini *et al.*[115] showed that during the delayed hypersensitivity reaction, induced with tuberculin or dinitrochlorobenzene, endothelial cell proliferation, as judged by ^{3}H thymidine labeling, coincided with the peak of monocytic infiltration.[115] Using a guinea pig cornea model to assess neovascularization, Polverini *et al.* then demonstrated that injection of activated macrophages from guinea pig or mouse consistently induced capillary proliferation (Fig. 2.3) and that this vascularization was not due to an immunological reaction induced by the injection of foreign cells.[116] It was further shown that intracorneal implantation of slow release polymers containing conditioned media from cultured activated macrophages produced a similar neovascular response.[116] Table 2.7 summarizes these data. Similar observations of macrophage-induced neovascularization have also been reported by Hunt and his coworkers using both cultured macrophages and wound fluids.[69, 144] It should be noted, however, that the presence of macrophages is not an absolute requirement for new blood vessel growth. For example, Sholley and Cotran,[137–139] using a thermal injury model of inflammation in leukopenic rats, observed endothelial proliferation in the virtual absence of monocytic infiltration. Further, granulomas which are replete with altered macrophages are relatively avascular. The point to make, however, is that macrophages are particularly good candidates for modulation of endothelial growth in inflammatory reactions since a number of factors influence synthesis and secretion of biologically active molecules by these ubiquitous cells.[147]

In subsequent studies *in vitro*, Martin *et al.*[102] showed that mouse peritoneal macrophages secrete a growth-promoting activity that stimulates the growth of 3T3 fibroblasts, vascular smooth muscle cells, and vascular endothelial cells in culture.[102] Production of this so-called macrophage-derived growth factor

TABLE 2.7. NEOVASCULARIZATION INDUCED BY MACROPHAGES AND MACROPHAGE-CONDITIONED MEDIUM IN GUINEA PIG CORNEA

Cell Preparations	No. of Corneas Tested	% Neovascular Response
Controls	24	0
Homologous resident	12	8
Homologous activated	18	78
Autologous activated	4	100
Isologous activated	8	75
Heterologous resident	12	8
Heterologous activated	25	68
Macrophage-conditioned medium*	23	65
Control media*	12	8

Reproduced with permission from P. J. Polverini *et al.*[115] For methods, see ref. 115.

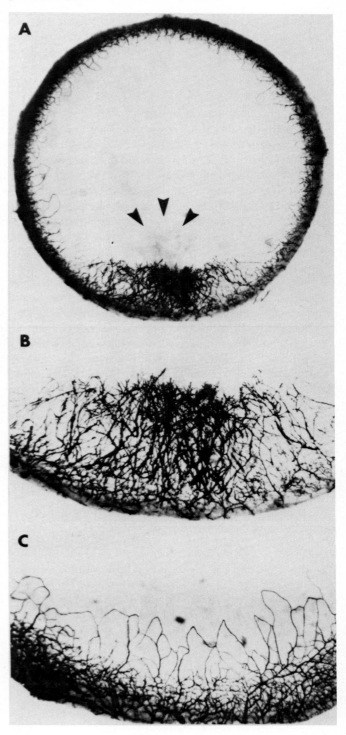

FIG. 2.3. (*A*) Whole mount preparation of guinea pig cornea showing growth of capillaries (labeled by intraarterial injection of colloidal carbon) towards site of injection of 5×10^5 homologous activated macrophages (*arrows*). (*B*) Higher magnification of capillary sprouts. (*C*) Normal vessels of control limbus. (Reproduced with permission from P. J. Polverini *et al.*[115].)

(MDGF) was directly related to the number of viable macrophages in culture and was independent of plasma-derived protein factors. Of particular interest is that treatment of cultured macrophages with activating agents, such as bacterial lipopolysaccharide, results in increased growth factor production. Preliminary biochemical characterization of MDGF indicates that it is a nondialyzable protein containing at least one essential disulfide bond and that it is not a serine protease. A similar growth factor has been since demonstrated in human monocytes, particularly after they are activated *in vitro*.[101, 103]

The capacity of macrophages to secrete a factor which causes the growth of endothelium, fibroblasts, and smooth muscle may be of critical importance in inflammatory neovascularization, fibroplasia, and atherosclerosis.

Much less is known of the stimuli for endothelial migration. Studies by Zetter[157] show that the conditioned medium from confluent sarcoma 180 cells induces significant endothelial migration *in vitro*, in addition to proliferation. More recently, Folkman's group has shown that mast cell heparin stimulates migration of capillary endothelial cells *in vitro*.[8] Mast cells are almost always found in increased numbers in pathological states associated with angiogenesis, such as chronic inflammation, immune rejection, tumor growth, and psoriasis.

Finally, mention should be made of recent studies by Castellot *et al.*[24] showing that conditioned medium from endothelial cell cultures causes inhibition of vascular smooth muscle cells *in vitro*. The material responsible for such inhibition is heparin-like, and indeed heparin can mimic the effects of such conditioned medium at doses of 10 ug/ml. Other endothelial products appear to stimulate vascular smooth muscle or endothelium.[7] All these experiments raise the possibility that endothelial cells may serve to control the growth and possibly other properties of vascular smooth muscle cells.[126]

REFERENCES

1. Altura, B. M. (ed.). Advances in the microcirculation, vascular endothelium and basement membranes. Basel, Karger, 1980.
2. Ashida, E. R., Johnson, A. R., and Lipsky, P. E. Human endothelial cell-lymphocyte interaction: endothelial cells function as accessory cells necessary for mitogen-induced human T lymphocyte activation *in vitro*. *J. Clin. Invest.* 67: 1490–1499, 1981.
3. Atherton, A. Growth stimulation of endothelial cells by simultaneous culture with sarcoma 180 cells in diffusion chambers. *Cancer Res.*, 37: 3619, 1977.
4. Ausprunk, D. H. Tumor angiogenesis. In *Chemical Messengers of the Inflammatory Process*. Edited by J. C. Houck, pp. 317–351. New York, North Holland Biomedical Press, 1979.
5. Ausprunk, D. H., Boudrian, C. L., and Nelson, D. A. Proteoglycans in the microvasculature. I. Histochemical localization in microvessels of the rabbit eye. *Am. J. Pathol. 103:* 353, 1981.
6. Ausprunk, D. H., and Folkman, J. Migration and proliferation of endothelial cells in preformed and newly formed vessels during tumor angiogenesis. *Microvasc. Res. 14:* 53, 1977.
7. Awbrey, B. J., Hoak, J. C., and Owen, W. G. Binding of human thrombin to cultured human endothelial cells. *J. Biol. Chem. 254:* 4092–4095.
8. Azizkhan, R. G., Azizkhan, J. C., Zetter, B. R., and Folkman, J. Mast cell heparin stimulates migration of capillary endothelial cells *in vitro*. *J. Exp. Med. 152:* 931–944, 1980.
9. Baenziger, N. L., Becherer, P. R., and Majerus, P. W. Characterization of prostacyclin synthesis in cultured human arterial smooth muscle cells, venous endothelial cells and skin fibroblasts. *Cell 16:* 967–974, 1979.
10. Baenziger, N. L., Dillender, M. J., and Majerus, P. W. Cultured human skin fibroblasts and arterial cells produce a labile platelet-inhibitory prostaglandin. *Biochem. Biophys. Res. Commun. 78:* 294–301, 1977.

11. Baldwin, W. M. III, Claas, F. H. J., van Es., L. A., and van Rood, J. J. HLA-A, -B, -DR and endothelial-specific antigens in kidney-graft rejection. *Immunol. Today, Dec:* 110–111, 1980.

12. Baldwin, W. M. III, Claas, F. H. J., van Es, L. A., and van Rood, J. J. Distribution of endothelial-monocyte and HLA antigens on renal vascular endothelium. *Transplant. Proc. 13:* 103–107, 1981.

13. Becker, C. G., and Harpel, P. C. α_2-macroglobulin on human vascular endothelium. *J. Exp. Med. 144:* 1–9, 1976.

14. Berman, M., Winthrop, D., Ausprunk, D., Rose, J., Langer, R., and Gage, J. Plasminogen activator (urokinase) causes vascularization of the cornea. *Invest. Ophthalmol. Vis. Sci.*, in press, 1982.

15. Birdwell, C. R., Gospodarowicz, D., and Nicolson, G. L. Factors from 3T3 cells stimulate proliferation of cultured vascular endothelial cells. *Nature 268:* 528–531, 1977.

16. Brenner, B. M., Hostetter, T. H., and Humes, H. D. The molecular basis of proteinuria of glomerular origin. *N. Engl. J. Med. 298:* 826, 1978.

17. Brown, R. A., Weiss, J. B., Tomlinson, I. W., Phillips, P., and Kumar, S. Angiogenic factor from synovial fluid resembling that from tumors. *Lancet 29:* 682–685, 1980.

18. Bundgaard, M. Transport pathways in capillaries—In search of pores. *Annu. Rev. Physiol. 42:* 325, 1980.

19. Buoanassisi, V. Sulfated micropolysaccharide synthesis and secretion in endothelial cell cultures. *Exp. Cell Res. 76:* 363, 1973.

20. Buoanassisi, V., and Venter, J. C. Hormone and neurotransmitter receptors in an established vascular endothelial cell line. *Proc. Natl. Acad. Sci. USA 73:* 1612–1616, 1976.

21. Burger, D. R., and Ford, D. M. Activation of human T cells by antigen presenting by HLA-DR compatible endothelial cells. In *17th Annual National Meeting, Reticuloendothelial Society*, 1980.

22. Busch, G. J., Reynolds, E. S., Galvanek, E. G., Braun, W. E., and Dammin, R. J. Human renal allografts: the role of vascular injury in early graft failure. *Medicine 50:* 29, 1971.

23. Caldwell, P. R. B., Seegal, B. C., Hsu, K. C., Das, M., and Soffer, R. L. Angiotensin-converting enzyme: vascular endothelial localization. *Science 191:* 1050, 1976.

24. Castellot, J. J. Jr., Addonizio, M. L., Rosenberg, R., and Karnovsky, M. J. Cultured endothelial cells produce a heparin-like inhibitor of smooth muscle cell growth. *J. Cell Biol. 90:* 372, 1981.

25. Castellot, J. J. Jr., Karnovsky, M. J., and Spiegelman, B. M. Potent stimulation of vascular endothelial cell growth by differentiated 3T3 adipocytes. *Proc. Natl. Acad. Sci. USA 77:* 6007–6011, 1980.

26. Chand, N., and Altura, B. M. Acetylcholine and bradykinin relax intrapulmonary arteries by acting on endothelial cells: role in lung vascular diseases. *Science 213:* 1376, 1981.

27. Chandler, A. B. *et al.* (eds.). *The Thrombotic Process in Atherogenesis.* New York, Plenum Press, 1978.

28. Cotran, R. S. The fine structure of the microvasculature in relation to normal and altered permeability. In *Physical Bases of Circulatory Transport.* Edited by E. B. Reeve and A. C. Guyton, pp. 249–275. Philadelphia, W. B. Saunders, 1967.

29. Cotran, R. S., and Majno, G. A light and electron microscopic analysis of vascular injury. *Ann. N. Y. Acad. Sci. 116:* 750, 1964.

30. Cotran, R. S., and Remensnyder, J. P. The structural basis of increased vascular permeability after graded thermal injury—Light and electron microscopic studies. *Ann. NY Acad. Sci. 150:* 495–509, 1968.

31. Curwen, K. D., Gimbrone, M. A., and Handin, R. I. *In vitro* studies of thromboresistance: the role of prostacyclin (PGI$_2$) in platelet adhesion to cultured normal and virally transformed human vascular endothelial cells. *Lab. Invest. 42:* 366–374, 1980.

32. Davies, P. F., Rennke, H. G., and Cotran, R. S. Influence of molecular charge upon the endocytosis and intracellular fate of peroxidase activity in cultured arterial endothelium. *J. Cell Sci. 49:* 69, 1981.

33. Davies, P. F., and Ross, R. Mediation of pinocytosis in cultured arterial smooth muscle and endothelial cells by platelet-derived growth factor. *J. Cell Biol. 79:* 663, 1978.

34. Davies, P. F., Selden, S. C., and Schwartz, S. M. Enhanced rates of fluid pinocytosis during exponential growth and monolayer regeneration by cultured arterial endothelial cells. *J. Cell Physiol. 102:* 119, 1980.

35. De Forrest, J. M., and Hollis, T. M. Shear stress and aortic histamine synthesis. *Am. J. Physiol.*

Δ8,11,14) by chain elongation. Finally, di-homo-γ-linolenic acid is converted to arachidonic acid (C20:4; Δ5,8,11,14) by another desaturation step forming one additional double bond (Fig. 3.1). Since linoleic and arachidonic acid represent the major dietary intake of essential fatty acids in Western diets, only prostaglandins of the 2-series will be discussed.

Arachidonic acid, following synthesis in the liver, is transported and esterified in cells into phospholipids, particularly in the 2-position of phosphatidylcholine, phosphatidylethanolamine, and phosphatidylinositol. The phospholipids are then incorporated into the lipid bilayers of most cellular membranes. In order for arachidonic acid to be utilized by cells to produce various prostaglandins and related products, it first must be liberated from the phospholipids. This is accomplished through activation of cellular phospholipases after stimulation of the cell, by mechanical, chemical, or radiation insult, or by other autacoids released by inflammatory cells (Fig. 3.2). Two mechanisms have been proposed for the liberation of arachidonic acid from cellular phospholipids (81) (Fig. 3.3). The first involves activation of cellular phospholipase A_2 (PLA$_2$), which then directly hydrolyses the arachidonic acid esterified in the 2 position, particularly in phosphatidylcholine and phosphatidylethanolamine. In certain cells, such as the platelet (2), recent evidence suggests that phospholipase C, with a unique specificity for phosphatidyl inositol, first attacks the phosphate ester in position 3. This results in the formation of a 1,2-diacyl-glycerol, which then is acted upon by a second enzyme, diglyceride lipase, which liberates arachidonic acid esterified in the 2 position. The result of either of the phospholipase pathways is the intracellular release of arachidonic acid, which can then be utilized by two types of specific microsomal enzymes that metabolize arachidonic acid into very diversified groups of highly biologically active autacoids.

Two major pathways of arachidonic acid metabolism are active in most cells involved in the acute and chronic inflammatory process (Fig. 3.4). The first involves a fatty acid cyclo-oxygenase enzyme, which converts arachidonic acid into the prostaglandin endoperoxide PGG$_2$ (15-hydroperoxy-9,11-peroxidoprosta-5,13-dienoic acid). Subsequently, PGG$_2$ is converted by enzymatic peroxidation into prostaglandin H$_2$ (PGH$_2$,15-hydroxy-9,11-peroxidoaprosta-5,13-dienoic acid) (28, 31, 59). During the conversion of PGG$_2$ to PGH$_2$, a free radical of oxygen is generated and may be involved in mediating some aspects of the inflammatory process and/or initiating tissue injury (see below). Following the formation of

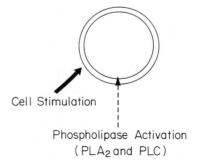

Fig. 3.2. Arachidonic acid to be made available in cells for the production of prostaglandins and their derivatives must first be released from phospholipids by the activation of specific phospholipases.

Cell Stimulation

Phospholipase Activation
(PLA$_2$ and PLC)

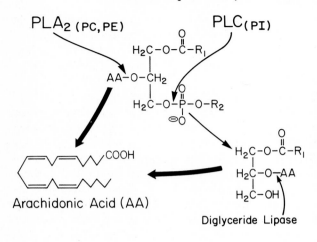

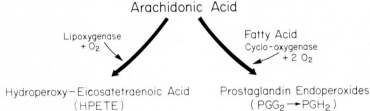

FIG. 3.3. Phospholipases involved in the liberation of arachidonic acid from phospholipids. Most arachidonic acid is derived from the second position of phospholipids by either *PLA₂* or by *PLC* and diglyceride lipase.

Arachidonic Acid

Lipoxygenase + O₂

Fatty Acid Cyclo-oxygenase + 2 O₂

Hydroperoxy–Eicosatetraenoic Acid (HPETE)

Prostaglandin Endoperoxides (PGG₂ → PGH₂)

FIG. 3.4. Two separate pathways are present in most cells for the intracellar metabolism of arachidonic acid. Cyclo-oxygenase converts arachidonic acid into the prostaglandin derivatives while lipoxygenase produces a second group of hydroperoxy- and hydroxyarachidonic acid derivatives.

PGH_2, it may be converted enzymatically into several products that have been implicated in the modulation of the inflammatory process.

A second set of intracellular enzymes called lipoxygenases converts arachidonic acid into a series of hydroperoxy fatty acid derivatives with the hydroperoxy group being placed at the 5 (9), 11 (72), 12 (27), or 15 (11) positions. Through subsequent peroxidative mechanisms, the hydroperoxy fatty acids may be transformed into their respective hydroxy derivatives, again with the formation of oxygen free radicals. Alternatively, the 5-hydroperoxy derivative may be converted into its epoxide derivative and subsequently into the leukotriene autacoids (see below).

Recently, a third mechanism of arachidonic metabolism has been reported (not shown in Fig. 3.4), whereby arachidonic acid may be converted into a potent mediator of the inflammatory process. This highly chemotactic product apparently is produced by peroxidation of arachidonic acid by oxygen-derived free radicals (64). Presently, the structure of this arachidonic acid-derived product is not known, but its chemotactic activity appears to be significantly greater than the products of the lipoxygenase pathway of arachidonic acid metabolism.

Thus, a number of highly biologically active products are derived through arachidonic acid metabolism. These highly potent lipid autacoids are thought to affect many aspects of the acute and chronic inflammatory process (*cf.* 19, 36, 51,

52, 76, 78, 81, 86). We will now review some of the products derived from the cyclo-oxygenase and lipoxygenase pathways of arachidonic acid metabolism.

CYCLO-OXYGENASE PRODUCTS OF ARACHIDONIC ACID METABOLISM

Arachidonic acid itself has been reported to participate in inflammation by inducing vasodilatation, edema, pain, platelet stimulation. However, it is likely that many of these biological activities can be explained by the subsequent metabolism of arachidonic acid into other biologically active molecules. As shown in Figure 3.4, fatty acid cyclo-oxygenase converts arachidonic acid into the prostaglandin endoperoxide PGG_2. Of significance was the finding that certain nonsteroidal anti-inflammatory drugs (*e.g.*, aspirin and indomethacin) specifically block cyclo-oxygenase (71, 84), thereby preventing the metabolism of arachidonic acid to PGG_2 and, thus, to other highly biologically active prostaglandins. These observations have provided one of the strongest arguments that products of arachidonic acid metabolism through the cyclo-oxygenase pathway are involved in the development of both acute and chronic inflammation. Following the intracellular production of PGG_2, it is then converted by peroxidation to PGH_2. During this process, oxygen-derived free radicals are produced and have been strongly implicated in mediating some aspects of the inflammatory process. Indeed, scavengers of these free radicals have been shown to significantly reduce certain inflammatory responses, such as the development of edema (41, 42). It is generally thought that various free radicals of oxygen also may affect tissue injury, which then would initiate further inflammatory responses. In addition, as described above, the production of oxygen-derived free radicals also can peroxidize liberated arachidonic acid with the subsequent production of a highly chemotactic, inflammatory mediator (64).

Following the intracellular production of PGH_2, two well-documented enzymatic pathways lead to the production of two potent autacoids with opposing biological properties. Thromboxane A_2 (TXA_2; 30, 71) is produced from PGH_2 enzymatically by the action of thromboxane synthetase (Fig. 3.5). TXA_2 has been

Prostaglandin Endoperoxide
PGH_2

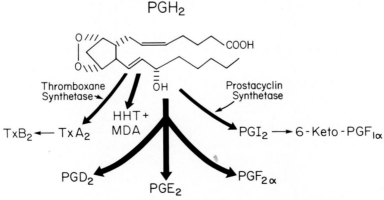

FIG. 3.5. Major products derived from the cyclo-oxygenase pathway of arachidonic acid metabolism.

shown to be one of the most potent platelet stimulators, inducing both platelet aggregation and the platelet release reaction. TXA_2 is produced in the platelet and has been shown to be responsible for the second wave of platelet aggregation induced by either ADP or collagen (47). TXA_2 also has potent vasoconstricting activities (18). Thus, the possible role of TXA_2 in the inflammatory process would be through its ability to activate the platelet as an inflammatory cell and to alter vascular hemodynamics, which secondarily could affect the inflammatory process.

Another product of arachidonic acid metabolism which strongly opposes TXA_2 is prostacyclin PGI_2 (39, 53) (Fig. 3.5). It, too, is produced from the prostaglandin endoperoxide PGH_2 by the enzyme prostacyclin synthetase. A major source for the production of PGI_2 is the vascular endothelium. It antagonizes the action of TXA_2 upon platelets by increasing the intracellular levels of cyclic AMP; PGI_2 is the most potent inhibitor of platelet aggregation and secretion known (47, 51, 52). In addition, PGI_2 also can elevate intracellular cyclic AMP levels in other cells, *e.g.*, PGI_2 inhibits neutrophil stimulation, as assessed both by chemotaxis and by secretion of lysosomal enzymes (86, 87). Thus, in this respect, PGI_2 would seem to serve as a "shutoff" mechanism with respect to inflammatory cell activation. On the other hand, the administration of PGI_2 has been shown to potentiate edema formation and produce hyperalgesia in association with other pain-inducing autacoids. Regarding enhancement of edema formation, PGI_2 is a potent vasodilator (51, 52) and it is likely that its vasodilatating effects are responsible for its ability to enhance edema formation.

Three other prostaglandin products, PGD_2 (28, 29), PGE_2 (1, 7, 75), and $PGF_{2\alpha}$ (1, 5, 6) also are derived directly from the prostaglandin endoperoxide PGH_2 (Fig. 3.5). Both PGE_2 and PGD_2 mimick some of the actions of PGI_2, although their relative biological potencies are decreased. Thus, both PGE_2 and PGD_2 cause vasodilatation and therefore potentiate edema induced by other autacoids, initiate hyperalgesia, and inhibit platelet aggregation by increasing intracellular cyclic AMP; in contrast, $PGF_{2\alpha}$ results in an increase in intracellular cyclic GMP and antagonizes the hyperalgesia induced by the other prostaglandins (19). Other products of arachidonic acid metabolism include HHT 12-L-hydroxy-5,8,10-heptadecatrienoic acid (HTT; 29, 89) and malondialdehyde (MDA). HHT has been reported to have chemotactic properties (23), and MDA may be cytotoxic through alterations in both proteins and cell membranes (47).

In summary, many of the products derived from the cyclo-oxygenase pathway of arachidonic acid metabolism appear to be involved in the modulation of the inflammatory process. Perhaps the strongest, although indirect, evidence for their involvement derives from the cyclo-oxygenase inhibitory activity by the nonsteroidal anti-inflammatory drugs. On the other hand, many prostaglandins (*i.e.*, PGI_2, PGD_2, and PGE_2) seem to attenuate inflammatory cell activation (primarily through stimulation of intracellular cyclic AMP), but inhibition of cyclo-oxygenase with nonsteroidal inflammatory drugs would also block their production. At the present time, this apparent enigma is difficult to explain; perhaps it is the oxygen-derived free radicals produced during conversion PGG_2 to PHG_2 that are primarily effectors of the inflammatory process (41, 42). Alternately, since products of arachidonic acid metabolism via the cyclo-oxygenase pathway are potent autacoids and possess many other potent pharmacologic properties, they may modulate various disease processes and thus secondarily affect the acute and chronic inflammatory responses. For example, certain of the prostaglandins have been implicated in the regulation of the immune response, bone resorption, chronic inflammation through fibroblastic proliferation, and protein synthesis, and are directly or indirectly involved in temperature regulation. A rigorous review of all these biological properties of the prostaglandin autacoids is beyond the scope of this chapter and has been covered more extensively by others (19, 52, 57).

LIPOXYGENASE PRODUCTS OF ARACHIDONIC ACID METABOLISM

Following the intracellular liberation of arachidonic acid, a second series of potent autacoids may be derived enzymatically (Fig. 3.4). This involves the conversion of arachidonic acid by fatty acid lipoxygenases with the subsequent development of the hydroperoxy derivatives, such as hydroperoxyeicosatetraenoic acid (HPETE). While in the platelet, 12-HPETE is the predominant hydroperoxide, 5 and 15-HPETE predominate in leukocytes due to differing specificities of the lipoxygenase enzymes of various cell types. The HPETE may undergo peroxidation to hydroxyeicosatetraenoic acid (HETE) with the release of oxygen-derived free radicals. Certain of the HPETE derivatives have been shown to induce vasoconstriction and hyperalgesia and to potentiate edema, although these properties again may be related to the production of oxygen-free radicals following HPETE peroxidation to HETE. HETE has been shown to be a relatively potent chemotactic stimulus for neutrophils (25, 83). As was the case with the products of the cyclo-oxygenase pathway of arachidonic acid metabolism, the lipoxygenase pathway is active in most inflammatory cells. Again, it is a bit puzzling as to why many nonsteroidal anti-inflammatory drugs (*e.g.*, aspirin and indomethacin), are so effective clinically since by blocking fatty acid cyclo-oxygenase but not lipoxygenase, arachidonic acid is shunted through the lipoxygenase pathway with the subsequent formation of highly active inflammatory autacoids.

LEUKOTRIENES

One of the most recent advances in the study of the lipoxygenase pathway of arachidonic acid metabolism has been the elucidation of the leukotrienes (76). It is now well established that the slow reacting substance of anaphylaxis (SRS-A) is derived from the lipoxygenase pathway of arachidonic acid metabolism. SRS-A was first reported in 1940 (40) due to its potent and prolonged ability to contract the guinea pig ileum. Only recently, however, has its structure been characterized and the molecule synthesized (77). As a result, a new class of potent arachidonic acid-derived lipid autacoids has been identified; additional biological properties of these arachidonic acid derivatives have now been characterized, some of which may be involved in the acute inflammatory process.

SRS-A was characterized to be a sulfur-containing polar lipid whose initial precursor was arachidonic acid and which was metabolized through the lipoxygenase pathway (63). Recently, structural analysis has demonstrated that SRS-A is composed of three structurally similar molecules called the leukotrienes C, D, and E (Fig. 3.6). The leukotrienes have been shown to be derived through the lipoxygenase pathway, subsequent to the formation of 5-HPETE. Subsequently,

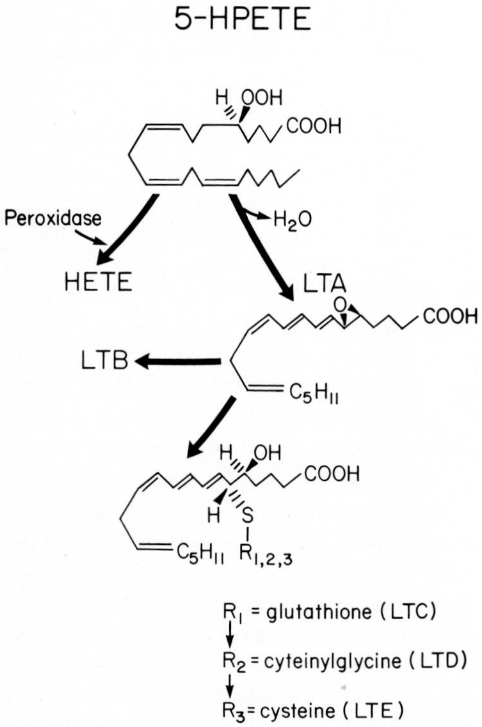

5-HPETE

Peroxidase

H₂O

HETE   LTA

LTB

FIG. 3.6. The leukotrienes are derived
through the lipoxygenase pathway of arachidonic acid metabolism. Fatty acid lipoxygenase
converts arachidonic acid into *5-HPETE*,
which then either forms *HETE* or the 5.6 epoxide derivative PTA. *LTA* then is further converted into either *LTB* or to *LTC, LTD*, and
LTE.

R_1 = glutathione (LTC)

R_2 = cyteinylglycine (LTD)

R_3 = cysteine (LTE)

an unstable 5,6 epoxide derivative, called leukotriene A (LTA) (12, 73), is formed
which then may be enzymatically converted to leukotriene B (LTB) (10), or to
leukotriene C (LTC, 5(S)-hydroxy-6(R)-S-glutathionyl-7,9-*trans*,11,14-*cis*-eico-
satetraenoic acid) (32, 33, 58), the latter by addition of a glutathione residue
through a thioether linkage at the 6 carbon. Leukotriene D (LTD) (54, 55, 62) is
identical to LTC, except for a conversion of the S-glutathionyl residue to S-
cysteinylglycine by γ-glutamyl transpeptidase. Subsequently, conversion of the
cysteinylglycine to the cysteinyl derivative results in the production of leukotriene
E (LTE) (44, 77). In addition to possessing relative potent SRS-A smooth muscle-
contracting activities, recent studies using synthetic leukotrienes have indicated
a possible role in their modulation of the acute inflammatory process. Thus, both
LTD and LTE have been shown to dramatically increase vascular permeability
whereas LTC initiates acute vasoconstriction (17, 43, 44). In addition LTB is a
potent neutrophil stimulator inducing both chemokinesis and neutrophil aggregation (21).

In summary, it would seem that many of the products derived from the
intracellular metabolism of arachidonic acid metabolism, either directly or indirectly, play important roles in the modulation of the acute and chronic inflammatory processes. Since within recent years the structures of arachidonic acid
metabolites have been elucidated and the molecules chemically synthesized, new
and interesting information should be forthcoming with respect to their involvement in the acute and chronic inflammatory processes. In addition, with the ever

increasing availability of specific antagonists and inhibitors of arachidonic acid metabolism, those products of arachidonic metabolism that are directly involved in inflammatory processes will be further defined in normal, as well as abnormal pathophysiologic states.

ACETYL GLYCERYL ETHER PHOSPHORYLCHOLINE (AGEPC)

The acetylated alkyl phosphoglycerides represent the most recently described and novel class of potent lipid autacoids. Biologically, their effect was observed over 10 years ago, when it was found that antigen stimulation of sensitized leukocytes resulted in stimulation of platelets (35). Subsequent studies demonstrated the release of a fluid-phase mediator from antigen stimulated, IgE-sensitized basophils which then stimulated the platelets to undergo the release reaction (3, 82); since the chemical structure of this fluid-phase mediator was not known, it was given the name *platelet-activating factor* (PAF; 3). The chemical structure of PAF has recently been documented (34) to be 1-*O*-hexadecyl/octadecyl-2-acetyl-*sn*-glyceryl-3-phosphorylcholine (AGEPC; Fig. 3.7); in addition, AGEPC has been synthesized in relatively large quantities (4, 8, 14). With the availability of this chemically pure autacoid, additional *in vivo* and *in vitro* studies have been performed which not only have documented its ability to stimulate human platelets (49), but have unveiled a spectrum of other potent biological activities. Indeed, while most other autacoids generally manifest only one or two biological activities associated with the inflammatory process, AGEPC would appear to be capable of evoking almost all of the well-known cardinal signs of acute inflammation (67, 69, 70).

Several *in vivo* investigations demonstrated that the intravenous infusion of 1-μg quantities of AGEPC into the rabbit or baboon (26, 48, 50, 68) reproduced all of the pathophysiologic sequelae of IgE-induced systemic anaphylactic shock (65) (Table 3.3). In addition, these *in vivo* studies suggested that AGEPC possessed biological activities over and above its ability to serve as a potent platelet stimulator. For example, the development of profound neutropenia after intravenous infusion of AGEPC (48, 50) indicated that AGEPC might induce neutrophil stimulation. Indeed, three separate studies (24, 61, 80) have shown

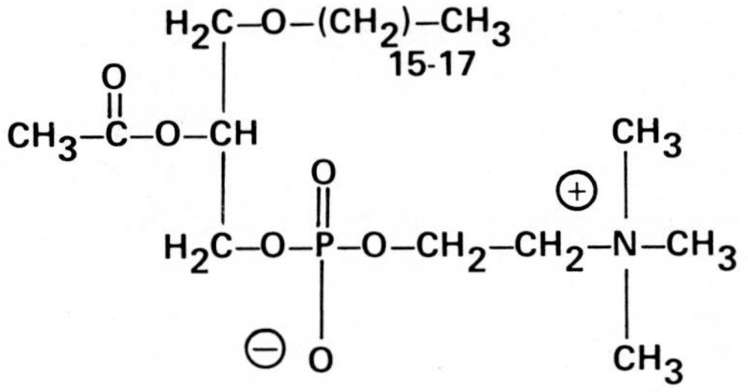

1—*O*—hexadecyl/octadecyl—2—acetyl—*sn*—glyceryl—3—phosphorylcholine (AGEPC)

Fig. 3.7. Chemical structure of acetyl glyceryl ether phosphorylcholine (*AGEPC*). Prior to its structural identification, AGEPC was known as PAF.

TABLE 3.3. BIOLOGICAL ACTIVITY OF AGEPC *IN VIVO*

Intravascular	Thrombocytopenia
	Neutropenia
	Basopenia
	Increased hematocrit
	Decreased total plasma protein
	PF4 secretion
	TxB_2 Release
Cardiovascular-Pulmonary	Elevated right ventricular and pulmonary artery pressures
	Systemic hypotension
	Increased pulmonary resistance
	Decreased dynamic lung compliance
	Decreased respiratory frequency
	Respiratory arrest and death
Cutaneous	Vasodilation
	Increased vascular permeability
	Vasoconstriction
	Neutrophil infiltrates

that AGEPC stimulates neutrophil aggregation, chemotaxis, secretion of azurophilic and specific granule enzymes, and the production of superoxide anion.

The various cardiovascular and pulmonary alterations induced by intravenous AGEPC infusion (26) (Table 3.3) indicated that AGEPC could also possess smooth muscle and vasoactive properties. Indeed, AGEPC has been shown to induce contraction of the guinea pig ileum (20) and parenchymal lung strips (60). With respect to contraction of the guinea pig ileum, the AGEPC-induced ileal contraction was independent from the stimulation of muscarinic, H1, or leukotriene receptors (20). Intracutaneous administration of AGEPC in human volunteers has also documented very potent vasoactive properties of this lipid autacoid (66, 67); thus on a molar basis AGEPC is between 100 and 1000 times more potent than histamine. In the guinea pig, AGEPC manifested even more potent vasoactive activities; intracutaneous administration of AGEPC induced increased vascular permeability with a potency between 1,000 and 10,000 times greater than the permeability observed with histamine or for LTD and LTE (37, 38). Thus as little as 0.5 pmole AGEPC initiated significant skin blueing in the guinea pig; at higher concentrations (50 pmoles), AGEPC initiated acute vasoconstriction, also previously reported to occur in man (37, 66). In addition to inducing erythema and edema in human skin, AGEPC commonly induced transient, severe burning pain (66). Thus, of the five cardinal signs of inflammation, AGEPC has been strongly implicated in four; its ability to induce fever is yet to be studied.

It is noteworthy to point out that, besides the spectrum of biological activity associated with AGEPC, this potent lipid autacoid is probably produced by a variety of inflammatory cells (69, 70). At the present time, however, all of the platelet-activating factors released from these cells cannot be equated to AGEPC, since their chemical structures await direct structure-proof elucidation. Nevertheless, the PAF released from human neutrophils and monocytes appears to have identical physicochemical and functional properties to AGEPC and probably is one and the same molecule (13, 45, 46). Thus, more extensive investigations must be conducted upon this unique class of acetylated alkyl phosphoglycerides.

SUMMARY

Significant progress has been made in the elucidation of the chemistry and biology of the products of arachidonic acid metabolism and the acetylated alkyl phosphoglycerides. While many of their biological properties make them tempting candidates as mediators of inflammation, their precise role in the acute and/or chronic inflammatory process remains to be proven. Thus, at present, it might be best to view these potent lipids not as *inflammatory mediators* but as *autacoids*. In the words of Douglas (16): "The very fact that the substances have been classified under the noncommittal title of *autacoids*, is, in a sense, a confession that the evidence does not at present permit a more precise functional classification such as, for example, hormone or neurohormone.... But the core of the matter is that, while the *autacoids* possess an astonishingly wide range of pharmacologic activities and in vanishing small amounts, there are comparatively few instances where a physiologic role can be stated with assurance." Hopefully, the coming years should prove to be exciting and fruitful for students of inflammation and immunopathology; if so, we may be able to unequivocally elucidate the precise role(s) of these fascinating lipid autacoids in modulating the inflammatory process. At that time, the term *autacoid* may no longer be appropriate, and a new, functional classification, perhaps *mediator*, can be instituted with assurance.

REFERENCES

1. Anggard, E. The isolation and determination of prostaglandins in lungs of sheep, guinea pig, monkey and man. *Biochem. Pharmacol. 14:* 1507–1516, 1965.
2. Bell, R. L., Stanford, N., Kennerly, D. A., and Majerus, P. W. Diglyceride lipase: A pathway for arachidonate release from human platelets. *Adv. Prostaglandin Thromb. Res. 6:* 219–224, 1980.
3. Benveniste, J., Henson, P. M., and Cochrane, C. G. Leukocyte-dependent histamine release from rabbit platelets. The role of IgE, basophils, and a platelet activating factor. *J. Exp. Med. 136:* 1356–1377, 1972.
4. Benveniste, J., Tence, M., Varenne, P., Bidault, J., Boullet, C., and Polonsky, J. Semi-synthese et structure porposee du facteur activant les plaquettes (P.A.F.): PAF-acether, un alkyl ether analogue de la lysophosphatidylcholine. *C. R. Acad. Sci. (Paris) 289:* 1037–1040, 1979.
5. Bergstrom, S., Dressler, F., Krabisch, L., Ryhage, R., and Sjovall, J. The isolation and structure of a smooth muscle stimulation factor in normal sheep and pig lungs. *Ark. Kemi. 20:* 63–66, 1962.
6. Bergstrom, S., and Sjovall, J. The isolation of prostaglandin F from sheep prostate glands. *Acta. Chem. Scand. 14:* 1693–1700, 1960.
7. Bergstrom, S., and Sjovall, J. The isolation of prostaglandin E from sheep prostate glands. *Acta. Chem. Scand. 14:* 1701–1705, 1960.
8. Blank, M. L., Snyder, F., Byers, L. W., Brooks, B., and Muirhead, E. E. Antihypertensive activity of an alkyl ether analogue of phosphatidylcholine. *Biochem. Biophys. Res. Commun. 90:* 1194–1200, 1979.
9. Borgeat, P., Hamberg, M., and Samuelsson, B. Transformation of arachidonic acid and homolinolenic acid by rabbit polymorphonuclear leukocytes. Mono-hydroxy acid from novel lipoxygenases. *J. Biol. Chem. 251:* 7816–7820, 1976.
10. Borgeat, P., and Samuelsson, B. Transformation of arachidonic acid by rabbit polymorphonuclear leukocytes. Formation of a novel dihydroxyeicosatetraenoic acid. *J. Biol. Chem. 254:* 2643–2646, 1979.

11. Borgeat, P., and Samuelsson, B. Arachidonic acid metabolism in polymorphonuclear leukocytes. Effects of ionophoroe A23187. *Proc. Natl. Acad. Sci. USA 76:* 2148–2152, 1979.

12. Borgeat, P., and Samuelsson, B. Arachidonic acid metabolism in polymorphonuclear leukocytes: Unstable intermediate in formation of dihydroxy acids. *Proc. Natl. Acad. Sci. USA 76:* 3213–3217, 1979.

13. Clark, P. O., Hanahan, D. J., and Pinckard, R. N. Physical and chemical properties of platelet-activating factor obtained from human neutrophils and monocytes and rabbit neutrophils and basophils. *Biochim. Biophys. Acta 628:* 69–75, 1980.

14. Demopoulos, C. A., Pinckard, R. N., and Hanahan, D. J. Platelet-activating factor. Evidence for 1-*O*-alkyl-2-acetyl-*sn*-glyceryl-3-phosphorylcholine as the active component (a new class of lipid chemical mediators). *J. Biol. Chem. 254:* 9355–9358, 1979.

15. Dormandy, T. L. Plasma antioxidant potential. In *Hemostatis, Prostaglandins and Renal Disease.* Edited by G. Remuzzi, G. Mecca, and G. de Gaetano, pp. 251–255, New York, Raven Press, 1980.

16. Douglas, W. W. Autacoids (1980). In *The Pharmacological Basis of Therapeutics.* Edited by A. G. Gilman, L. S. Goodman, and A. Gilman, pp. 608–646, New York, MacMillan, 1980.

17. Drazen, J. M., Austen, K. F., Lewis, R. A., Clark, D. A., Goto, G., Marfat, A., and Corey, E. J. Comparative airway and vascular activities of leukotrienes C-1 and D *in vivo* and *in vitro*. *Proc. Natl. Acad. Sci. USA 77:* 4354–4358, 1980.

18. Dusting, G. J., Moncada, S., and Vane, J. R. Vascular actions of arachidonic acid and its metabolites in perfused mesenteric and femoral beds of the dog. *Eur. J. Pharmacol. 49:* 65–72, 1978.

19. Ferreira, S. H. Prostaglandins. In *Chemical Messengers of the Inflammatory Process.* Edited by J. C. Houck, pp. 113–151, Elsevier/North Holland Biochemical Press, Amsterdam, 1979.

20. Findlay, S. R., Lichtenstein, L. M., Hanahan, D. J., and Pinckard, R. N. The contraction of guinea pig ileal smooth muscle by acetyl glyceryl ether phosphorylcholine. *Am. J. Physiol. 241:* C130–134, 1981.

21. Ford-Hutchinson, A. W., Bray, M. A., Doig, M. V., Shipley, M. E., and Smith, M. J. H. Leukotriene B: A potent chemokinetic and aggregating substance released from polymorphonuclear leukocytes. *Nature 286:* 264–265, 1980.

22. Garattini, S., DiMinno, G., and de Gaetano, G. Modulation of arachidonic acid metabolism: Dietary and pharmacological perspectives. In *Hemostatis, Prostaglandins and Renal Disease.* Edited by G. Remuzzi, G. Mecca, and G. de Gaetano, pp. 217–233, New York, Raven Press, 1980.

23. Goetzl, E. J., and Gorman, R. R. Chemotactic and chemokinetic stimulation of human eosinophil and neutrophil polymorphonuclear leukocytes by 12-L-hydroxy-5,8,10-heptadecatrienoic acid (HHT). *J. Immunol. 120:* 526–531, 1978.

24. Goetzl, E. J., Derian, C. K., Tauber, A. I., and Valone, F. H. Novel effects of 1-*O*-hexadecyl-2-acyl-*sn*-glycero-3-phosphorylcholine mediators on human leukocyte function: Delineation of the specific roles of the acyl substituents. *Biochem. Biophys. Res. Commun. 94:* 881–888, 1980.

25. Goetzl, E. J., Woods, J. M., and Gorman, R. R. Stimulation of human eosinophil and neutrophil polymorphonuclear leukocyte chemotaxis and random migration by 12-L-hydroxy-5,8-11,14-eicosatetraenoic acid. *J. Clin. Invest. 59:* 179–183, 1977.

26. Halonen, M., Palmer, J. D., Lohman, I. C., McManus, L. M., and Pinckard, R. N. Respiratory and circulatory alterations induced by acetyl glyceryl ether phosphorylcholine (AGEPC), a mediator of IgE anaphylaxis in the rabbit. Am. Rev. Resp. Dis. *122:* 915–924, 1980.

27. Hamberg, M., and Samuelsson, B. Prostaglandin endoperoxides. Novel transformations of arachidonic acid in human platelets. *Proc. Natl. Acad. Sci. USA 71:* 3400–3404, 1974.

28. Hamberg, M., and Samuelsson, B. Detection and isolation of an endoperoxide intermediate in prostaglandin biosynthesis. *Proc. Natl. Acad. Sci. USA 70:* 899–903, 1973.

29. Hamberg, M., Svensson, J., and Samuelsson, B. A new concept concerning the mode of action and release of prostaglandins. *Proc. Natl. Acad. Sci. USA 71:* 3824–3828, 1974.

30. Hamberg, M., Svensson, J., and Samuelsson, B. Thromboxanes: A new group of biologically active compounds derived from prostaglandin endoperoxides. *Proc. Natl. Acad. Sci. USA 72:* 2994–2998, 1975.

31. Hamberg, M., Svensson, J., Wakabayashi, T., and Samuelsson, B. Isolation and structure of two

prostaglandin endoperoxides that cause platelet aggregation. *Proc. Natl. Acad. Sci. USA 71:* 345–349, 1974.

32. Hammarstrom, S., Murphy, R. C., Samuelsson, B., Clark, D. A., Mioskowski, C., and Corey, E. J. Structure of leukotriene C. Identification of the amino acid part. *Biochem. Biophys. Res. Commun. 91:* 1266–1272, 1979.

33. Hammarstrom, S., Samuelsson, B., Clark, D. A., Goto, G., Marfat, A., Mioskowski, C., and Corey, E. J. Stereochemistry of leukotriene C-1. *Biochem. Biophys. Res. Commun. 92:* 946–953, 1980.

34. Hanahan, D. J., Demopoulos, C. A., Liehr, J., and Pinckard, R. N. Identification of platelet-activating factor isolated from rabbit basophils as acetyl glyceryl ether phosphorylcholine. *J. Biol. Chem. 225:* 5514–5516, 1980.

35. Henson, P. M. Release of vasoactive amines from rabbit platelets induced by sensitized mononuclear leukocytes and antigen. *J. Exp. Med. 131:* 287–306, 1970.

36. Higgs, G. A., Moncada, S., and Vane, J. R. The role of arachidonic acid metabolites in inflammation. *Adv. Inflammation Res. 1:* 413–418, 1979.

37. Humphrey, D. M., McManus, L. M., Hanahan, D. J., and Pinckard, R. N. Vasoactive properties of 1-*O*-alkyl-2-acetyl-*sn*-glyceryl-3-phosphorylcholine (AGEPC), submitted for publication, 1981.

38. Humphrey, D. M., Pinckard, R. M., McManus, L. M., and Hanahan, D. J. Intradermal neutrophil infiltrates induced by 1-*O*-alkyl-2-acetyl-*sn*-glyceryl-3-phosphorylcholine (AGEPC). *Fed. Proc. 40:* 1003, 1981.

39. Johnson, R. A., Morton, D. R., Kinner, J. H., Gorman, R. R., McGuire, J. C., Sun, F. F., Whittaker, N., Bunting, S., Salmon, J., Moncada, S. and Vane, J. R. The chemical structure of prostaglandin X (prostacyclin). *Prostaglandins 12:* 915–928, 1976.

40. Kellaway, C. H., and Trethewie, E. R. The liberation of a slow-reacting smooth muscle-stimulating substance in anaphylaxis. *J. Exp. Physiol. 30:* 121–145, 1940.

41. Kuehl, F. A., Humes, J. L., Ham, E. A., Egan, R. W., and Dougherty, H. W. Inflammation: The role of peroxidase-derived products. *Adv. Prostaglandin Thromb. Res. 6:* 77–86, 1980.

42. Kuehl, F. A., Humes, J. L., Torchiana, M. L., Ham, E. A., and Egan, R. W. Oxygen-centered radicals in inflammatory processes. *Adv. Inflammation Res. 1:* 419–430, 1979.

43. Lewis, R. A., Austen, K. F., Drazen, J. M., Clark, D. A., Marfat, A., and Corey, E. J. Slow reacting substances of anaphylaxis: Identification of leukotrienes C-1 and D from human rat and sources. *Proc. Natl. Acad. Sci. USA 77:* 3710–3714, 1980.

44. Lewis, R. A., Drazen, J. M., Austen, K. F., Clark, D. A., and Corey, E. J. Identification of the C(6)-S-conjugate of leukotriene A with cysteine as a naturally occurring slow reacting substance of anaphylaxis (SRS-A). Importance of the 11-*cis*-geometry for biological activity. *Biochem. Biophys. Res. Commun. 96:* 271–277, 1980.

45. Lotner, G. Z., Lynch, J. M., Betz, S. J., and Henson, P. M. The release of a platelet-activating factor by stimulated rabbit neutrophils. *J. Immunol. 124:* 676–684, 1980.

46. Lynch, J. M., Lotner, G. Z., Betz, S. J., and Henson, P. M. The release of a platelet-activating factor by stimulated rabbit neutrophils. *J. Immunol. 123:* 1219–1226, 1979.

47. Marcus, A. J. The role of prostaglandins in platelet function. *Prog. Hematol. 11:* 147–171, 1979.

48. McManus, L. M., Hanahan, D. M., Demopoulos, C. A., and Pinckard, R. N. Pathobiology of the intravenous infusion of acetyl glyceryl ether phosphorylcholine (AGEPC), a synthetic platelet-activating factor (PAF), in the rabbit. *J. Immunol. 124:* 2919–2924, 1980.

49. McManus, L. M., Hanahan, D. J., and Pinckard, R. N. Human platelet stimulation by acetyl glyceryl ether phosphorycholine (AGEPC). *J. Clin. Invest. 67:* 903–906, 1981.

50. McManus, L. M., Pinckard, R. N., Fitzpatrick, F. F., O'Rourke, R. A., Crawford, M. H., and Hanahan, D. J. Acetyl glyceryl ether phosphorylcholine (AGEPC): Intravascular alterations following intravenous infusion in the baboon. *Lab. Invest. 45:* 303–307, 1981.

51. Moncada, S. Prostacyclin and thromboxane A$_2$ in the regulation of platelet-vascular interactions. In *Hemostasis, Prostaglandins and Renal Disease.* Edited by G. Remuzzi, G. Mecca, and G. de Gaetano, pp. 175–188. New York, Raven Press, 1980.

52. Moncada, S., Flower, R. J., and Vane, J. R. Prostaglandins, prostacyclin and thromboxane A$_2$. In *The Pharmacological Basis of Therapeutics.* Edited by A. G. Gilman, L. Goodman, and A. Gilman, pp. 668–681, New York, MacMillan, 1980.

53. Moncada, S., Gryglewski, R., Bunting, S., and Vane, J. R. An enzyme isolated from arteries

transforms prostaglandin endoperoxides to an unstable substance that inhibits platelet aggregation. *Nature 263:* 663–665, 1976.

54. Morris, H. R., Taylor, G. W., Piper, P. J., Samhoun, M. N., and Tippins, J. R. Slow reacting substances (SRS-s): The structure identification of SRS-s from rat basophil leukemia (RBL-1) cells. *Prostaglandins 19:* 185–201, 1980.

55. Morris, H. R., Taylor, G. W., Rokach, J., Girard, Y., Piper, P. J., Tippins, J. R., and Samhoun, M. N. Slow reaction substance of anaphylaxis, SRS-A: Assignment of the stereochemistry. *Prostaglandins 20:* 601–607, 1980.

56. Movat, H. Z. Kinins and the kinin system as inflammatory mediators. In *Chemical Messengers of the Inflammatory Process.* Edited by J. C. Houck, pp. 47–112. Amsterdam, Elsevier/North Holland Biomedical Press, 1979.

57. Murota, S., Chang, W-C., Tsurufuji, S., and Morita, I. The possible roles of prostacyclin (PGI₂) and thromboxanes in chronic inflammation. *Adv. Inflammation Res. 1:* 439–455, 1979.

58. Murphy, R. C., Hammarstrom, S., and Samuelsson, B. Leukotriene C.: A slow-reacting substance from murine mastocytoma cells. *Proc. Natl. Acad. Sci. USA 76:* 4275–4279, 1979.

59. Nugteren, D. H., and Hazelhof, E. Isolation and properties of intermediates in prostaglandin biosynthesis. *Biochim. Biophys. Acta 326:* 448–461, 1973.

60. O'Flaherty, J. T., Lees, J. C., and Stimler, N. P. Anaphylatoxic and polymorphonuclear neutrophil (PMN)-stimulating actions of platelet activating factor (PAF). *Fed. Proc. 40:* 1015, 1981.

61. O'Flaherty, J. T., Wykle, R. L., Miller, C. H., Lewis, J. C., Waite, M., Bass, D. A., McCall, C. E., and DeChatetlet, L. R. 1-*O*-alkyl-*sn*-glyceryl-3-phosphorylcholines. A novel class of neutrophil stimulants. *Am. J. Pathol. 103:* 70–78, 1981.

62. Orning, L., Hammarstrom, S., and Samuelsson, B. Leukotriene D.: A slow reacting substance from rat basophilic leukemia cells. *Proc. Natl. Acad. Sci. USA 77:* 2014–2017, 1980.

63. Parker, C. W., Jakschik, B. A., Huber, M. G., and Falkenhein, S. F. Characterization of slow reacting substance as a family of thiolipids derived from arachidonic acid. *Biochem. Biophys. Res. Commun. 89:* 1186–1192, 1979.

64. Perez, H. D., Weksler, B. B., and Goldstein, I. M. Generation of a chemotactic lipid from arachidonic acid by exposure to a superoxide-generating system. *Inflammation 4:* 313–328, 1980.

65. Pinckard, R. N., Farr, R. S., and Hanahan, D. J. Physicochemical and functional identity of platelet-activating factor (PAF) released *in vivo* during IgE anaphylaxis with PAF released *in vitro* from IgE sensitized basophils. *J. Immunol. 123:* 1847–1857, 1979.

66. Pinckard, R. N., Kniker, W. T., Lee, L., Hanahan, D. J., and McManus, L. M. Vasoactive effects of 1-*O*-alkyl-2-acetyl-*sn*-glyceryl-3-phosphorylcholine (AcGEPC) in human skin. *J. Allergy Clin. Immunol. 65:* 196, 1980.

67. Pinckard, R. N., McManus, L. M., Demopoulos, C. A., Halonen, M., Clark, P. O., Shaw, J. O., Kniker, W. T., and Hanahan, D. J. Molecular pathobiology of acetyl glyceryl ether phosphorylcholine (AGEPC): Evidence for the structural identify with platelet-activating factor. *J. Reticuloendothel. Soc. 28:* 95–103S, 1980.

68. Pinckard, R. N., McManus, L. M., O'Rourke, R. A., Crawford, M. H., and Hanahan, D. J. Intravascular and cardiovascular effects of acetyl glyceryl ether phosphorylcholine (AGEPC) infusion in the baboon. *Clin. Res. 28:* 258A, 1980.

69. Pinckard, R. N., McManus, L. M., Halonen, M., and Hanahan, D. J. Immunopharmacology of acetyl glyceryl ether phosphorylcholine (AGEPC). In *Immunopharmacology of the Lung.* Edited by H. H. Newball, New York, Marcel Dekker, in press, 1982.

70. Pinckard, R. N., McManus, L. M., and Hanahan, D. J. Chemistry and biology of acetyl glyceryl ether phosphorylcholine (platelet-activating factor). *Adv. Inflammation Res.,* in press, 1981.

71. Piper, P. J., and Vane, J. R. Release of additional factors in anaphylaxis and its antagonism by anti-inflammatory drugs. *Nature 223:* 29–35, 1969.

72. Porter, N. A., Wolf, R. A., Pagels, W. R., and Marnett, L. J. A test for the intermediacy of 11-hydroperoxyeicosa-5,8,12,14-tetraenoic acid (11-HPETE) in prostaglandin biosynthesis. *Biochem. Biophys. Res. Commun. 92:* 349–355, 1980.

73. Radmark, O., Malmsten, C., Samuelsson, B., Clark, D. A., Goto, G., Marfat, A., Mioskowski, C., and Corey, E. J. Leukotriene A: Stereochemistry and enzymatic conversion to leukotriene B. *Biochem. Biophys. Res. Commun. 92:* 954–961, 1980.

74. Ryan, G. B., and Majno, G. Acute inflammation. A review. *Am. J. Pathol. 86:* 185–276, 1977.
75. Samuelsson, B. Isolation and identification of prostaglandins from human seminal plasma. *J. Biol. Chem. 238:* 3229–3234, 1963.
76. Samuelsson, B., Borgeat, P., Hammarstrom, S., and Murphy, R. C. Leukotrienes: A new group of biologically active compounds. *Adv. Prostaglandin Thromb. Res. 6:* 1–18, 1980.
77. Samuelsson, B., and Hammarstrom, S. Nomenclature for leukotrienes. *Prostaglandins 19:* 645–648, 1980.
78. Samuelsson, B., Hammarstrom, S., Murphy, R. C., and Borgeat, P. Leukotrienes and slow reacting substance of anaphylaxis. *J. Allergy 35:* 375–381, 1980.
79. Schafer, E. A. *The Endocrine Organs: An Introduction to the Study of Internal Secretion.* New York, Longmans, Green & Co., 1916.
80. Shaw, J. O., Pinckard, R. N., Ferrigni, K. S., McManus, L. M., and Hanahan, D. J. Activation of human neutrophils with 1-*O*-hexadecyl/octadecyl-2-acetyl-*sn*-glyceryl-3-phosphorylcholine or platelet-activating factor. *J. Immunol.,* in press, 1981.
81. Silver, M. J., Smith, J. B., McKean, M. L., and Bills, T. K. Prostaglandins and thromboxanes: Current concepts. In *Hemostasis, Prostaglandins and Renal Disease.* Edited by G. Remuzzi, G. Messa, and G. de Gaetano, pp. 159–173, New York, Raven Press, 1980.
82. Siraganian, R. P., and Osler, A. G. Destruction of rabbit platelets in the allergic response of sensitized leukocytes. I. Demonstration of a fluid phase intermediate. *J. Immunol. 106:* 1244–1251, 1971.
83. Turner, S. R., Tainer, J. A., and Lynn, W. S. Biogenesis of chemotactic molecules by the arachidonate lipoxygenase system of platelets. *Nature 257:* 680–681, 1975.
84. Vane, J. R. Inhibition of prostaglandin biosynthesis as mechanisms of action for aspirin-like drugs. *Nature 231:* 232–235, 1971.
85. Ward, P. A., Hugli, T. E., and Chenoweth, D. E. Complement and chemotaxis. In *Chemical Messengers of the Inflammatory Process.* Edited by J. C. Houck, pp. 153–196, Amsterdam, Elsevier/North-Holland Biochemical Press, 1979.
86. Weissmann, G., Smolen, J. E., and Korchak, H. Prostaglandins and inflammation: Receptor/cyclase coupling as an explanation of why PGEs and PGI_2 inhibit functions of inflammatory cells. *Adv. Prostaglandin Thromb. Res. 8:* 1637–1653, 1980.
87. Weksler, B., Knapp, J. M., and Jaffe, E. A. Prostacyclin (PGI_2) synthesized by cultured endothelial cells modulate polymorphonuclear leukocyte functions. *Blood* (Suppl. 1) *50:* 287, 1977.
88. Wiggins, R. C., and Cochrane, C. G. Hageman factor and the contact activation system. In *Chemical Messengers of the Inflammatory Press.* Edited by J. C. Houck, Amsterdam, Elsevier/North-Holland Biochemical Press, pp. 179–196, 1979.
89. Wlodawer, P., and Samuelsson, B. On the organization and mechanism of prostaglandin synthesis. *J. Biol. Chem. 248:* 5673–5678, 1973.

Chapter 4

The Chemotaxis System*

PETER A. WARD

INTRODUCTION

Over the past two decades, there has been what can only be described as a revolution in experimental approaches to a study of the inflammatory response. It is probably fair to say that during this period more progress in delineating basic mechanisms of inflammation has been made than has occurred in the past century. The recent emphasis has involved both a structural definition of the inflammatory mediators, as well as a detailed analysis of the cell biology of the inflammatory response. Information emanating from a large number of laboratories will surely result in the next few years in totally new and different strategies for manipulating inflammatory responses in patients. Nowhere is the likelihood of this prediction more evident than in the rapid progress that is being made in the biochemical definition of products of the prostaglandin system and in the rapid development of inhibitors and analogues of the prostaglandins.

Our own studies, as well as those of many others, have focused on the cell biology and the mediators of the acute inflammatory response. It is now possible to separate factors responsible for vasopermeability change from those mediators that will trigger chemotactic responses of leukocytes. This chapter will deal broadly with the chemotactic system of humans.

THE CELL BIOLOGY OF THE CHEMOTACTIC SYSTEM

For all intents and purposes, it seems likely the emigration of leukocytes from the vascular compartment is under control of chemotactic mediators generated beyond the confines of the vascular compartment. In the absence of chemotactic mediators, cells will remain within the vascular space. The ability of leukocytes to respond to chemotactic mediators is first and foremost related to the presence of specific chemotactic *receptors* in the cell membranes of inflammatory cells (Fig. 4.1). Neutrophils, eosinophils, monocytes, and macrophages have been directly demonstrated to contain receptors for the complement-derived chemotactic peptide, C5a, and for synthetic oligopeptides, of which N-formyl-methionyl-leucyl-phenylalanine (FMLP) is the most widely studied peptide (1, 15). Estimates of the number of receptors on neutrophils vary from 10,000 to 20,000/cell. Recent

---

* This work was supported in part by NIH Grants 7RO1 AI17690-01, 1RO1 GM28499-01, and CA29551-02.

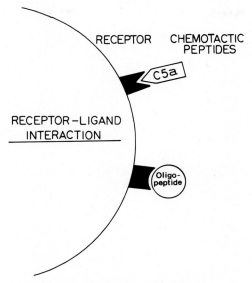

FIG. 4.1. The chemotactic mechanism—1.

evidence suggests that chemotactic receptors on the surfaces of neutrophils can be differentiated by the presence of low affinity and high affinity receptors. The receptor for each class of chemotactic peptide is different; binding of C5a to its receptor does not affect the ability of the synthetic oligopeptide to affix to its own receptor. Nor can one of the chemotactic peptides displace another chemotactic peptide bound to its own receptor.

The binding of the ligand to the receptor is characterized by being rapid, reversible, and displaceable. A direct relationship exists between the extent of ligand binding to the receptor and the subsequent cell response. Based on rough calculations, it would appear that a maximal cell reponse occurs when 20% of the receptors are occupied by chemotactic peptide.

Occupancy of the receptor on the leukocyte with a chemotactic peptide results in a series of events, the precise sequence of which has not been determined. *Cationic fluxes* occur both across the cell membrane as well as across membranes within the cell (10). Na^+ and Ca^{2+} are moved to the interior of the cell (Fig. 4.2). Ca^{2+} is also mobilized from membranes within the cell, resulting in an increase in ionic calcium within the cytosol. This is thought to be a key event that is ultimately linked to assembly of the contractile apparatus, namely, actin filaments, within the cell. Simultaneously, however, there is clear evidence that chemotatic peptide-receptor interaction also initiates activation of the intracellular metabolism of arachidonic acid via both the cyclo-oxygenase and the lipoxygenase pathways of the prostaglandin system (Fig. 4.3; reviewed in ref. 4). The ratio of the identifiable reaction products for each pathway is roughly 1:10, respectively. Identification of the activation products of these two pathways resulting in facilitation of the response of the leukocyte to the chemotactic stimulus is uncertain. For instance, blocking of the cyclo-oxygenase pathway by indomethacin will prevent a variety of repsonses of the cell to the chemotactic

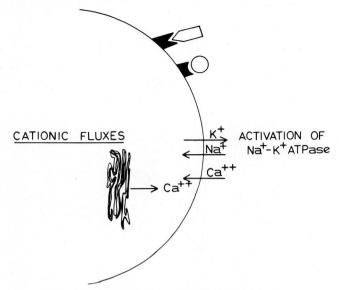

FIG. 4.2. The chemotactic mechanism—2.

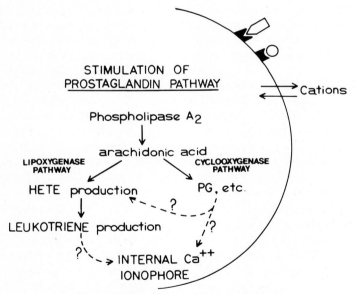

FIG. 4.3. The chemotactic mechanism—3.

stimulus, including motility, aggregation, and adherence changes. On the other hand, nondihydroguaretic acid, which is thought to be a specific inhibitor of the lipoxygenase pathway, also abruptly terminates the response of the leukocyte to a chemotactic stimulus (12). These observations are limited by inherent difficulties in assumptions that the effects of inhibitors are highly specified and exclusive to the functions under study. Using a different approach, which is akin to "force-feeding" the prostaglandin system by incubating leukocytes in the presence of arachidonic acid, reproduces to a limited degree the functional responses of the same cells to a chemotactic stimulus (11). As would be expected, analogues of archidonic acid will interfere with leukocytic responses to chemotactic stimuli. In summary, accumulated data implicate the prostaglandin system as an important intermediary in facilitating the ability of a leukocyte to respond to a chemotactic stimulus. Precisely how the prostaglandin system is involved and the nature of the critical product(s) is not known.

Activation of the leukocytic lipoxygenase pathway by a chemotactic stimulus also results in the generation of a series of lipids that have varying biological activities (4). For instance, monohydroxyeicosatetraenoic acid (5-HETE) and a dihydroxy-HETE product (also known as leukotriene B_4) are chemotactic lipids, the latter being approximately 1000-fold more active. Precisely what role the production of chemotactic lipids by cells activated with a chemotactic peptide plays in the inflammatory response is unclear. This could be an amplification process for mobilization of leukocytes. Activation of the lipoxygenase pathway also leads to generation of other leukotrienes, some of which undergo glutathione adduction, resulting in the formation of slow reacting substance (SRS). The chief biological activities of the SRS leukotrienes appear to be smooth muscle contraction and increased vasopermeability. Whether any of the lipids described above are essential and critical products for facilitation of the chemotactic response of the leukocyte is not presently known. The only overriding observation would appear to be the fact that interruption of the prostaglandin system blocks the cell response to a chemotactic peptide. All else is speculation.

Coincidental Leukocytic Responses to Chemotactic Peptides

Binding of a chemotactic peptide with its receptor not only leads to increases in both random and directed (chemotactic) motility, but the event also results in at least two other functional responses. Those include secretory release of lysosomal enzymes and production of oxygen metabolites (Fig. 4.4) (5, 14). The former involves a nonspecific release of lysosomal products, although contents of secondary granules are released before those of azurophilic granules. It is possible to quantitate the enzyme release response of the neutrophil to a chemotactic stimulus, provided the stimulus is a peptide. Chemotactic lipids will not induce enzyme secretion. Also, it should be pointed out that chemotactic peptides induce changes in cell motility but do not cause secretory release of granule contents from eosinophils. Thus, enzyme release is not a necessary concomitant of the response of the leukocyte to a chemotactic stimulus.

The other potentially important concomitant of the leukocyte response to a chemotactic stimulus is activation of NADP(H) oxidase and the subsequent production of a series of oxygen products, including O_2^-, $OH\cdot$, $^1O_2$ and H_2O_2. The first three of these are extremely unstable products; O_2^-, $OH\cdot$, H_2O_2 can participate in peroxidative reactions, the result of which may lead to direct structural changes in lipids, proteins, and carbohydrates, as well as inactivation of antiproteases (α_1-antiproteinase) and the oxidation of arachidonic acid resulting in a chemotactic lipid. It has been demonstrated under *in vitro* conditions that oxygen products from activated leukocytes can directly inflict cell injury on red cells,

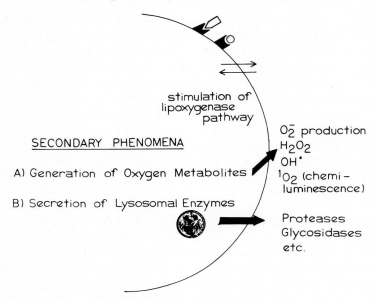

FIG. 4.4. The chemotactic mechanism—4.

fibroblasts, tumor cells, and endothelial cells, depending on the particular experimental circumstances (reviewed in ref. 8). Thus, oxygen metabolites generated
from leukocytes have a wide potential for causing cell injury, amplification of the
inflammatory response, and impairment of defenses against leukocytic proteases.
In recent studies of acute immune complex-induced lung injury, direct evidence
has been obtained that oxygen products (presumably from leukocytes) play a
major role in lung damage, via O_2^- generation, which intensifies the inflammatory
response, and H_2O_2, which is directly related to tissue injury (11).

It should be emphasized that, like enzyme release, the production of oxygen
products from chemotactically stimulated leukocytes is not an essential step
required for the chemotactic response of the cell, since granulocytes from patients
with chronic granulomatous disease of childhood demonstrate normal chemotactic function, even though these cells are incapable of generating oxygen
metabolites (reviewed in ref. 1). This defect appears to be due to the failure in
activation of NADP(H) oxidase after cell contact with a chemotactic stimulus.

REGULATION OF CHEMOTACTIC PEPTIDES

In view of the extraordinary degree of biological activity possessed by chemotactic peptides (in the range of 10^{-7} to 10^{-10} M), it is not surprising that highly
efficient control mechanisms exist. These are of two types and involve either
plasma inhibitors or cell regulators. The plasma inhibitors include chemotactic
factor inactivators (reviewed in ref. 1) and the anaphylatoxin inactivator (reviewed in ref. 15) The latter is a carboxypeptidase N of serum which cleaves the
C terminal residue (arginine) from C5a (and from bradykinin), resulting in its
biological inactivation. C5a des arg, however, can apparently interact with an
acidic cofactor protein in plasma, resulting in restoration and stabilization of
biological (chemotactic) activity. However, the anaphylatoxin activity (identified
by smooth muscle contracting activity and histamine releasing activity for baso-

phils and mast cells) is not restored in the process. The chemotactic factor inactivator(s) probably represents a family of enzyme-like substance in plasma (or serum). One of these, which has been purified to homogeneity, has the ability to inactivate irreversibly both C5a and C5a des arg. A second inactivator present in human plasma or serum has the ability to bring about hydrolysis and, thus, inactivation of the synthetic chemotactic oligopeptides. Imbalances in the levels of the chemotactic factor inactivator result in perturbed inflammatory responses (reviewed in ref. 1). Deficiencies of the inactivator are associated with excess generation of chemotactic activity in complement-activated serum while excess levels of the inactivator are associated with depressed amounts of chemotactic activity generated in complement-activated serum. Patients with lepromatous leprosy, as a rule, have high levels in serum of the chemotactic factor inactivator. In these individuals, skin inflammatory reactions result in an accumulation of neutrophils that is approximately half of what has been observed quantitatively in patients with tuberculoid leprosy, a condition in which the inactivator levels are normal (2). Experimentally it has been demonstrated that, in animals developing acute immune complex-induced alveolitis, the presence of small (micrograms) quantities of purified human chemotactic factor inactivator will markedly suppress the inflammatory reaction, presumably through the ability of the inactivator to rapidly destroy chemotactic signals in tissue generated from immune complex activation of the complement system (6).

There are also leukocyte-related mechanisms that regulate chemotactic factors bound to cell surface receptors. For instance, the binding of the synthetic chemotactic peptide N-formyl-Met-Leu-Phe is associated with a rapid hydrolysis of the peptide, presumably due apparently to the presence of an ectoenzyme on the surface of the leukocyte (reviewed in ref. 1). Once bound to the receptor, any nonhydrolyzed chemotactic peptide is rapidly internalized, apparently within pinocytic vesicles. This occurs both in the case of FMLP as well as C5a. The fate of the internalized peptide is not known, although there is preliminary evidence of peptide hydrolysis. The internalization process not only results in removal of receptor-bound chemotactic peptide but also in removal of the chemotactic receptor, leading to a diminished density of surface bound receptors and a form of "down regulation" of chemotactic receptors. To date, nothing can be said regarding turnover of chemotctic receptors under "resting" (nonoccupancy) conditions and "activation" (receptor occupancy) conditions. There are some hints that nonsteroidal anti-inflammatory drugs cause reduction in density of chemotactic receptors on neutrophils, but whether this is related to the clinical (anti-inflammatory) effects of the drugs is not presently known.

CLINICALLY RELEVANT DEFECTS OF THE CHEMOTACTIC SYSTEM

Over the past decade there have been an enormous number of reports of chemotactic defects in humans, some associated clinically with profound, recurrent life-threatening bacterial infections, others being incidental observations, and many lying between these two extremes (reviewed in ref. 3). Interestingly, there is no evidence that chemotactic defects are associated with an increased incidence of viral infections, suggesting that mobilization of blood leukocytes may not be critical in host defenses to pathogenic viruses. Many surveys of chemotactic defects have been presented and will not be repeated here. From a mechanistic point of view, however, chemotactic defects can be divided into three broad categories: those with *cell associated defects*, those due to *deficiencies* of *substrates* for the generation of chemotactic factors. and, finally, those related to the presence of *serum inhibitors.*

The first category (cell defects) comprises both familial and acquired defects, although the latter greatly outnumber the former. Familial defects of chemotaxis include the Chediak-Higashi syndrome and the actin-dysfunction syndrome, both of which are associated with combined chemotactic and phagocytic defects (reviewed in ref. 3). The basis of the dysfunction in the Chediak-Higashi syndrome is thought to be due to defective microtubules, while in the actin dysfunction syndrome the problem appears to be related to a protein cofactor required for actin filament integrity. Acquired chemotactic defects are numerous and occur in relation to viral infectious diseases, metabolic disorders (diabetes mellitus, uremia), neoplastic states, prematurity, and a large number of other circumstances. In general, the cell biological or biochemical basis for these defects is not usually known, although the chemotactic defect found in leukocytes from neonatal individuals has been related to diminished cell membrane deformability. With the ability to measure receptor density on leukocyte cell membranes, it is possible that the basis for many of the acquired chemotactic defects will be related to diminished numbers of chemotactic receptors on leukocytes.

Defects involving deficiency of substrates related to generation of chemotactic peptides may be of more theoretical than practical significance. For instance, the overriding problem in humans genetically deficient in the fifth component of complement (C5) is a relative inability to deal with bacterial infections due to *Neisseria sp.* It has been assumed that the basis for this problem is the inability to generate the cytotoxic unit (membrane attack complex, C5–9) which appears to be critical for defenses against these bacteria. However, it should be pointed out that disturbance of chemotactic mechanisms in these individuals has not been ruled out. A genetically determined deficiency of C3 appears to be incompatible with survival, although whether the key problem here is the loss of sequential activation leading to fragmentation products of C5, or the loss of opsonic function of C3 products, is not known.

The last category of chemotactic defects in humans is related to the presence of abnormal levels of serum inhibitors. It should be emphasized that these inhibitors exist normally in human serum in very low concentrations; they appear to be natural regulators of the chemotactic system, providing a modulating influence and preventing runaway activation of the inflammatory response. One of the inhibitors, the chemotactic factor inactivator (CFI) of C5-related chemotactic peptides, has been described above. In sera that are deficient in the usual low concentration of this CFI (seen, curiously, in patients with a genetic deficiency of α_1 antiproteinase), complement activation results in supernormal levels of chemotactic activity generated in serum. Patients with this defect could be predicted to have excessive expression of inflammatory reactions. The much more common abnormality in CFI is elevated levels, which are commonly found in sera from patients with Hodgkin's disease, pulmonary sarcoidosis, hepatic cirrhosis, and lepromatous leprosy. Complement activation of sera from these individuals produces much lower levels of chemotactic activity when compared to the levels generated in normal serum. In general, elevated serum levels of CFI are associated with depressed skin reactions to cutaneously injected stimuli (antigens from bacteria or fungi) and are also associated with a diminished mobilization of neutrophils into nonspecifically irritated epidermal areas.

The other naturally occurring regulator of the chemotaxis system is the cell directed inhibitor (CDI), which is present in the IgG fraction of serum (9). CDI reversibly impairs chemotactic function of both neutrophils and monocytes and also reversibly inhibits phagocytic function of neutrophils. Assuming that CDI is a subfraction of serum IgG, the inhibitory activity appears to be associated with the Fc rather than Fab portion of the molecule, ruling out that CDI is simply a type of autoantibody to leukocytes. Elevated levels of CDI occur in patients with malignant tumors and in a variety of other conditions which frequently prevent unusual infectious diseases (*e.g.*, *Listeria* meningitis).

Understanding the chemotactic system has resulted in many new insights into the inflammatory process. As rapid progress continues in the area of inflammation, it can be predicted that new and novel approaches to suppressing the inflammatory system are just beyond the horizon.

REFERENCES

1. Becker, E. L., and Ward, P. A. Chemotaxis. In *Clinical Immunology*. Edited by C. Parker, pp. 272–297. Philadelphia, W. B. Saunders, 1980.
2. Bullock, W. E., Ho, M. F., and Chen, M. J. Quantitative and qualitative studies of the local cellular exudative response in leprosy. *J. Reticuloendothelial Soc. 16:* 259–268, 1974.
3. Clark, R. A. Disorders of granulocyte chemotaxis. In *Leukocyte Chemotaxis: Methods, Physiology and Clinical Implications*. Edited by J. I. Gallin and P. G. Quie, pp. 329–356. New York, Raven Press, 1978.
4. Goetzl, E. J. Mediators of immediate hypersensitivity derived from arachidonic acid. *N. Engl. J. Med. 14:* 822–825, 1980.
5. Goldstein, I. M., Cerqueira, M., Lind, S., and Kaplan, H. B. Evidence that the superoxide-generating system is associated with the cell surface. *J. Clin. Invest. 59:* 249–254, 1977.
6. Johnson, K. J., Anderson, T. P., and Ward, P. A. Suppression of immune complex-induced inflammation by the chemotactic factor inactivator. *J. Clin. Invest. 59:* 951–958, 1977.
7. Johnson, K. J., and Ward, P. A. The role of oxygen metabolites in acute immune complex induced injury of the lung. *J. Immunol.*, in press, 1982.
8. Klebanoff, S., and Clark, R. A. *The Neutrophil: Function and Clinical Disorders*. New York, North Holland, 1978.
9. Maderazo, E. G., Ward, P. A., Woronick, C. L., and Quintilliani, R. A cell directed inhibitor of leukotaxis. *J. Lab. Clin. Med. 89:* 192–199, 1977.
10. Naccache, P. H., Showell, H. J., Becker, E. L., and Sha'afi, R. I. Sodium, potassium and calcium transport across rabbit polymorphonuclear leukocyte membranes: Effect of chemotactic factor. *J. Cell Biol. 73:* 482–444, 1977.
11. O'Flaherty, J. T., Showell, H. J., Becker, E. L., and Ward, P. A. Arachidonic acid aggregate neutrophils. *Inflam. 3:* 431–436, 1979.
12. O'Flaherty, J. T., Showell, H. J., Ward, P. A., and Becker, E. L. A possible role of arachidonic acid in human neutrophil aggregation and degranulation. *Am. J. Pathol. 95:* 799–810, 1979.
13. Perez, H. D., Goldstein, I. M., Webster, R. O., and Henson, P. M. Enhancement of the chemotactic activity of human C5a des arg by an anionic polypeptide ("cochemotaxin") in normal serum and plasma. *J. Immunol. 126:* 800–804, 1981.
14. Showell, H. J., Freer, R. J., Zigmond, S. H., Schiffmann, E., Aswanilsumar, S., Corcoran, B., and Becker, E. L. The structure activity relations of synthetic peptides as chemotactic factors and inducers of lysosomal enzyme secretion from neutrophils. *J. Exp. Med. 143:* 1154–1169, 1976.
15. Ward, P. A., Hugli, T. E., and Chenaveth, D. E. Complement and chemotaxis. In *Chemical Messengers of the Inflammatory Process, Handbook of Inflammation*, Vol. I, pp. 153–178, 1979.

Chapter 5

Proteases, Antiproteases, and Oxidants: Pathways of Tissue Injury during Inflammation*

AARON JANOFF AND HARVEY CARP†

INTRODUCTION

Human leukocytes contain potentially harmful substances within their cyto-plasmic granules, including proteases capable of degrading connective tissue components (44). Polymorphonuclear neutrophils (PMN) accumulate at sites of acute inflammation, and their lysosomal enzymes may escape to the outside of the cells with subsequent damage to surrounding connective tissue structures (38). In addition, mononuclear phagocytes which accumulate at sites of chronic inflammation are able to secrete neutral proteases with similar potential for degrading connective tissue macromolecules (96, 97). There is, however, a system of antiproteases in the circulation and tissue fluids that inactivates proteases released from PMN (69). Alpha 1-proteinase inhibitor (α1-PI, alpha 1-antitrypsin) is an important component of the antiprotease system in man and is responsible for over 90% of the inhibitory capacity of normal human serum for neutrophil elastase (69). A different antiprotease, not present in the circulation but secreted locally by mucous epithelium of selected organs, is a second important inhibitor of PMN elastase (25). The local balance between inflammatory cell proteases and mucus and circulating antiproteases is probably of great importance in controlling the degree of tissue injury resulting from inflammation.

Recent studies have shown that oxidation inactivates both α1-PI and the mucous inhibitor (12, 14, 15, 19, 61). This is attributed, in the case of α1-PI, to oxidation of methionine residues in or near the active site of the antiprotease (49, 50). Because leuckocytes produce and release several reactive oxygen species during phagocytosis (2), the local balance between proteases and antiproteases may be further disrupted during inflammation by the oxidative inactivation of proteinase inhibitors in the microenvironment of these cells. In this event, tissue components adjacent to leukocytes at sites of inflammation would be even more susceptible to damage by proteases simultaneously released from the phagocytes.

In the present chapter, we will first review some of the proteases of inflam-matory leukocytes and then briefly discuss those endogenous inhibitors which

* This work was supported, in part, by USPHS Grant HL-14262 and by Grant 1143 from The Council for Tobacco Research-U.S.A., Inc.

† H. Carp is a Postdoctoral Fellow of The National Insitute of Environmental Health Sciences (grant 5-T32-07088).

are important regulators of these enzymes. We will then summarize some of the metabolic pathways involved in the generation of reactive oxygen species by leukocytes and follow this with observations on the inactivation of antiproteases by these agents. Evidence will be presented to show that phagocyte-derived oxidants can suppress the activity of α1-PI and the mucous inhibitor. Finally, these divergent observations will be gathered into a composite scheme, and a tentative hypothesis will be offered to account for tissue injury at sites of inflammation.

Detailed reviews of selected aspects of this subject can be found in Havemann and Janoff (36), Baggiolini *et al.* (3, on the neutral proteases of PMN), Fritz *et al* (26, on endogenous antiproteases), and Babior (2) and Klebanoff and Clark (55, on phagocyte oxidizing systems).

PROTEASES OF INFLAMMATORY CELLS

ACID PROTEASES OF PMN

In the period from 1960 to 1970, the acid proteases of PMN (cathepsins D and E) were extensively studied as potential mediators of tissue injury in inflammation (18, 57, 66, 94). The hydrogen ion concentration in the bulk phase of an inflammatory exudate is not sufficiently low to permit these proteases to reach optimal activity (63). However, their contribution to tissue injury is still an open question because the degree of acidity in the *microspace* between phagocytically active neutrophils and connective tissue structures has never been accurately determined. Nevertheless, most workers presently assume that the activity of PMN acid cathepsins is primarily limited to intracellular digestion of phagocytosed protein, since the concentration of hydrogen ions required for acid-cathepsin activity is more likely to be attained within the confines of cytoplasmic vacuoles than in the extracellular space.

With respect to the mediation of tissue injury by inflammatory leukocytes, attention has shifted in recent years to the neutral pH active proteases of these cells (see Table 5.1). In the following two sections, we will discuss those neutral proteases of PMN and macrophages that have been especially implicated in the mediation of tissue damage. Particular emphasis will be placed on the elastases of leukocytes. Potential tissue targets of these enzymes will also be indicated.

TABLE 5.1. NEUTRAL PROTEASES OF NEUTROPHILIC LEUKOCYTES AND MACROPHAGES

Cell	Species	Enzyme	Class	Subcellular Localization
PMN	Man	Elastase	Serine	Azurophil granule
		Cathepsin G	Serine	Azurophil granule
		Unspecified	Serine	Azurophil granule
		Collagenases	Metallo	Specific granule
Macrophage	Mouse	Elastase	Metallo	Secretory product
		Procollagenase	Metallo	Secretory product
		Plasminogen-activator	Serine	Secretory product

a See text for details and references.

NEUTRAL PROTEASES OF PMN AND THEIR TISSUE TARGETS

The polymorphonuclear neutrophil contains preformed proteases in its cytoplasmic lysosomal granules. These enzymes are discharged when the cell encounters objects to be phagocytosed or undergoes postmortem autolysis. For a recent discussion of the mechanisms of lysosomal enzyme discharge by viable PMN, see Weismann *et al.* (95) and Chapter 6 in this volume.

The protease content of the cytoplasmic granules of human PMN has been reviewed by Baggiolini and coworkers (1978). The azurophil granules of these cells contain three proteases active at neutral pH: elastase, cathepsin G (which is responsible for the chymotrypsin-like activity first described in PMN by Mounter and Atiyeh (65) and characterized by Rindler *et al.* (75)), and a third enzyme which (like the aforementioned two) is also a serine-protease (3). (In addition, azurophil granules of human PMN contain small amounts of the carboxyl protease cathepsin D, active at acid pH, as well as the thiol protease cathepsin B.) Two neutral metallo-proteases are contained in the specific granules of human PMN, of which one is the specific collagenase originally described by Lazarus *et al.* (58). Thus, all four families of proteolytic enzymes (aspartic acid, cysteine, serine, and metallo) are represented in the two granule classes of human PMN.

Of the various PMN proteases mentioned above, the elastase has attracted the greatest attention because of its broad substrate specificity. Human PMN elastase is a well-characterized enzyme which has been purified and described by many different workers (8, 22, 45, 71, 79, 83, 90). The enzyme has a molecular weight of about 33,000 and is a glycoprotein with variably reported carbohydrate content. PMN elastase is a serine protease which is inhibited by diisopropyl fluorophosphate and by active site-directed chloromethyl ketone inactivators of pancreatic elastase, including those with high specificity for the latter enzyme, but the two proteases can be distinguished by immunologic and other criteria, as well as on the basis of their different molecular weights. Studies by Blow (10) showed preferential cleavage of the oxidized insulin B chain by PMN elastase at peptide bonds to which valine contributes the carboxyl group.

A wide variety of proteins can be readily hydrolyzed by PMN elastase. In addition to solubilizing elastin (47, 48), this enzyme can attack cartilage proteoglycan (7, 46, 52) and several types of collagen molecules (28, 59, 82). Types I and II collagen are apparently cleaved by PMN elastase at the nonhelical, telopeptide region of the molecules, which contain the intermolecular cross-links. Resultant depolymerization and denaturation facilitates further nonspecific proteolytic attack. By contrast, types III and IV collagen (the latter is present primarily in basement membranes) are cleaved by PMN elastase across the helical portion of the tropocollagen molecules, randomly in the case of type IV collagen but at a single cleavage site in type III collagen. This site has been localized to a peptide bond which is only four amino acid residues away from the specific cleavage site of true mammalian collagenases (60).

In addition to the foregoing structural tissue components, a variety of functionally important molecules usually present at sites of inflammation can be degraded by PMN elastase. These include immunoglobulins (23, 74) and intermediates of the kinin, complement, fibrinolytic, and clotting cascades (for a review, see Havemann and Janoff (36)).

Cathepsin G, the second major neutral protease of the human PMN, is also a serine protease, but with chymotrypsin-like properties (75). This enzyme has been purified and characterized (76, 79). Cathepsin G attacks the microfibrillar component of the elastic fiber and even degrades amorphous elastin, albeit weakly (86). Proteoglycan molecules can also be hydrolyzed by this enzyme (52) as well as certain components of the complement, fibrinolytic, and clotting cascades (reviewed in Havemann and Janoff (36)).

The extent to which specific-granule collagenases and the unidentified serine protease of azurophil granules (see Table 5.1) contribute to PMN-mediated tissue injury is presently unclear.

NEUTRAL PROTEASES OF MACROPHAGES AND THEIR TISSUE TARGETS

A considerable body of evidence has accumulated recently showing that stimulated macrophages secrete a variety of neutral proteases in cell culture systems. Protease secretion can be induced by a phagocytic challenge (32), by nonspecific inflammatory stimuli (96, 97), or by lymphokines secreted from thymus-derived lymphocytes after exposure to specific antigens (31, 56, 68, 92, 93). Most of this evidence derives from studies of peritoneal exudative macrophages of mice, but secretion of elastase by mouse alveolar macrophages has also been recently demonstrated (99). The enzymes produced by mouse peritoneal exudative macrophages include a serine-dependent plasminogen-activator with trypsin-like specificity (91) and a metalloenzyme with specific collagenolytic activity (96), which is secreted in proenzyme form and can be activated by trypsin or plasmin (98). Mouse macrophages also secrete an elastolytic protease that appears to be quite different from other known mammalian elastases.

Murine macrophage elastase is a calcium-dependent metalloenzyme (4, 96, 100) with a molecular weight of 21,000 to 28,000 (100). Mouse macrophage elastase appears to be resistant to inhibition by human alpha 1-proteinase inhibitor (100) and, in fact, can degrade this inhibitor (6). Using the oxidized B chain of insulin as substrate, Kettner et al. (53) showed that the enzyme preferentially hydrolyzed peptide bonds to which leucine contributes the amino group (the major cleavage sites being Ala-Leu and Tyr-Leu).

The elastase secreted by murine macrophages slowly hydrolyzes insoluble elastin, but the rate of elastin solubilization can be markedly enhanced if the particulate substrate is first complexed with anionic detergents like sodium dodecyl sulfate (SDS) (97, 99). Kagan and Lerch (51) have suggested that the increased susceptibility of SDS-elastin to elastolytic attack may be due to enhancement of charge complementarity between enzyme and substrate when the latter bears negatively charged SDS ligands. Mouse macrophage elastase can also degrade proteoglycan molecules (White and McDevitt, personal communication) and immunoglobulins (5).

However, secretion of an elastase by *human* macrophages is not yet clearly established. De Cremoux and his colleagues (21) reported secretion of an elastase-like enzyme by human and monkey alveolar macrophages, and Green et al. (33) observed elastolytic activity produced by alveolar macrophages of dogs and man. Rodriguez et al.[77] also detected elastase secretion from cultured alveolar macrophages of human smokers, but not from those of nonsmokers. However, Hinman and coworkers (39) showed that the hydrolysis of insoluble elastin by human alveolar macrophages is probably due to polymorphonuclear neutrophil elastase previously sequestered in the macrophages. These workers also detected a second enzyme in human macrophages which hydrolyzed a synthetic amide substrate of elastase and which was clearly different from the PMN enzyme. However, this second enzyme was secreted in very small amounts and did not hydrolyze insoluble elastin. Thus, its biological significance remains to be determined. In support of Hinman's findings, the elastolytic enzyme of human alveolar macrophages described by Green *et al.* (33) closely resembles human PMN elastase (a serine protease) and differs markedly from mouse macrophage elastase (a metalloenzyme). Furthermore, there is direct evidence that human alveolar macrophages can endocytose human PMN elastase (11). For these reasons, it is still too early to say with certainty that a true elastase is synthesized and secreted by human macrophages.

ENDOGENOUS INHIBITORS OF INFLAMMATORY CELL PROTEASES (Table 5.2)

ALPHA 1-PROTEINASE INHIBITOR (ALPHA 1-ANTITRYPSIN)

In man, α1-PI is a glycoprotein with a molecular weight of 52,000, and it is synthesized primarily in hepatocytes. Alpha 1-PI in tissues is derived mainly from the circulation as a component of plasma transudate. The molecule is a relatively broad spectrum proteinase inhibitor, but its principal physiologic role appears to be the inhibition of elastase released from phagocytically active or dying PMN throughout the body (69). Macrophage elastase, by contrast, resists inhibition by

TABLE 5.2. SOME ENDOGENOUS INHIBITORS OF PMN NEUTRAL PROTEASES

Inhibitor	Source(s)	Molecular Weight (daltons, $\times 10^{-3}$)	Physiological Regulators	References
Alpha 1-proteinase inhibitor	Liver	52	PMN elastase	Ohlsson (69); Johnson and Travis (49); Gadek *et al.* (27)
Alpha 1-antichymotrypsin	Liver	68	PMN cathepsin G	Aronsen *et al.* (1); Ohlsson and Akesson (70); Travis *et al.* (86); Travis *et al.* (87); Beatty *et al.* (9)
Alpha 2-macroglobulin	Liver mainly (also macrophage)	725	PMN elastase, cathepsin G, and collagenase	Ohlsson and Olsson (72); Starkey and Barrett (81); White *et al.* (100)
Mucous proteinase inhibitors	Mucous epithelium	10	PMN elastase and cathepsin G	Hochstrasser *et al.* (42); Ohlsson *et al.* (73); Tegner (84); Fritz *et al.* (25); Hochstrasser (40)

a Major physiological regulator.

α1-PI (5, 100). The active site structure of this inhibitor has recently been determined by Johnson and Travis (49), who showed that it contains a methionine-serine peptide bond. It is apparently this bond which is cleaved by elastase early in a series of reactions that ultimately leads to formation of highly stable complexes between 1 mole of protease and 1 mole of antiprotease. The high stability of this complex (which allows α1-PI to act as a "pseudoirreversible" inhibitor) may be based on either a very low dissociation constant or on covalent bonding or tetrahedral complex formation between the enzyme's active center serine residue and a carbonyl group at the active site of the inhibitor (20, 64). In any event, the inhibition of elastase by α1-PI depends on cleavage of a methionine-serine bond in the inhibitor by the enzyme, and this dependence will figure prominently in our later discussion of the effects of phagocyte-derived oxidants on α1-PI function at sites of inflammation.

ALPHA 1-ANTICHYMOTRYPSIN

Alpha-1-antichymotrypsin (37) is also synthesized in the liver and reaches inflamed tissues via the circulation. Like α1-PI, α1-antichymotrypsin (α1-ACHY) is an acute phase reactant protein, but plasma concentrations of α1-ACHY increase more rapidly and to higher levels following injury than do those of α1-PI. Although the normal plasma molar concentration of α1-ACHY is only about one-fifth that of α1-PI, the concentration of the former inhibitor may double within 8 hours after injury whereas α1-PI elevation requires 24 to 48 hours to reach peak values and, even then, seldom reaches 150 percent of its base line concentration (1). The rapid and large acute phase response of α1-ACHY suggests an important protective function for this agent in inflammatory reactions, and this function may be to inhibit PMN cathepsin G (the chymotrypsin-like enzyme of the azurophil granules in human PMN) (9, 69, 70). In addition, other chymotrypsin-like enzymes in tissues, for example, mast cell "chymase," may be regulated by α1-ACHY. Further details of the properties and reactions of this inhibitor can be found in recent articles by Travis and his coworkers (87, 88).

ALPHA 2-MACROGLOBULIN

In contrast to the two plasma inhibitors just discussed, alpha-2-macroglobulin (α-2M) possesses quite different properties. This liver-synthesized molecule has the broadest enzyme inhibitory spectrum of all the circulating antiproteases, being active against many enzymes of bacterial, plant, and animal origin (81). In addition, α-2M has two combining sites for many mammalian enzymes, including PMN elastase, so that 1 mole of α-2M can inhibit 2 moles of the PMN enzyme (72). Third, α-2M does not form a rigid structural complex with proteases involving covalent bonding* or tetrahedral complex formation between active centers of enzyme and inhibitor. Instead, following cleavage by the enzyme of susceptible peptide bonds in the inhibitor, the latter undergoes a conformational change which "traps" the protease within its confines, sterically hindering further interaction of the enzyme with its substrates (81). The degree of inhibition,

---

* Recently, however, some evidence has been obtained suggesting that α2M-protease complexes may be partly stabilized by covalent bonds. Nevertheless, these bonds do not involve the active center of the enzyme (78a).

however, is dependent on substrate size; small synthetic substrates are readily hydrolyzed, and even some high molecular weight substrates can be degraded by α-2Mprotease complexes under certain circumstances. Thus, tropoelastin, soluble elastin, and even insoluble elastin have been reported to undergo attack by α-2Melastase complexes (29, 30). Finally, as might be predicted from the fact that an "endopeptidase-trapping" mechanism of inhibition requires conformational changes, α-2M is a very large molecule (725,000 in molecular weight). This last feature probably accounts for the very low molar concentration of α-2M in plasma transudates in comparison to α1-PI and α1-ACHY, except when inflammation with attendant increased vascular permeability is present. Monocytes and macrophages may be capable of synthesizing small amounts of α-2M (43, 101).

LOCAL MUCOUS PROTEINASE INHIBITORS

Human mucous secretions, including bronchial mucus, contain locally produced inhibitors of leukocyte proteases (Fritz *et al.*, 1978). The inhibitors present in seminal plasma, cervical mucus, and bronchial secretions have been purified and appear identical in their immunological and antiprotease activities, although some differences may exist in their primary amino acid sequences (40). In contrast to the circulating inhibitors, the local mucous proteinase inhibitors are low molecular weight and acid-stable, and they are found in only trace amounts in the circulation (micrograms per deciliter).

The low molecular weight, acid-stable proteinase inhibitor present in human bronchial mucus (BMPI) was first described by Hochstrasser *et al.* (41) and, later, was isolated and partly characterized by Ohlsson *et al.* (73). This substance is a cationic polypeptide with a molecular weight of 10,322. It is thought to represent the major antiprotease (on a molar basis) protecting the upper, mucus-lined airways against the destructive effects of inflammatory cell proteases (84). Both PMN elastase and cathepsin G are well-inhibited by this agent; by contrast, macrophage elastase appears to resist inhibition by BMPI (Carp and White, unpublished observations).

The precise cellular source of the low molecular weight mucous inhibitors is presently uncertain. In the case of BMPI, immunoperoxidase staining techniques have demonstrated its presence in the seromucous glands of tracheal and maxillary-sinus mucosa (85). The serous cells of bronchial mucous glands as well as goblet cells and Clara cells have also been suggested as possible sources of BMPI (24). Gadek and colleagues (27) reported undetectable levels of BMPI in bronchioalveolar lavage fluids of humans, obtained by washing below the major airways. They suggested that BMPI is present in only small amounts in peripheral airways and that its primary function is to protect the upper airways (bronchi, trachea, and nasopharynx) against proteolytically mediated injury.

OXIDATIVE INACTIVATION OF α1-PI AND BMPI

In an earlier section, the molecular mechanism of elastase inhibition by α1-PI was briefly discussed, and it was pointed out that an important early step in the process involves cleavage of a methionyl-seryl bond in the active site of the inhibitor (49). All subsequent steps leading to the formation of stable complexes between the protease and the antiprotease depend on hydrolysis of this peptide bond. In their more recent work, Johnson and Travis (49) showed that selective, chemical oxidation of the active site methionine thioether side chain to methionine sulfoxide prevents the cleavage of the adjacent peptide bond by elastase (a prerequisite for inhibition of the enzyme). Oxidized α1-PI interacts with PMN elastase at only 1/2000th of the rate given by the native inhibitor (9). Similar findings have been obtained with synthetic elastase substrates containing methionine in the P_1 position. Oxidation of the methionine side chain in these synthetic peptides also prevents hydrolysis of adjacent amide or ester bonds by PMN elastase (67).

The active site structure of BMPI is not presently known; however, oxidizable residues also appear to be present close to the reactive center of this inhibitor (Fritz, personal communication). (A closely related, low molecular weight, acid-stable inhibitor in dog submandibular glands contains a methionyl aspartyl bond in its elastase and chymotrypsin-directed reactive center (41).) As might be expected, BMPI can also be inactivated by chemical oxidants *in vitro* (14).

Thus, oxidants generated by inflammatory cells could theoretically inactivate two important components of the tissue antiprotease "screen", namely, α1-PI and locally produced mucous proteinase inhibitors. In the next section, we will identify some inflammatory cell oxidants which could act in this way.

OXIDANTS GENERATED BY INFLAMMATORY CELLS

The oxidizing systems of phagocytes, which participate in microbial killing by these cells, have recently been reviewed in some detail (2, 55). According to present knowledge, the main features of oxygen metabolism in PMN (and, with some modification, in monocytes and macrophages) are as follows. Upon phagocytosis or exposure to certain membrane-active agents, phagocytes undergo a "respiratory burst" characterized by increased oxygen consumption, increased production of hydrogen peroxide, and increased utilization of glucose via the hexose monophosphate shunt. The increase in oxygen consumption may be related to activation of a cyanide-insensitive, membrane-bound NAD(P) H-dependent oxidoreductase which catalyzes the single electron reduction of molecular oxygen to the superoxide radical, as in equation a: $2\ O_2 + NAD(P)\ H \rightarrow 2\ O_2^- + NAD(P)^+ + H^+$. The NAD(P) generated in this reaction stimulates the hexose monophosphate shunt, since NAD(P) is a substrate in the first step of this metabolic pathway. In this first step, glucose-6-phosphate is converted to 6-phosphogluconate by glucose-6-phosphate dehydrogenase. At the same time, NAD(P) is converted to NAD(P)H, thus replenishing the substrate required by the membrane oxidase in equation a above. NAD(P)H generated by the shunt is also utilized by glutathione reductase. (The latter enzyme, together with glutathione peroxidase, functions to detoxify any excess hydrogen peroxide produced by PMN in the course of the "respiratory burst.")

The superoxide radical formed in equation a can serve as an oxidant directly, or this radical can generate more powerful activated oxygen species (†) or oxygen free radicals (‡) by the reactions shown in equations b and c:

Equation b (dismutation reaction)§:
$P_2^- + O_2^- + 2H^+ \rightarrow H_2O_2$ (†) $+ O_2$ (or singlet O_2?) (†)
Equation c (Haber-Weiss type reaction, trace metal catalyzed):
$O_2^- + H_2O_2 \rightarrow OH^-$ (‡) $+ OH^- + O_2$ (or singlet O_2?) (†)

---

§ Evidence is presently lacking to confirm the production of singlet oxygen by phagocytic cells in equations b and c.

Theoretically, these activated oxygen species and oxygen free radicals could inactivate α1-PI and BMPI within the phagocytic vacuole or in the immediate environment of the phagocytic cell.

In addition to the reaction shown in equation *c*, hydrogen peroxide can participate in other oxidative processes by serving as a cofactor for myeloperoxidase of PMN and monocytes. A second cofactor, usually a halide such as chloride or iodide anion, is also required. (Thyroid hormones can seve as a source of iodide for PMN.) In these myeloperoxidase-catalyzed reactions, hypohalous acids (*e.g.*, HOCl) or free halogens (*e.g.*, iodine) can be formed, and these, in turn, are powerful oxidizing agents.

Activation of the membrane-oxidase which initiates the foregoing series of reactions (see equation *a*) appears to require a limited proteolysis step mediated by a serine enzyme with chymotrypsin-like activity (54). However, PMN and monocytes of individuals with chronic granulomatous disease appear incapable of activating the membrane-oxidase during phagocytosis. In these subjects, a normal "respiratory burst" does not accompany the endocytic event. This condition is one of several in which phagocyte oxidative reactions are impaired, with serious consequences for host antimicrobial defense.

It seems reasonable to propose that stimulated phagocytes might be capable of inactivating proteinase inhibitors by virtue of oxidative reactions described above. Evidence to support this will be presented next.

INACTIVATION OF α1-PI AND BMPI BY PHAGOCYTE-DERIVED OXIDANTS

Carp and Janoff (13) showed that human PMN, phagocytosing opsonized antigen-antibody complexes adsorbed to the outer surface of dialysis membranes, produce diffusible substances which are capable of suppressing the elastase-inhibiting capacity of whole serum of purified α1-PI present within the membrane-bound compartment (Fig. 5.1). Superoxide dismutase (which catalyzes the dismutation of superoxide radical to hydrogen peroxide), catalase (which breaks down hydrogen peroxide to water and oxygen), and mannitol (a scavenger of hydroxyl radical (OH·)) partly protected serum against inactivation, suggesting that products of the "respiratory burst" were responsible for the observed results (Table 5.3). An artificial superoxide radical-generating system, involving xanthine and xanthine oxidase, could be substituted for phagocytosing PMN with similar results (Table 5.4).

More recently, the same authors (15) extended their observations to human mononuclear phagocytes (blood monocytes and alveolar macrophages) in addition to PMN, and they activated the cells with a nonphagocytic stimulus (cell membrane excitation with phorbol myristate acetate). Under these conditions, "respiratory-burst" products are formed without bulk release of azurophil granule constituents (Fig. 5.2). Such stimulated cells also released reactive oxygen species able to suppress elastase inhibition by human serum (Table 5.5). Immunoelectrophoretic analysis of the enzyme-serum reaction mixtures showed decreased α1-PI-elastase complexes and free elastase (Fig. 5.3). Treatment of phagocyte-inactivated serum with dithiothreitol (a reducing agent) resulted in significant recovery of inhibitory activity (Fig. 5.3) suggesting that, originally, α1-PI had been

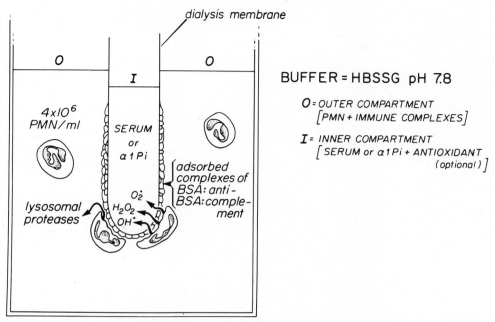

FIG. 5.1. Experimental system for assaying the effect of oxidants released from phagocytosing PMN upon serum proteinase inhibitors. Opsonized immune complexes (bovine serum albumin + anti-bovine serum albumin) are adsorbed to the external surface of the dialysis membranes and serve as a phagocytic stimulus for PMN present in the external compartment (dialysate). Low molecular weight oxygen-free radicals, activated oxygen species, and activated halides can diffuse into the dialysis membrane-bound inner compartment (dialysand) containing the proteinase inhibitors. Higher molecular weight lysosomal proteases (which also consume inhibitors by complex-formation) cannot penetrate the membrane and so are prevented from entering. Free radical scavengers such as suproxide dismutase and mannitol or other protective agents such as catalase can be added to the inner compartment in selected experiments.

oxidatively inactivated. Again, superoxide dismutase and catalase were partly protective (Table 5.5). Catalase was more effective than dismustase, possibly because elimination of H_2O_2 blocks both OH^- formation *and* myeloperoxidase-dependent reactions (see below). PMN and monocytes from a patient with chronic granulomatous disease (which do not undergo a "respiratory burst"), as expected, failed to produce detectable levels of superoxide anion following stimulation with phorbol ester, and these cells also failed to suppress serum elastase inhibition (Table 5.5).

Matheson *et al.* (61) demonstrated the inactivation of α1-PI by PMN myeloperoxidase acting in a cell-free system. More recently, these investigators succeeded in isolating human myeloperoxidase and they extended their characterization of the inactivation of human α1-PI by the homologous peroxidatic enzyme (Travis, personal communication). Carp and Janoff (15) confirmed Matheson's finding of α1-PI inactivation by purified myeloperoxidase and showed that the reaction is dependent on H_2O_2 and a halide cofactor and that it can take place at neutral pH (see Fig. 5.3). They also implicated myeloperoxidase in the inactivation of α1-PI by phagocytosing PMN (13) and by PMN and monocytes stimulated

TABLE 5.3. INACTIVATION OF PURIFIED α1 AND SERUM ELASTASE INHIBITING CAPACITY (EIC) BY PHAGOCYTOSING PMN

Dialysate Contents[a]			Dialysand Contents[b]			Assay Results (%)	
Opsonized BSA (anti-BSA complexes)[c]	PMN	NaN$_3$	Serum	α1-PI	Protective agent	O$_2'$ in dialysand[d]	EIC of dialysand[e]
+	−	−	−	−	−	0	0
+	−	−	+	−	−	0	100
+	+	−	+	−	−	100	64 ± 2.3
−	+	−	+	−	−	0	100 ± 3.1
+	+	−	+	−	SOD	0	81 ± 1.9
+	+	−	+	−	Catalase	97 ± 2.3	84 ± 2.0
+	+	−	+	−	Mannitol	98 ± 2.9	83 ± 1.9
+	+	−	+	−	SOD + catalase + mannitol	0	81 ± 1.8
+	+	−	+	−	HISOD	97 ± 3.5	60 ± 2.4
+	+	−	+	−	HI catalase	103 ± 3.5	58 ± 3.2
+	−	−	−	+	−	NT	100
+	+	−	−	+	−	NT	46 ± 2.1
+	+	−	−	−	SOD + catalase + mannitol	NT	0[f]
+	+	−	−	−	−	NT	0[f]
+	+	+	−	−	−	NT	0[f]
+	+	+	+	−	−	103 ± 2.8	79 ± 3 2

(Data reproduced with permission from H. Carp and A. Janoff (13).)

[a] Concentrations: PMN, 4×10^6/ml; NaN$_3$, 2 mM. The buffer was Hanks' balanced salt solution + 0.2% glucose (HBSSG), pH 7.8.

[b] Concentrations: SOD and heat-inactivated (HI) SOD, 280 units/ml; catalase and HI catalase, 50 units/ml; mannitol, 20 mM; pure α1-PI, 0.075 μg/μl; human serum, 2.5% (vol/vol). The buffer was HBSSG, pH 7.8.

[c] The immune complexes were adsorbed to the external surfaces of the dialysis bags.

[d] The results (mean of three experiments ± 1 SEM) are expressed as a percentage of O$_2'$ detected under standard conditions (immune complexes, 4×10^6 PMN/ml). 100% corresponds to 2.6 nM of O$_2'$.

[e] The results (mean of three experiments ± 1 SEM) are expressed as a percentage of EIC of serum or pure α1-PI not exposed to phagocytosing PMN. EIC = elastase standard (elastase + inhibitor)/ elastase standard × 100.

[f] Control for effects of all reagents used on the enzymatic activity of elastase (EIC = 0 represents 100% enzyme activity).

with phorbol ester (15). The latter conclusions were based on the finding that azide (an inhibitor of myeloperoxidase and other heme enzymes) partly protected serum elastase-inhibition against inactivation by the phagocytes (Tables 5.3 and 5.5).

Two low molecular weight mucous inhibitors, human BMPI and a closely related inhibitor present in human seminal plasma (HUSI-I), were also shown to lose activity following *in vitro* exposure to myeloperoxidase, hydrogen peroxide, and chloride anion (14). These last results are shown in Table 5.6. Tsan and Chen (89) recently demonstrated oxidation of free methionine by PMN and ascribed the effect to myeloperoxidase-mediated reactions and singlet oxygen.

TABLE 5.4. INACTIVATION OF PURIFIED α1-PI AND SERUM EIC BY XANTHINE-XANTHINE OXIDASE

Dialysate Contents[a]		Dialysand Contents[b]			Assay Results (%)	
Xanthine	Xanthine oxidase	Serum	α1-PI	Protective agent	O$_2$ in dialysand[c]	EIC of dialysand[d]
−	−	−	−	−	0	0
−	−	+	−	−	0	100
+	−	+	−	−	0	100 ± 3.0
−	+	+	−	−	0	99 ± 2.4
+	+	+	−	−	100	63 ± 1.6
+	+	+	−	SOD	0	102 ± 2.4
+	+	+	−	Catalase	98 ± 2.3	103 ± 2.1
+	+	+	−	Mannitol	97 ± 2.1	97 ± 3.5
+	+	+	−	HISOD	100 ± 1.5	62 ± 1.5
+	+	+	−	HI catalase	102 ± 3.1	64 ± 3.1
+	+	−	−	−	NT	0[e]
+	+	−	−	SOD	NT	0[e]
+	+	−	−	Catalase	NT	0[e]
+	+	−	−	Mannitol	NT	0[e]
−	−	−	+	−	NT	100
+	+	−	+	−	NT	44 ± 2.1

(Data reproduced with permission from Carp, H. and A. Janoff (13).)

[a] Concentrations: xanthine, 50 μM; xanthine oxidase, 0.6 μM. The buffer was Hanks' balanced salt solution (HBSS), pH 7.8.

[b] Concentrations: the same as in Table 5.3. The buffer was HBSS, pH 7.8.

[c] The results (mean of three experiments ±1 SEM) are expressed as a percentage of O$_2$ detected under standard conditions (only xanthine and xanthine oxidase in the dialysate). 100% corresponds to 3.4 nM of O$_2$.

[d] The results (mean of three experiments ±1 SEM) are expressed as a percentage of EIC of serum or pure α1-PI not exposed to xanthine-xanthine oxidase reaction.

[e] Controls for effects of all reagents used on the enzymatic activity of elastase (see Table 5.3).

Thus, oxidants generated by phagocytically active or metabolically stimulated phagocytes at sites of acute (PMN) or chronic inflammation (monocytes, macrophages) may cause local functional decreases in the activity of elastase inhibitors such as BMPI and HUSI-I and α1-Pi. These reactions could alter the balance between inflammatory cell proteases and tissue antiproteases in favor of the enzymes.

OTHER ACTIONS OF PHAGOCYTE-DERIVED OXIDANTS AT SITES OF INFLAMMATION

In addition to their actions on proteinase inhibitors, the oxidizing agents generated by leukocytes and macrophages can also influence the inflammatory reaction by acting upon a variety of other host cells and molecules. It may be worthwhile to pause briefly to consider some of these additional effects.

Chemotactic peptides, thought to play a role in attracting PMN and monocytes to sites of inflammation, can be inactivated by oxidants generated by the responding cells. Both C5a and N-formyl-methionyl peptides are affected by oxidants (17). This may constitute an important feedback mechanism for self-regulation of leukocyte chemotactic responses at sites of inflammation.

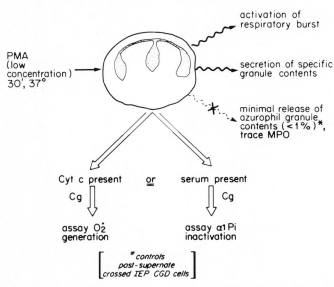

FIG. 5.2. Experimental system for assaying the effect of oxidants released from *PMN*, monocytes (*MNC*), or macrophages stimulated with phorbol myristate acetate (*PMA*) upon serum proteinase inhibitors (*Pi*). At the low concentrations of phorbol ester used, products of the "respiratory burst" are formed, but bulk release of azurophil granule proteases does not take place. Therefore, physical separation of proteinase inhibitors from cells (as in Fig. 5.1) is not necessary. The stimulated cells are either incubated with cytochrome c (and O_2^- production is then measured), or with proteinase inhibitor (and effects upon elastase inhibitory capacity (EIC) are then determined). A variety of experiments ruled out inactivation of proteinase inhibitors by bulk release of lysosomal proteases (crossed antigen-antibody electrophoresis, short-lived potency of inactivating factor(s), failure of chronic granulomatous disease (*CGD*) leukocytes to be effective, protection by antioxidants). In addition, direct measurement of azurophil granule enzymes in the incubation medium revealed <1% release of granule contents.

Oxidant cytotoxicity can decrease viability of a variety of cell types present at inflammatory foci (16, 17), even including the leukocytes responsible for oxidant generation (78).

Host connective tissue macromolecules can also be altered by oxygen free radicals and other reactive oxygen species. For example, gelation of collagen at 37° can be inhibited, if the collagen is first preincubated with xanthine oxidase and hypoxanthine (a superoxide anion generating system). The inhibitory effect is dependent upon production of the superoxide radical during conversion of hypoxanthine to uric acid by the oxidase and is completely blocked by addition of superoxide dismutase or catalase (34). Also, superoxide anion and other secondary oxygen-derived free radicals (produced either by xanthine oxidase or from stimulated polymorphonuclear neutrophils) can depolymerize hyaluronic acid, as reflected in its decreased viscosity and the appearance of glycosaminoglycans of lower molecular weight. The depolymerized hyaluronic acid is then more susceptible to degradation by beta-*N*-acetylglucosaminidase (35). Again, radical scavengers block all of the foregoing changes (35, 62).

Thus, chemotactic mediators, platelets, leukocytes, and extracellular supportive structures can all be altered by phagocyte-derived oxidants at sites of inflamma-

TABLE 5.5. INACTIVATION OF SERUM ELASTASE INHIBITORY CAPACITY (EIC) BY REACTIVE OXYGEN SPECIES FROM PMA*-STIMULATED PHAGOCYTES

Phagocytic Cell (Human)	Phorbol Ester (ng/ml)	Protective Agent	Superoxide Anion Produced (nM/1.6×10^6 cells)	Serum EIC (% of control)
PMN	0	–	0	97 ± 9
PMN	1.5	–	37 ± 7	45 ± 6
PMN	1.5	SOD	0	64 ± 7
PMN	1.5	HISOD	36 ± 8	42 ± 6
PMN	1.5	CAT	35 ± 6	89 ± 5
PMN	1.5	HICAT	36 ± 7	47 ± 5
PMN	1.5	NaN_3	35 ± 7	75 ± 6
CGD-PMN	1.5	–	0	97 ± 9
Monocyte	0	–	2 ± 1	95 ± 5
Monocyte	1.5	–	22 ± 5	52 ± 8
Monocyte	1.5	SOD	0	70 ± 6
Monocyte	1.5	CAT	21 ± 5	95 ± 7
Monocyte	1.5	NaN_3	22 ± 4	77 ± 6
CGD-monocyte	1.5	–	0	96 ± 8
Macrophage	0	–	4 ± 2	90 ± 11
Macrophage	100	–	18 ± 4	55 ± 5

(Data modified from Carp and Janoff (15).)

* PMA, phorbol myristate acetate (phorbol ester); SOD, superoxide dismutase (400 units/ml); CAT, catalase (1500 units/ml); NaN_3, sodium azide (0.3 mM); CGD, chronic granulomatous disease; HI, heat-inactivated. Data are expressed as the mean of three experiments $\pm$ 1 SEM.

tion, in addition to the balance between proteases and proteinase inhibitors. Each of these disturbances may influence the progression of tissue injury at the inflamed site. In the final section, below, the effect of protease-antiprotease imblance will be considered.

SUMMARY AND CONCLUSIONS

The major hypothesis put forward in this article can now be integrated and summarized. Inflammatory leukocytes (PMN in acute reactions, monocytes and macrophages in chronic reactions) liberate a variety of proteolytic enzymes into the surrounding connective tissues in the course of their phagocytic activity. In the case of PMN these include both acid and neutral proteases, of which the latter are more likely to be determinants of extracellular damage. PMN neutral proteases are preformed and stored in azurophil and specific granules and include elastase, cathepsin G, collagenase and a fourth serine-protease with trypsin-like activity. Macrophage neutral proteases are secreted by stimulated cells and include an elastase (different from the PMN enzyme), procollagenase, and plasminogen activator. Connective tissue targets of this array of enzymes include amorphous elastin and associated microfibrils, types I, II, III, and IV collagen, and matrix proteoglycans. A system of proteinase inhibitors is present in tissue fluids which can protect connective tissue macromolecules against attack by phagocyte-derived proteases, but at least two of these inhibitors, α1-PI and locally produced mucous PI, are susceptible to inactivation by oxidants. Reactive oxygen species generated by PMN, monocytes, and macrophages and liberated into the extracellular environment at the same time as the enzymes are capable of

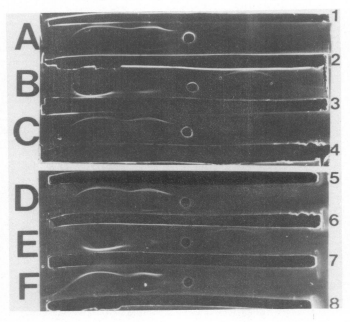

FIG. 5.3. Immunoelectrophoretic analysis of mixtures of elastase and serum under various experimental conditions. Troughs 1, 3, 5, and 7 contain rabbit antiserum to human α1-Pi. Troughs 2, 4, 6, and 8 contain rabbit antiserum to porcine pancreatic elastase. Anode to the left, cathode to the right. *A.* Elastase added to control serum that had been incubated with unstimulated PMN. Note the presence of free α1-PI migrating toward the anode, followed by complexes of α1-PI and elastase. No free elastase was detected. *B.* Elastase added to serum that had been incubated with phorbol ester-stimulated PMN. Note increased free α1-PI, decreased α1-PI-elastase complexes, and uncomplexed elastase migrating toward the cathode. *C.* Elastase added to serum that had been previously treated as in *B*, followed by treatment with dithiothreitol (a reducing agent). In contrast to *B*, no free elastase was detected, and increased α1-PI-elastase complexes were present. *D.* Elastase added to control serum that had been previously incubated with glucose oxidase (as a source of hydrogen peroxide) + Cl$^-$. Note the presence of α1-PI elastase complexes. No free elastase was detected. *E.* Elastase added to serum that had been previously incubated with myeloperoxidase + glucose oxidase + Cl$^-$. Note decreased α1-PI-elastase complexes and uncomplexed elastase migrating toward the cathode. *F.* Elastase added to serum that had been previously treated as in *E*, followed by treatment with dithiothreitol. In contrast to *E*, no free elastase was detected, and increased α1-PI-elastase complexes were present. (Reproduced with permission from H. Carp and A. Janoff (15).

inactivating α1-PI and mucous PI. Oxidants formed by the myeloperoxidase H_2O_2 and halide system of PMN and monocytes are also able to destroy the functional activity of these inhibitors. Since α1-PI and mucous PI are the most effective endogenous regulators of extracellular PMN elastase, some of this enzyme, released at sites of inflammation, may remain free to act on elastin, collagen, and proteoglycan if high enough concentrations of phagocyte-oxidants are present. In this way, a pathway for tissue injury can be visualized (see Fig. 5.4) in which proteases, antiproteases, and oxidants interact to play a key role.

TABLE 5.6. SUPPRESSION OF THE ELASTASE INHIBITORY CAPACITY (EIC) OF TWO LOW MOLECULAR WEIGHT MUCOUS INHIBITORS BY THE MYELOPEROXIDASE-HYDROGEN PEROXIDE-HALIDE SYSTEM

Incubation Mixture					Assay Results
MPO[a] (20 mU/ml)	Glucose-Oxidase (H_2O_2 Source, 50 mU/ml)	Cl⁻ (0.15 M)	Inhibitor (0.5 $\mu g/\mu l$)	Protective Agent	EIC (Mean of 3 Trials ±1 SEM)
−	−	−	HUSI-I	−	100
+	+	+	HUSI-I	−	39 ± 8
−	+	+	HUSI-I	−	97 ± 8
+	−	+	HUSI-I	−	101 ± 9
+	+	−	HUSI-I	−	97 ± 6
+	+	+	HUSI-I	NaN_3	104 ± 9
+	+	+	HUSI-I	CAT	96 ± 10
−	−	−	BMPI	−	100
+	+	+	BMPI	−	54 ± 8
−	+	+	BMPI	−	102 ± 9
+	−	+	BMPI	−	98 ± 10
+	+	−	BMPI	−	98 ± 9
+	+	+	BMPI	NaN_3	97 ± 7
+	+	+	BMPI	CAT	103 ± 7
−	−	−	−	−	0*
+	+	+	−	−	0*
+	+	+	−	NaN_3	0*
+	+	+	−	CAT	0*

(Data modified from Carp and Janoff (14).)

[a] MPO, myeloperoxidase; HUSI-I, human seminal plasma inhibitor; BMPI, human bronchial mucous inhibitor; CAT, catalase (2500 units/ml); NaN_3, sodium azide (2 mM); +, present; −, absent; EIC, human PMN elastase standard (elastase + inhibitor)/elastase standard × 100. Data are expressed as percent of control EIC given by inhibitor alone. *, control for effect of reagent on elastase (EIC = 0, enzyme unaffected).

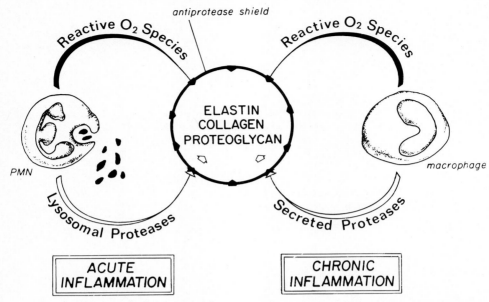

FIG. 5.4. A proposed pathway of tissue injury at sites of inflammation. Proteases, antiproteases, and oxidants interact to modulate the degree of connective tissue destruction which ensues. The major physiologic regulators of PMN elastase (α1-PI and BMPI) are susceptible to inactivation by reactive oxygen species generated at sites of acute inflammation. However, the endogenous regulators of macrophage elastase, an enzyme which may be secreted at sites of chronic inflammation, have not yet been identified (see text). Therefore, it is not known if these inhibitors would also be susceptible to oxidative inactivation. Possible regulation of the overall pathway by tissue antioxidants remains to be explored.

REFERENCES

1. Aronson, K. F., Ekelund, G., Kindmark, C. O., and Laurell, C. B. Sequential changes of plasma proteins after surgical trauma. *Scand. J. Clin. Lab. Invest. 29* (Suppl. 124): 127–136, 1972.
2. Babior, B. M. Oxygen-dependent microbial killing by phagocytes. *N. Engl. J. Med. 298:* 659–668, 721–725, 1978.
3. Baggiolini, M., Bretz, V., Dewald, B., and Feigensen, M. E. The polymorphonuclear leukocyte. *Agents Actions 8* (1–2): 3–10, 1978.
4. Banda, M. J., and Werb, Z. Purification and characterization of macrophage elastase (abstr.) *Fed. Proc. 38* (Part 2): 1339, 1979.
5. Banda, M. J., and Werb, Z. Macrophage elastase degradation of immunoglobulins regulates binding to macrophage Fc receptors. *Fed. Proc. 39* (Part 1): 799, 1980.
6. Banda, M. J., Clark, E. J., and Werb, Z. Limited proteolysis by macrophage elastase inactivates human alpha-1-proteinase inhibitor *J. Exp. Med. 152:* 1563–1570, 1980.
7. Barrett, A. J. The possible role of neutrophil proteinases in damage to articular cartilage. *Agents Actions 8:* 11–18, 1978.
8. Baugh, R. J., and Travis, J. Human leukocyte granule elastase: Rapid isolation and characterization. *Biochemistry 15:* 836–841, 1976.
9. Beatty, K., Bieth, J., and Travis, J. Kinetics of association of serine proteinases with native and oxidized α-1-proteinase inhibitor and α-1-antichymotrypsin. *J. Biol. Chem. 255:* 3931–3934, 1980.
10. Blow, A. M. J. Action of human lysosomal elastase on the oxidized B chain of insulin. *Biochem. J. 161:* 13–16, 1977.
11. Campbell, E. J., White, R. R., Senior, R. M., Rodriguez, R. J., and Kuhn, C. Receptor-mediated binding and internalization of leukocyte elastase by alveolar macrophages *in vitro. J. Clin. Invest. 64:* 824–833, 1979.

12. Carp, H., and Janoff, A. Possible mechanisms of emphysema in smokers. *In vitro* suppression of serum elastase-inhibitory capacity by fresh cigarette smoke and its prevention by anti-oxidants. *Am. Rev. Respir. Dis. 118:* 617–621, 1978.

13. Carp, H., and Janoff, A. *In vitro* suppression of serum elastase-inhibitory capacity by reactive oxygen species generated by phagocytosing polymorphonuclear leukocytes. *J. Clin. Invest. 63:* 793–797, 1979.

14. Carp, H., and Janoff, A. Inactivation of bronchial mucous proteinase inhibitor by cigarette smoke and phagocyte-derived oxidants. *Exp. Lung Res. 1:* 225–237, 1980a.

15. Carp, H., and Janoff A. Potential mediator of inflammation. Phagocyte-derived oxidants suppress the elastase-inhibitory capacity of alpha 1-proteinase inhibitor *in vitro*. *J. Clin. Invest. 66:* 987–995, 1980b.

16. Clark, R. A. Toxic effects of myeloperoxidase and H_2O_2 secreted by neutrophils exposed to a soluble stimulus (abstr.). *Clin. Res. 27:* 209A, 1979.

16a. Clark, R. A., and Klebanoff, S. J. Neutrophil-mediated release of serotonin from human platelets: role of myeloperoxidase and H_2O_2 (abstr.). *Clin. Res. 25:* 474A, 1977.

17. Clark, R. A., and Klebanoff, S. J. Chemotactic factor inactivation by the myeloperoxidase-hydrogen peroxide-halide system. An inflammatory control mechanism. *J. Clin. Invest. 64:* 913–920, 1979.

18. Cochrane, C. G., and Aiken, B. S. Polymorphonuclear leukocytes in immunologic reactions. *J. Exp. Med. 124:* 733–752, 1966.

19. Cohen, A. B. The effects of *in vivo* and *in vitro* of oxidative damage to purified α-1-antitrypsin and to the enzyme-inhibiting activity of plasma. *Am. Rev. Resp. Dis. 119:* 953–960, 1979.

20. Cohen, A. B., Gruenke, L. D., Craig, J. C., and Geczy, D. Specific lysine labeling by [18]OH— during alkaline cleavage of the α-1-antitrypsin-trypsin complex. *Proc. Natl. Acad. Sci. U.S.A. 74:* 4311–4314, 1977.

21. De Cremoux, H., Hornebeck, W., Jaurand, M., Bignon, J., and Robert, L. Partial characterization of an elastase-like enzyme secreted by human and monkey alveolar macrophages. *J. Pathol. 125:* 171–177, 1978.

22. Feinstein, G., and Janoff, A. A rapid method of purification of human granulocyte cationic neutral proteases: purification and further characterization of human granulocyte elastase. *Biochim. Biophys. Acta 403:* 493–505, 1975.

23. Folds, J. D., Prince, H. E., and Spitznagel, J. K. Limited cleavage of human immunoglobulins by elastase of human neutrophil polymorphonuclear granulocytes: possible modulator of immune complex disease. *Lab. Invest. 39:* 313–321, 1978.

24. Franken, C., Kramps, J. A., Meyer, C. J. C. M., and Dijkman, J. H. Localization of the low molecular weight proteinase inhibitor in the respiratory tract. In: *Biochemistry, Pathology and Genetics of Pulmonary Emphysema*. Edited by P. Sadoul and J. Bignon, Paris, Pergamon Press, 1980.

25. Fritz, H., Schiessler, H., and Geiger, R. Naturally occurring low molecular weight inhibitors of neutral proteinases from PMN-granulocytes and of kallikreins. *Agents Actions 8:* 57–64, 1978.

26. Fritz, H., Tschesche, H., Greene, L. J., and Truscheit, E. (eds.). *Proteinase Inhibitors* (Bayer Symposium V). New York, Springer-Verlag, 1974.

27. Gadek, J. E., Fells, G. A., Wright, D. G., and Crystal, R. G. Human neutrophil elastase functions as a type III collagen collagenase. *Biochem. Biophys. Res. Commun. 95:* 1815–1822, 1980.

28. Gadek, J., Fells, G., Zimmerman, R., and Crystal, R. The antielastase screen of the human lower respiratory tract: an assessment of the alpha 1-antitrypsin hypothesis (abstr.). *Am. Rev. Resp. Dis. 121* (part 2): 341, 1980.

29. Galdston, M. Enhanced activity of human neutrophil elastase complexed to alpha 2-macroglobulin in serum of alpha 1-antitrypsin deficient individuals. In *Neutral Proteases of Human Polymorphonuclear Leukocytes*. Edited by K. Havemann and A. Janoff. Baltimore, Urban & Schwarzenberg, 1978.

30. Galdston, M., and Levgtska, V. Enhanced proteolysis of ^{3}H-labelled insoluble elastin by human neutrophil elastase bound to alpha 2-macroglobulin in MM and ZZ (Pi) phenotype sera for alpha 1-antitrypsin (abstr.). *Am. Rev. Resp. Dis. 117* (Part 2): 117, 1978.

31. Gordon, S., Newman, W., and Bloom, B. Macrophage proteases and rheumatic diseases: Regulation of plasminogen activator by thymus-derived lymphocytes. *Agents Actions 8* (1–2): 19–26, 1978.

32. Gordon, S., Unkeless, J. C., and Cohn, Z. A. Induction of macrophage plasminogen activator by

endotoxin stimulation and phagocytosis. Evidence for a two-stage process. *J. Exp. Med. 140:* 995–1010, 1974.

33. Green, M. R., Lin, J. S., Berman, L. B., Osman, M. M., Cerreta, J. M., Mandl, I., and Turino, G. M. Elastolytic activity of alveolar macrophages in normal dogs and human subjects. *J. Lab. Clin. Med. 94:* 549–562, 1979.

34. Greenwald, R. A., and Moy, W. W. Inhibition of collagen gelation by action of the superoxide radical. *Arthritis Rheum. 22:* 251–259, 1979.

35. Greenwald, R. A., and Moy, W. W. Effect of oxygen-derived free radicals on hyaluronic acid. *Arthritis Rheum. 23:* 455–463, 1980.

36. Havemann, K., and Janoff, A. (eds.): *Neutral Proteases of Human Polymorphonuclear Leukocytes.* Baltimore, Urban & Schwarzenberg, 1978.

37. Heimburger, M., and Haupt, H. Karacterisierung von Alpha 1-X-Glycoprotein abs Chymotrypsin inhibitor des Human-plasma. *Clin. Chim. Acta 12:* 116–118, 1965.

38. Henson, P. M. The immunologic release of constituents from neutrophil leukocytes. I. The role of antibody and complement on nonphagocytosable surfaces or phagocytosable particles. *J. Immunol. 107:* 1535–1546, 1971.

39. Hinman, L. M., Stevens, C. A., Matthay, R. A., and Gee, J. B. L. Elastase and lysozyme activities in human alveolar macrophages. Effects of cigarette smokking. *Am. Rev. Resp. Dis. 121:* 263–271, 1980.

40. Hochstrasser, K. Low molecular weight proteinase inhibitors in the respiratory tract. Biochemistry and function. In *Biochemistry, Pathology and Genetics of Pulmonary Emphysema.* Edited by P. Sadoul and J. Bignon. Paris, Pergamon Press, 1980.

41. Hochstrasser, K., Bretzel, G., Wachter, E., and Heindl, S. The amino acid sequence of the double-headed proteinase inhibitor from canine submandibularis glands. *Hoppe-Seyler's Z. Physiol. Chem. 356:* 1865–1877, 1975.

42. Hochstrasser, K., Reichert, R., Schwarz, S., and Werle, E. Isolierung und Characterisierung eines Proteaseninhibitors ans menschlichem Bronchialsekret. *Hoppe-Seyler's Z. Physiol. Chem. 353:* 221–226, 1972.

43. Hovi, T., Mosher, D. F., and Vaheri, A. Cultured human monocytes synthesize and secrete α2-macroglobulin. *J. Exp. Med. 145:* 1580–1589, 1977.

44. Janoff, A. Neutrophil proteases in inflammation. *Annu. Rev. Med. 23:* 177–189, 1972.

45. Janoff, A. Purification of human granulocyte elastase by affinity chromatograph. *Lab. Invest. 29:* 458–464, 1973.

46. Janoff, A., Feinstein, G., Malemud, C. J., and Elias, J. M. Degradation of cartilage proteoglycan by human leukocyte granule neutral proteases—a model of joint injury. I. Penetration of enzyme into rabbit articular cartilage and release of $^{35}SO_4$-labelled material from the tissue. *J. Clin. Invest. 57:* 615–624, 1976.

47. Janoff, A., Sandhaus, R. A., Hospelhorn, V. D., and Rosenberg R. Digestion of lung proteins by human leukocyte granules *in vitro. Proc. Soc. Exp. Biol. Med. 140:* 516–519, 1972.

48. Janoff, A., Sloan, B., Weinbaum, G., Damiano, V., Sandhaus, R. A., Elias, J., and Kimbel, P. Experimental emphysema induced with purified human neutrophil elastase: Tissue localization of the instilled protease. *Am. Rev. Resp. Dis. 115:* 461–478, 1977.

49. Johnson, D., and Travis, J. Structural evidence for methionine at the reactive site of human alpha 1-proteinase inhibitor. *J. Biol. Chem. 253:* 7142–7144, 1978.

50. Johnson, D., and Travis, J. The oxidative inactivation of human alpha 1-proteinase inhibitor: further evidence for methionine at the reactive center. *J. Biol. Chem. 254:* 4022–4026, 1979.

51. Kagan, H. M., and Lerch, R. M. Amidated carboxyl groups in elastin. *Biochim. Biophys. Acta 434:* 223–232, 1976.

52. Kaiser, H., Greenwald, R. A., Feinstein, G., and Janoff, A. Degradation of cartilage proteoglycan by human leukocyte granule neutral porteases—a model of joint injury. II. Degradation of isolated bovine nasal cartilage proteoglycan. *J. Clin. Invest. 57:* 625–632, 1976.

53. Kettner, C., Shaw, E., White, R., and Janoff, A. The specificity of macrophage elastase on the insulin B-chain. *Biochem. J. 195:* 369–372, 1981.

54. Kitagawa, S., Takaku, F., and Sakamoto, S. Evidence that proteases are involved in superoxide production by human PMN leukocytes and monocytes. *J. Clin. Invest. 65:* 74–81, 1980.

55. Klebanoff, S. J., and Clark, R. A. *The Neutrophil: Function and Clinical Disorders.* Elsevier/North Holland, Amsterdam, 1978.

56. Klimetzek, V., and Sorg, C. Lymphokine-induced secretion of plasminogen activator by murine macrophages. *Eur. J. Immunol. 7:* 185–187, 1977.

57. Lapresle, C., and Webb, T. *Biochem. J. 84:* 455, 1962.

58. Lazarus, G. S., Daniels, J. R., Brown, R. S., Bladen, H. A., and Fullmer, H. M. Degradation of collagen by human granulocyte collagenolytic system. *J. Clin. Invest. 47:* 2622–2629, 1968.

59. Mainardi, C. L., Dixit, S. N., and Kang, S. H. Degradation of type IV basement membrane collagen by a proteinase isolated from human polymorphonuclear leukocyte granules. *J. Biol. Chem. 255:* 5435–5441, 1980a.

60. Mainardi, C. L., Hasty, D. L., Sayer, J. M., and Kang, A. H. Specific cleavage of human type III collagen by human polymorphonuclear leukocyte elastase. *J. Biol. Chem. 255:* 12006–12010, 1980b.

61. Matheson, N. R., Wong, P. S., and Travis, J. Enzymatic inactivation of human alpha-1-proteinase inhibitor by neutrophil myeloperoxidase. *Biochem. Biophys. Res. Commun. 88:* 402–409, 1979.

62. McCora, J. M. Free radicals and inflammation: protection of synovial fluid by superoxide dismutase. *Science 185:* 529–531, 1974.

63. Menkin, V. Studies on inflammation. X. The cytological picture of an inflammatory exudate in relation to its hydrogen ion concentration. *Am. J. Pathol. 10:* 193–210, 1934.

64. Moroi, M., and Yamasaki, M. Mechanism of interaction of bovine trypsin with human $\alpha 1$-antitrypsin. *Biochim. Biophys. Acta 359:* 130–141, 1974.

65. Mounter, L. A., and Atiyeh, W. Proteases of human leukocytes. *Blood 15:* 52–59, 1960.

66. Movat, H. Z., Vkada, K., and Takeuchi, Y. *Thromb. Diath. Haemmorrh. 40* (Suppl.)*:* 211, 1970.

67. Nakajima, K., Powers, J. C., Ashe, B. M., and Zimmerman, M. Mapping the extended substrate binding site of cathepsin G and human leukocyte elastase. Studies with peptide substrates related to the α-1-protease inhibitor reactive site. *J. Biol. Chem. 254:* 4027–4032, 1979.

68. Noguiera, N., Gordon, S., and Cohn, Z. Trypanosoma cruzi: the immuunological induction of macrophage plasminogen activator requires thymus-derived lymphocytes. *J. Exp. Med. 146:* 172–183, 1977.

69. Ohlsson, K. Interaction of granulocyte neutral proteases with alpha 1-antitrypsin, alpha 2-macroglobulin and alpha 1- antichymotrypsin. In: *Neutral Proteases of Human Polymorphonuclear Leukocytes.* Edited by K. Havemann and A. Janoff, pp. 167–177. Baltimore, Urban & Schwarzenberg, 1978.

70. Ohlsson, K., and Akesson, V. Alpha 1-antichymotrypsin interaction with cationic proteins from granulocytes. *Clin. Chim. Acta 73:* 285–291, 1976.

71. Ohlsson, K., and Olsson, I. The neutral proteases of human granulocytes: Isolation and partial characterization of granulocyte elastases. *Eur. J. Biochem. 42:* 519–527, 1974a.

72. Ohlsson, K., and Olsson, I. Neutral proteases of human granulocytes. III. Interaction between human granulocyte elastase and plasma protease inhibitors. *Scand. J. Clin. Lab Invest. 34:* 349–355, 1974b.

73. Ohlsson, K., Tegner, T., and Akesson, U. Isolation and partial characterization of a low molecular weight acid stable protease inhibitor from human bronchial secretion. *Hoppe-Seyler's Z. Physiol. Chem. 358:* 583–589, 1977.

74. Prince, H. E., Folds, J. D., and Spitznagel, J. K. Interaction of human polymorphonuclear leukocyte elastase with human IgM. *In vitro* production of an Fabμ-like fragment. *Mol. Immunol. 16:* 301–306, 1979.

75. Rindler, R., Hortnagl, H., Schmaltz, F., and Braunsteiner, H. Hydrolysis of a chymotrypsin substrate and of naphthol AS-D chloroacetate by human leukocyte granules. *Blut 26:* 239–249, 1973.

76. Rindler-Ludwig, R., Bretz, U., and Baggiolini, M. Cathepsin G: the chymotrypsin-like enzyme of human polymorphonuclear leukocytes. In: *Neutral Proteases of Human Polymorphonuclear Leukocytes.* Edited by K. Havemann and A. Janoff, pp. 138–149. Baltimore, Urban & Schwarzenberg, 1978.

77. Rodriguez, R. J., White, R. R., Senior, R. M., and Levine, E. A. Elastase release from human alveolar macrophages: comparison between smokers and non-smokers. *Science 198:* 313–314, 1977.

78. Salin, M. L., and McCord, J. M. Free radicals and inflammation. Protection of phagocytosing leukocytes by superoxide dismutase. *J. Clin. Invest. 56:* 1319–1322, 1975.

78a. Salvesen, G. S., and Barrett, A. J. Covalent binding of proteinases in their reaction with $\alpha 2$-

macroglobulin. *Biochem. J. 187:* 695–701, 1980.

79. Schmidt, W., and Havemann, K. Isolation of elastase-like and chymotrypsin-like neutral proteases from human granulocytes. *Hoppe-Seyler's Z. Physiol. Chem. 355:* 1077–1082, 1974.

80. Schmidt, W., and Havemann, K. Chymotrypsin-like neutral proteases from lysosomes of human polymorphonuclear leukocytes. In: *Neutral Proteases of Human Polymorphonuclear Leukocytes.* Edited by K. Havemann and A. Janoff, pp. 150–160. Baltimore, Urban & Schwarzenberg, 1978.

81. Starkey, P. M., and Barrett, A. J. α-2 Macroglobulin, a physiological regulator of proteinase activity. In: *Proteinases in Mammalian Cells and Tissues.* Edited by A. J. Barrett. New York, North Holland, 1977.

82. Starkey, P. M., Barrett, A. J., and Burleigh, M. C. The degradation of articular collagen by neutrophil proteinases. *Biochim. Biophys. Acta 483:* 386–397, 1977.

83. Taylor, J. C., and Crawford, I. P. Purification and preliminary characterization of human leukocyte elastase. *Arch. Biochem. Biophys. 169:* 91–101, 1975.

84. Tegner, H. Quantitation of human granulocyte protease inhibitors in non-purulent bronchial lavage fluids. *Acta Otolaryngol. 85:* 282–289, 1978.

85. Tegner, H., and Ohlsson, K. Localization of a low molecular weight protease inhibitor to tracheal and maxillary sinus mucosa. *Hoppe-Seyler's Z. Physiol. Chem. 358:* 427–429, 1977.

86. Travis, J., Baugh, R., Giles, P. J., Johnson, D., Bowen, J., and Reilly, C. F. Human leukocyte elastase and cathepsin G: Isolation, characterization and interaction with plasma proteinase inhibitors. In: *Neutral Proteases of Human Polymorphonuclear Leukocytes.* Edited by K. Havemann and A. Janoff, pp. 118–128. Baltimore, Urban & Schwarzenberg, 1978.

87. Travis, J., Bowen, J., and Baugh, R. Human α-1-antichymotrypsin: interaction with chymotrypsin-like proteinases. *Biochemistry 17:* 5651–5656, 1978.

88. Travis, J., Garner, D., and Bowen, J. Human α-1-antichymotrypsin: purification and properties. *Biochemistry 17:* 5647–5651, 1978.

89. Tsan, M. F., and Chen, J. W. Oxidation of methionine by human polymorphonuclear leukocytes. *J. Clin. Invest. 65:* 1041–1050, 1980.

90. Twumasi, D. Y., and Liener, I. E. Proteases from purulent sputum: purification and properties of the elastase and chymotrypsin-like enzymes. *J. Biol. Chem. 252:* 1917–1926, 1977.

91. Unkeless, J. C., Gordon, S., and Reich, E. Secretion of plasminogen activator by stimulated macrophages. *J. Exp. Med. 139:* 834–850, 1974.

92. Vassali, J. D., and Reich, E. Macrophage plasminogen activator: induction by products of activated lymphoid cells. *J. Exp. Med. 145:* 429–437, 1977.

93. Wahl, L. M., Wahl, S. M., Mergenhagen, S. E., and Martin, G. R. Collagenase production by lymphokine-activated macrophages. *Science 187:* 261–263, 1975.

94. Wasi, S., Murray, R. K., Macmorine, D. R. L., and Movat, H. Z. *Br. J. Exp. Pathol. 47:* 411, 1966.

95. Weissmann, G., Smolen, J. E., and Korchak, H. M. Release of inflammatory mediators from stimulated neutrophils. *N. Engl. J. Med. 303:* 27–34, 1980.

96. Werb, Z., and Gordon, S. Secretion of a specific collagenase by stimulated macrophages. *J. Exp. Med. 142:* 346–360, 1975a.

97. Werb, Z., and Gordon, S. Elastase secretion by stimulated macrophages. *J. Exp. Med. 142:* 361–377, 1975b.

98. Werb, Z., Mainardi, C. L., Vater, C. A., and Harris, E. D., Jr. Endogenous activation of latent collagenase by rheumatoid synovial cells: evidence for a role of plasminogen-activator. *N. Engl. J. Med. 296:* 1017–1023, 1977.

99. White, R. R., Lin, H. S., and Kuhn, C. Elastase secretion by peritoneal exudative and alveolar macrophages. *J. Exp. Med. 146:* 802–808, 1977.

100. White, R. R., Norby, D., Janoff, A., and Dearing, R. Partial purification and characterization of mouse peritoneal exudative macrophage elastase. *Biochim. Biophys. Acta 612:* 233–244, 1980a.

101. White, R., Janoff, A., and Godfrey, H. P. Secretion of alpha-2-macroglobulin by human alveolar macrophages. *Lung 158:* 9–14, 1980b.

Chapter 6

Activation of the Human Neutrophil: The Roles of Lipid Remodeling and Intracellular Calcium*

HELEN M. KORCHAK,† CHARLES N. SERHAN,‡ AND
GERALD WEISSMANN

STIMULUS-RESPONSE COUPLING IN POLYMORPHONUCLEAR NEUTROPHILS (PMN)

The mature neutrophil is highly specialized for its primary function, the phagocytosis, killing, and digestion of microrganisms. Appropriate opsonized particles elicit the aggregation, ingestion, killing, and degranulation response. In conditions where these functions are defective, the host is subject to recurrent infections. Neutrophils are also commonly found at sites of inflammation and, through release of their granule contents, active oxygen species, and arachidonate derivatives (5-HPETE, leukotrienes, and thromboxanes), are probably responsible for the development and amplification of the inflammatory response and its associated tissue destruction (95).

The release of granule contents and superoxide anion ($O_2 \cdot^-$) normally occurs into the closed phagocytic vacuole. Closure of the phagocytic vacuole can be prevented by the addition of cytochalasin B. Under these conditions the neutrophil is converted into a secretory cell. The physiology of the neutrophil can therefore be treated in a fashion analogous to the secretory responses of endocrine and exocrine organs.

The binding of specific ligands such as immune complexes, chemotactic peptides, and lectin concanavalin A initiates a prompt change in membrane potential, reflecting the importance of ion fluxes in the activation process (41, 69, 72, 88, 97).

Calcium appears to play a role as a second messenger, as it does in other systems (15, 16, 59), since the calcium ionophore A23187 can bypass the receptor ligand step and initiate degranulation and $O_2 \cdot^-$ generation (24). Mobilization of

* This work was aided by grants AM-11949 and HL-19721 from the National Institutes of Health and the Arthritis Foundation, respectively.

† Helen M. Korchak is a Fellow of the Arthritis Foundation and the recipient of a Cystic Fibrosis Foundation grant.

‡ Charles N. Serhan is the recipient of a predoctoral Fellowship, CA-09161, Department of Pathology.

membrane-associated Ca^{2+} appears to be most critical in the activation sequence since the Ca^{2+} mobilization inhibitor TMB-8 completely inhibits the secretory response (79, 80). This rapid Ca^{2+} influx apparently serves as an amplifying mechanism, since removal of all extracellular Ca^{2+} had only a small inhibitory effect (40).

Cyclic AMP is a second messenger in many secretory systems. In the neutrophil, exogenous cAMP is *not* sufficient to activate the secretory response. Cyclic AMP, but not GMP, is transiently elevated in activated neutrophils, a process that is greatly amplified in the presence of the prostaglandins PGE and PGI (30, 33, 39, 77, 81). Cyclic AMP appears to act as a feedback inhibitor in neutrophils since agents that elevate cAMP also inhibit secretion (94, 101). Ligand receptor interaction, as well as the calcium ionophore A23187, provokes the generation of prostaglandins, thromboxanes, and derivatives of the lipoxygenase pathway hydroxyeicosatetraenoic acid, and hydroperoxyeicosatetraenoic acid (5-HETE, 5-HPETE, leukotrienes) (7, 8, 25, 26, 76, 78, 96, 99, 100). The observation that several prostaglandins added *in vitro* inhibit phagocytosis and lysosomal enzyme release (78, 94, 96) indicates that these products play a regulatory role in neutrophil activation, possibly by elevating intracellular cAMP.

MEMBRANE LIPIDS AND PMN RESPONSES

A number of different ligands (complement components, chemotactic peptides, immune complexes, and lectins) can react with specific receptors on the plasma membrane and initiate the activation of such cell responses as chemotaxis, aggregation, phagocytosis, degranulation, and $O_2 \cdot^-$ generation. These receptors are embedded in the plasmalemmal lipid bilayer. The membrane phospholipids are not merely an inert matrix of these membrane proteins and a barrier to water-soluble substance; rather, there is a dynamic interaction between membrane proteins and lipids (13, 73). Perturbation of the membrane by treatment with surface active agents such as deoxycholate, digitonin, and saponin stimulates a respiratory burst in a manner similar to that of phagocytosis (27, 63, 98). Phospholipase C treatment of neutrophils results in a similar respiratory burst (36, 56). A change in the lipoprotein structure of the plasma membrane was proposed as the stimulus for this cell activation.

The activation sequence of the neutrophil involves a series of steps in which the lipoprotein structure of the membrane is probably of importance in: (*a*) binding of a ligand with a plasmalemmal receptor; (*b*) translocation of ions, the most critical being Ca^{2+}, across the plasmalemma; (c) activation of a membrane-associated enzyme adenylate cyclase; (d) release of arachidonic acid for further metabolism via the cyclooxygenase and lipoxygenase pathways; and (e) fusion of granule membrane with the plasmalemma.

PHOSPHOLIPID METABOLISM AND Ca^{2+} TRANSLOCATION

In many tissues, the addition of hormones or other ligands that stimulate Ca^{2+} entry results in an increased break-down of phosphatidyl inositol (PI) to diglyceride (DG), phosphorylation to phosphatidic acid (PA) and finally a resynthesis of PI (Fig. 6.1) (4, 9, 12, 18–20, 22, 23, 29, 32, 34, 35, 43, 50, 51, 55, 61, 92) including neutrophils (10, 11, 37, 38, 83, 85, 86). It has been proposed that the PI breakdown induced by ligand-receptor interaction might be directly involved in controlling

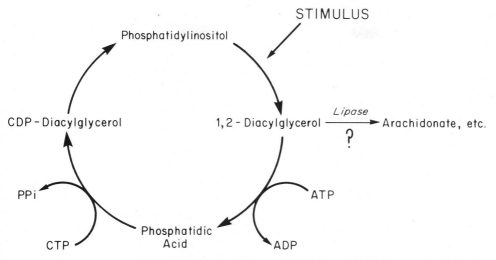

FIG. 6.1. The phosphatidyl inositol/phosphatidate cycle. *PPi*, inorganic phosphate (pyrophosphate).

calcium entry into the cell. In order for the PI/PA cycle to qualify as a regulator of the cell's gating mechanism it must fulfill several criteria: (a) the breakdown of PI must be rapid and precede both secretion and the Ca^{2+} influx; (b) it must be triggered specifically by binding of the ligand to the receptor; (c) it should not be dependent on the presence of extracellular Ca^{2+}. In most tissues studied, these criteria appear to be fulfilled. In the neutrophil, however, the PI/PA cycle is inhibited by the absence of extracellular calcium (10, 11) under conditions in which cell activation occurs. This may be because the neutrophil is so highly dependent on intracellular Ca^{2+}.

The precise role of the PI/PA cycle is the sequence of events that leads from the receptor-ligand interaction is not known. Recently, Berridge and Fain (4) proposed a model which physically links the induction of PI metabolism to a hypothetical Ca^{2+} gate located in the plasma membrane, which "opens" and "closes" in response to PI turnover. Although the proposed model helps visualize the relationship between Ca^{2+} gating and PI turnover, no sound experimental evidence for a protein Ca^{2+} "channel" or "gate" has been provided in the literature.

An alternative to the "protein calcium channel" model is the concept that the cell produces its own "endogenous Ca^{2+} ionophore" via remodeling of its membranes (28, 87). This ionophore would theoretically be capable not only of transporting Ca^{2+} across the plasmalemma, but also of mobilizing intracellular calcium. There is a precedent for this concept in the natural ionophores produced by fungi and bacteria. A classical example of a naturally occurring Ca^{2+} ionophore is the compound A23187.

It has recently been suggested that the phosphatidic acid which is formed in the PI/PA cycle could act in the cell as a Ca^{2+} translocator (60, 67, 70) since it has been shown to act as a calcium ionophore in liposomes and in a Pressman chamber. There are, however, other candidates for an endogenous ionophore. On the basis of inhibitor studies a role for lipoxygenase pathway mediator(s) has been proposed for Ca^{2+} translocation in the neutrophil (75, 89, 91). In support of this concept it has been demonstrated in liposomes that a polymeric prostaglandin derivative (PGB_x) translocates Ca^{2+} (70) and that PGB_x can also activate $O_2 \cdot^-$ generation and degranulation (71). Although PGB_x is not a natural derivative and is an unlikely candidate for a naturally occurring ionophore, it does serve as a useful model.

PHOSPHOLIPID TURNOVER AND THE ARACHIDONIC ACID CASCADE

Stimulated neutrophils actively generate oxygenated arachidonic acid derivatives which can serve to modulate cell function. Since the size of the free arachidonic acid pool serves to regulate the rate of production of these products (42), it is of considerable interests to define the source of the free arachidonate and the metabolic path leading to its release. The scheme initially proposed for the release of arachidonate involved the action of phospholipase A_2 (6, 14, 17, 44, 46, 47, 62, 64–66, 68, 84, 90) in cleaving arachidonate from the C-2 position of a phosphatidate. A phospholipase A_2 activity has been demonstrated in neutrophils (17, 62), but the substrate phosphatidate for release of arachidonate has not been rigorously established (17) nor have free lysophosphatides been demonstrated, suggesting that if this pathway is active, a rapid reacylation must occur. Indeed, endogenous lysolecithin is converted to lecithin in the presence of neutrophils (21), indicating the possibility of an active deacylation-reacylation cycle. This type of recycling could explain the fatty acid remodeling observed in phagocytosing neutrophils (49, 74, 82). In addition, the calcium requirement of both phospholipase A_2 and the generation of arachidonate make this a plausible pathway.

An alternative pathway for arachidonate release involving the action of PI-specific phospholipase C has been proposed by researchers working with platelets (1–3, 9, 23, 48, 58). PI would be cleaved to DG, which would then be deacylated in the 2-position by the action of a diglyceride lipase, liberating arachidonate. Recent studies by Broekman et al. (9) have provided evidence for two pathways for the release of arachidonate from platelet phospholipids: one involves a phospholipase with phosphatidyl ethanolamine as principal substrate. The accumulation of appropriate lysophosphatides was demonstrable. The other pathway involves the cleavage of PI by a phospholipase C as suggested by Bell and Majerus (2). The rate of PA accumulation was less than the rate of PI cleavage, suggesting the loss of an intermediate, such as cleavage of DG, to give MG + AA or, alternatively, the cleavage of PA itself. The latter possibility has been suggested for platelets (5) and neutrophils stimulated with A23187 (45). In the platelet, it has been suggested (5) that the Ca^{2+}-independent phospholipase C is activated first, possibly by exposure of membrane PI. This step would lead to the rapid production of PA and induction of phospholipase A_2 activity and cleavage of arachidonic acid. This type of scheme can be tested by an extension of the kinetic analysis we have used for the neutrophil activation scheme. If the scheme of Billah et al. (5) were to operate in the neutrophil, then receptor ligand interaction, but not A23187, should lead to a turnover in PI. The breakdown of

PI should initiate a rapid influx of Ca which would in turn activate the phospholipase A_2 lead to the generation of prostanoids which would in turn modulate the activation response. If however, the hypothesis that a lipoxygenase product is responsible for Ca^{2+} translocation (75, 89, 91) is correct, then Ca^{2+} mobilization would follow arachidonate release. By this type of temporal analysis it should thus be possible to gain further insight into the mechanisms of the signaling process in neutrophil activation. Since Ca^{2+} translocation is central in the activation scheme, it is essential to obtain a better understanding of how this Ca^{2+} translocation is accomplished (*i.e.*, "the cell's own ionophore"). Such studies are now in progress.

A BIOLOGICALLY RELEVANT ASSAY FOR Ca^{2+} IONOPHORES

The hypothesis that increments in activity of intracellular calcium mediate stimulus-response coupling in a wide variety of tissues is strongly supported by experiments with ionophores of microbial origin such as A23187 and ionomycin. These agents bypass the initial ligand-receptor step in the activation of a variety of cells which use calcium as a second messenger. The fungal ionophores, which promote the directional translocation of Ca^{2+} across cellular and intracellular membranes, also move calcium from aqueous solution into nonpolar solvents such as chloroform or carbon tetrachloride. Both properties, that of translocating calcium across membranes and that of promoting the transfer of calcium into organic solvents, have also been attributed to several membrane phospholipids, proteins, bile acids and prostaglandins, each of which could then be described as an "endogenous calcium ionophore."

Before investigating the possible role of an endogenous Ca^{2+} ionophore in the stimulus-response sequence of the human neutrophil, it was necessary to devise a sensitive and relatively discriminating method for the detection of iontophoretic activity. The system popularized by Pressman, which consists of the translocation of $^{45}Ca^{2+}$ from an aqueous into a simple organic phase, does not constitute the most discriminating model for a biomembrane, since there is no membrane involved.

Based on these considerations, it was necessary to establish strict criteria for a proposed endogenous calcium ionophore. The ionophore should:

(a) translocate Ca^{2+} from an aqueous phase, across an intact lipid bilayer, into another aqueous compartment,
(b) act at micromolar concentrations when added in the aqueous phase, or, alternately, when preincorporated in the bilayer, should act at molar ratios (of putative ionophore: bulk lipid) comparable to those of natural membranes,
(c) should be permselective with respect to the two major divalent cations of physiological fluids (*i.e.*, $Ca^{2+} \gg Mg^{2+}$) and, finally,
(d) should not lyse the membrane.

For this purpose, multilamellar (MLV) and large unilamellar (LUV) liposomes have been prepared with the metallochromic dye arsenazo III (AIII) entrapped in their aqueous compartments. Since AIII displays a spectral shift when complexed with Ca^{2+}, the translocation of Ca^{2+} across the liposomal bilayer can readily be quantitated. By this means it was possible to detect 1 dimer of A23187 per liposome upon preincorporation of 10 nM A23187 when added externally.

Permselectivity can be established by this method, since other divalent cations also form complexes with AIII. Moreover, the integrity of the liposomes after Ca^{2+} translocation can also be monitored, by either the addition of EGTA or rechromatography of the liposomes. By the use of this highly sensitive assay, and with the criteria for a putative endogenous ionophore in mind, it was possible to examine a number of phospholipids, fatty acids, prostaglandins (both stable and endoperoxide analogues), prostaglandin derivatives (PGB_x), oxidation products of fatty acids, and retinoids to determine whether they might serve the function of endogenous calcium ionophores. It was also possible to compare the activity of these compounds in this assay system with that of the known Ca^{2+} ionophores, A23187, and ionomycin (70).

Of the compounds tested, only PGB_x (a polymeric derivative of prostaglandin B_1), phosphatidic acid, oxidative products derived from linoleic acid, linolenic acid, and two eicosatrienoic acids provoked Ca^{2+} influx into the liposomes. Phosphatidic acid was shown to translocate calcium at a rate of 3 mmoles Ca^{2+}/ mole membrane lipid/minute, while a variety of other phospholipids, *e.g.*, phosphatidyl serine; fatty acids, *e.g.*, arachidonic acid; prostaglandins, *e.g.*, PGE_1 and PGB_1; retinoids; and "platelet activating factors" were without effect. The results of these studies suggested that phosphatidic acid and/or oxidation products derived from trienoic acids which could act as calcium ionophores in model lipid bilayers could serve as "endogenous ionophores" in cells (70).

After describing the ionophoretic properties of PGB_x (a water-soluble derivative of prostaglandin B_1) in liposomes, the interactions of PGB_x with human neutrophils was studied. PBG_x provoked $O_2^- \cdot$ generation and degranulation in cytochalasin B-treated neutrophils in the presence of extracellular divalent cations (Ca^{2+}, Sr^{2+}, Mg^{2+}, Mn^{2+}, Ba^{2+}). Kinetic and dose-response studies showed that PGB_x mimicked the action of the ionophore A23187 in the neutrophil. Both ionophores induced $O_2^- \cdot$ generation and release of granule-associated enzymes without eliciting the release of the cytoplasmic marker enzyme lactic dehydrogenase. In contrast, the precursor of PGB_x and PGB_1, as well as arachidonic acid, did not mimic ionophore-induced stimulation of human neutrophils. PGB_x induced enzyme release in the presence of either Ca^{2+} or Ba^{2+}, whereas A23187 showed specificity for Ca^{2+}. This selectivity in the neutrophil paralleled the permselectivity shown by the respective ionophores in the liposome system. These studies provide additional evidence that increments in the intracellular level of divalent cations (Ca^{2+}) serve as a signal in the stimulus response sequence of human neutrophils.

SUMMARY

The stimulus-response coupling sequence of neutrophils has been partially elucidated, and a temporal order for some of the initial events in PMN activation has been established; membrane potential, Ca^{2+} motivation, Ca^{2+} influx, cAMP pulse, aggregation, $O_2^- \cdot$ generation and degranulation. Receptor-ligand interaction is followed by membrane hyperpolarization and the mobilization of Ca^{2+} from intracellular loci. In common with other secretory cells, neutrophils utilize Ca^{2+} as a second messenger to mediate cellular responses. For optimal activation, neutrophils require an influx of extracellular Ca^{2+}. However, the mechanism by which Ca^{2+} enters neutrophils or other cells is not known. In view of our recent findings that phosphatidic acid and oxidized trienoic acids can translocate Ca^{2+} in lipid bilayers, it should be apparent that a study of phospholipid metabolism (particularly changes in phosphatidyl inositol and phosphatidic acid) in human neutrophil activation together with a temporal analysis of Ca^{2+} influx will contribute to an understanding of the mechanism of stimulus-secretion coupling. Since arachidonic acid metabolites play an important role in inflammation and have recently been suspected of modulating stimulus-secretion coupling, studies of the release of arachidonic acid from membrane phospholipids are important because all prostaglandins and hydroxy acids are derived from this initial step. Finally, the generation, by neutrophils, of free arachidonic acid and its oxygenation products might serve as a model system for other tissues in addition to their important role in inflammation.

REFERENCES

1. Bell, R. L., Kennerly, D. A., Stanford, N., and Majerus, P. W. Diglyceride lipase: a pathway for arachidonate release from human platelets. *Proc. Natl. Acad. Sci. USA 76:* 3238–3241, 1979.
2. Bell, R. L., and Majerus, P. W. Thrombin-induced hydrolysis of phosphatidyl inositol in human platelets. *J. Biol. Chem. 255:* 1790–1792, 1980.
3. Bell, R. L., Stanford, N., Kennerly, D. A., and Majerus, P. Diglyceride lipase: a pathway for arachidonate release from human platelets. *Adv Prostaglandin Thromb Res 6:* 219–229, 1980.
4. Berridge, M. J., and Fain, J. N. Inhibition of phosphatidyl inositol synthesis and the inactivation of calcium entry after prolonged exposure of the blowfly salivary gland to 5-hydroxytryptamine. *Biochem. J. 178:* 58–69, 1979.
5. Billah, M. M., Lapetina, E. G., and Cuatrecasas, P. Phospholipase A_2 and phospholipase C activities of platelets. Differential substrate specificity, Ca^{2+} requirement pH dependence and cellular localization. *J. Biol. Chem.* 255:10227–10231, 1980.
6. Bills, T. K., Smith, J. B., and Silver, M. J. Selective release of arachidonic acid from the phospholipids of human platelets in response to thrombin. *J. Clin. Invest. 60:* 1–6, 1977.
7. Borgeat, P., Hamberg, M., and Samuelsson, B. Transformation of arachidonic acid and homo-γ-linolenic acid by rabbit polymorphonuclear leukocytes. *J. Biol. Chem. 251:* 7816–7820, 1976.
8. Borgeat, P., and Samuelsson, B. Arachidonic acid metabolism in polymorphonucler leukocytes: effects of ionophore A23187. *Proc. Natl. Acad. Sci. USA 76:* 2148–2152, 1979.
9. Broekman, M. J., Ward, J. W., and Marcus, A. J. Phospholipid metabolism in stimulated human platelets: changes in phosphatidyl inositol, phosphatidic acid and lysophospholipids. *J. Clin. Invest. 66:* 275–283, 1980.
10. Cockcroft, S., Bennett, J. P., and Gomperts, B. D. F-Met-Leu Phe-induced phosphatidyl inositol turnover in rabbit neutrophils is dependent on extracellular calcium. *FEBS Letters 110:* 115–118, 1980.
11. Cockcroft, S., Bennett, J. P., and Gomperts, B. D. Stimulus-secretion coupling in rabbit neutrophils is not mediated by phosphatidyl inositol breakdown. *Nature 288:* 275–277, 1980.
12. Cockcroft, S., and Gomperts, B. D. Evidence for a role of phosphatidyl inositol turnover in stimulus secretion coupling: studies with rat peritoneal mast cells. *Biochem. J. 178:* 681–687, 1979.
13. Cronan, J. E., Jr., and Gelmann, E. P. Physical properties of membrane lipids: biological relevance and regulation. *Bacteriol. Rev. 39:* 232–256, 1975.
14. Derksen, A., and Cohen, P. Patterns of fatty acid release from endogenous substrates by human platelet homogenates and membranes. *J. Biol. Chem. 250:* 9342–9347, 1975.
15. Douglas, W. W. Stimulus-secretion coupling: the concept and clues from chromaffin and other cells. *Br. J. Pharmacol. 34:* 451–474, 1968.
16. Douglas, W. W. Involvement of calcium in exoytosis and the exocytosis-vesiculation sequence. *Biochem. Soc. Symp. 39:* 1–28, 1974.
17. Elsbach, P., and Weiss, J. Lipid metabolism by phagocytic cells In: *The Reticuloendothelial*

System. A Comprehensive Treatise. Edited by A. J. Sbarra and R. R. Strauss, Vol. 2, pp. 91–119. New York, Plenum Press, 1980.

18. Fain, J. N., and Berridge, M. J. Relationship between hormonal activation of phosphatidyl inositol hydrolysis, fluid secretion and calcium flux in the blowfly salivary gland. *Biochem. J. 178:* 45–58, 1979.

19. Fain, J. N., and Berridge, M. J. Relationship between phosphatidyl inositol synthesis and recovery of 5-hydroxytryptamine-responsive Ca^{2+} flux in blowfly salivary glands. *Biochem. J. 180:* 655–661, 1979.

20. Fain, J. N., and Garcia-Sainz, J. A. Role of phosphatidyl inositol turnover in alpha$_1$ and of adenylate cyclase inhibition in alpha$_2$ effects of catecholamines. *Life Sciences 26:* 1183–1194.

21. Franson, R., Weiss, J., Martin, L., Spitznagel, J. K., and Elsbach, P. Phospholipase A activity associated with the membranes of human polymorphonuclear leukocytes. *Biochem. J. 167:* 839, 1977.

22. Garcia-Saine, J. A., and Fain, J. N. Effect of adrenergic amines on phosphatidyl inositol labeling and glycogen synthase activity in fat cells from euthyroid and hypothyroid rats. *Mol. Pharmacol. 18:* 72–77, 1980.

23. Garcia-Saine, J. E., Hoffman, B. B., Li, S-Y., Lefkowitz, R. J., and Fain, J. N. Role alpha, adrenoceptors in the turnover of phosphatidyl-inositol and of alpha$_2$ adrenoceptors in the regulation of cyclic AMP accumulation in hamster adipocytes. *Life Sci. 27:* 953–961, 1980.

24. Goldstein, I. M., Horn, J. K., Kaplan, H. B., and Weissmann, G. Calcium-induced lysozyme secretion from human polymorphonuclear leukocytes. *Biochem. Biophys. Res. Commun. 60:* 807–812, 1974.

25. Goldstein, I. M., Malmsten, C. L., Kindahl, H., Kaplan, H. B., Rådmark, O., Samuelsson, B., and Weissmann, G. Thromboxane generation by human peripheral blood polymorphonuclear leukocytes. *J. Exp. Med. 148:* 787–792, 1978.

26. Goldstein, I. M., Malmsten, C. S., Samuelsson, B., and Weissmann, G. Prostaglandins, thromboxanes, and polymorphonuclear leukocytes: mediation and modulation of inflammation. *Inflammation 2:* 309–317, 1977.

27. Graham, R. C., Jr., Karnovsky, M. J., Shafer, A. W., Glass, E. A., and Karnovsky, M. L. Metabolic andmorphological observations on the effect of surface-active agents on leukocytes. *J. Cell Biol. 32:* 629–647, 1967.

28. Green, D. E., Fry, M., and Blondin, G. Phospholipids as the molecular instruments of ion and solute transport in biological membranes. *Proc. Natl. Acad. Sci. USA 77:* 257–261, 1980.

29. Hanley, M. R., Lee, C. M., Jones, L. M., and Michell, R. H. Similar effects of substance P and related peptides on salivation and on phosphatidyl inositol turnover in rat salivary glands. *Mol. Pharmacol. 18:* 78–83, 1980.

30. Herlin, T., Petersen, C. S. and Esmann. V. The role of calcium and cyclic adenosine 3′,5′-monophosphate in the regulation of glycogen metabolism in phagocytizing human polymorphonuclear leukocytes. *Biochim. Biophys. Acta 542:* 63–76, 1978.

31. Hoffstein, S. T. Ultrastructural demonstration of calcium loss from local regions of the plasma membrane of surface-stimulated human granulocytes. *J. Immunol. 123:* 1395–1402, 1979.

32. Hokin, M. R., and Hokin, L. E. Metabolism and Physiological Significance of Lipids. Edited by R. M. C. Dawson and D. N. Rhodes p. 423. London, John Wiley, 1964.

33. Jackowski, S., and Sha'afi, R. I. Response of adenosine cyclic-3′,5′-monophosphate level in rabbit neutrophils to the chemotactic peptide formyl-methionyl-phenylalanine. *Mol. Pharmacol. 16:* 473–481, 1979.

34. Jafferji, S., and Michel, R. H. Effects of calcium-antagonistic drugs on the stimulation by carbamoyl choline and histamine of phosphatidyl inositol turnover in longitudinal smooth muscle of guinea pig ileum. *Biochem. J. 160:* 163–169, 1976.

35. Jones, L. M., Cockcroft, S., and Michell, R. H. Stimulation of phosphatidyl inositol turnover in various tissues by cholinergic and adrenergic agonists, by histamine and by caerulein. *Biochem. J. 182:* 669–676, 1979.

36. Kaplan, S. S., Finch, S. C. and Basford, R. E. Polymorphonuclear leukocyte activation: Effects of phospholipase C. *Proc. Soc. Exp. Biol. 140:* 540–543, 1972.

37. Karnovsky, M. L., Shafer, A. W., Cagan, R. H., Graham, R. C., Karnovsky, M. J., Glass, E. A. and Saito, K. Membrane function and metabolism in phagocytic cells. *Trans. N. Y. Acad. Sci. 28:* 778–787, 1966.

38. Karnovsky, M. L., and Wallach, D. F. H. The metabolic basis of phagocytosis. III. Incorporation of inorganic phosphate into various classes of phosphatides during phagocytosis. *J. Biol. Chem. 236:* 1895–1901, 1961.

39. Keller, H. U., Gerisch, G., and Wissler, J. H. A transient rise in cyclic AMP levels following chemotactic stimulation of neutrophil granulocytes. *Cell Biol. Int. Rep. 3:* 759–765, 1979.

40. Korchak, H. M., Smolen, J. E., Serhan, C., and Weissmann, G. Calcium and the neutrophil (PMN): prostaglandins as the cells own ionophore. *Clin. Res. 28:* 512a, 1980.

41. Korchak, H. M., and Weissmann, G. Changes in membrane potential of human granulocytes antecede the metabolic responses to surface stimulation. *Proc. Natl. Acad. Sci. USA 75:* 3818–3822, 1978.

42. Kunze, H., and Vogt, W. Significance of phospholipase A for prostaglandin formation. *Ann. N. Y. Acad. Sci. 180:* 123–125, 1971.

43. Jones, L. M., Cockcroft, S., and Michel, R. H. Stimulation of phosphatidyl inositol turnover in various tissues by cholinergic and adrenergic agonists, by histamine and by caerulein. *Biochem. J. 182:* 669–676, 1979.

44. Lands, W. E. M., and Rome, L. H. Inhibition of prostaglandin synthesis. In: *Prostaglandins: Chemical and Biochemical Aspects.* Edited by S. M. M. Karim, pp. 87–138. London, MTP, 1976.

45. Lapetina, E. G., Billah, M. M., and Cuatrecasas, P. Rapid acylation and deacylation of arachidonic acid into phosphatidic acid of horse neutrophils. *J. Biol. Chem. 255:* 10966–10970, 1980.

46. Lapetina, E. G., and Cuatrecasas, P. Stimulation of phosphatidic acid production in platelets precedes the formation of arachidonate and parallels the release of serotonin. *Biochim. Biophys. Acta 573:* 394–402, 1979.

47. Marshall, P. J., Boatman, D. E., and Hokin, L. E. Direct demonstration of the formation of prostaglandin E_2 due to phosphatidyl inositol breakdown associated with stimulation of enzyme secretion in the pancreas. *J. Biol. Chem. 256:* 844–847, 1981.

48. Marshall, P. J., Dixon, J. F., and Hokin, L. C. Evidence for a role in stimulus-secretion coupling of prostaglandins derived from release of arachidonoyl residues as a result of phosphatidyl inositol breakdown. *Proc. Natl. Acad. Sci. USA 77:* 3292–3296, 1980.

49. Mason, R. J., Stossel, T. P., and Vaughan, M. Lipids of alveolar macrophages, polymorphonuclear leukocytes, and their phagocytic vesicles. *J. Clin. Invest. 51:* 2399–2407, 1972.

50. Michell, R. H. Inositol phospholipids and cell surface receptor function. *Biochim. Biophys. Acta 415:* 81–147, 1975.

51. Michel, R. H. Inositol phospholipids in membrane function. *Trends Biochem. Sci. 4:* 128–131, 1979.

52. Naccache, P. H., Showell, H. J., Becker, E. L., and Sha'afi, R. I. Sodium, potassium and calcium transport across rabbit polymorphonuclear leukocyte membranes. *J. Cell Biol. 73:* 428–444, 1977.

53. Naccache, P. H., Showell, H. J., Becker, E. L., and Sha'afi, R. I. Changes in ionic movements across rabbit polymorphonuclear leukocyte membranes during lysosomal enzyme release. *J. Cell Biol. 75:* 635–649, 1977.

54. Naccache, P. H., Showell, H. J., Becker, E. L., and Sha'afi, R. I. Involvement of membrane calcium in the response of rabbit neutrophils to chemotactic factors as evidenced by the fluorescence of chlorotetra. *J. Cell Biol. 83:* 179–186, 1979.

55. Oron, Y., Lowe, M., and Selinger, Z. Incorporation of inorganic [^{32}P] phosphate into rat parotid phosphatidylinositol. Induction through activation of alpha adrenergic and cholinergic receptors and relation to K^+ release. *Mol. Pharmacol. 11:* 79–86, 1975.

56. Patriarca, P., Zatti, M., Cramer, R., and Rossi, F. Stimulation of the respiration of polymorphonuclear leucocytes by phospholipase C. *Life Sci. 9:* 841–849, 1970.

57. Petroski, R. J., Naccache, P. H., Becker, E. L., and Sha'afi, R. I. Effect of chemotactic factors on the calcium levels of rabbit neutrophils. *Am. J. Physiol. 237*C43–C49, 1979.

58. Prescott, S. M., and Majerus, P. W. The fatty acid composition of phosphatidyl inositol from thrombin-stimulated human platelets. *J. Biol. Chem. 256:* 579–582, 1981.

59. Putney, J. E. Stimulus-permeability coupling: role of calcium in the receptor regulation of membrane permeability. *Pharmacol. Rev. 30:* 209–245, 1979.

60. Putney, J. R., Jr., Weiss, S. J., van de Walle, C. M., and Haddas, R. A. Is phosphatidic acid a calcium ionophore under neurohumoral control? *Nature 284:* 345–347, 1980.

61. Rittenhouse-Simmons, S. Production of diglyceride from phosphatidyl inositol in activated human platelets. *J. Clin. Invest. 63:* 580–587, 1977.

62. Rittenhouse-Simmons, S., and Deykin, D. The mobilization of arachidonic acid in platelets exposed to thrombin or ionophore A23187. *J. Clin. Invest. 60:* 495–498, 1977.

63. Rossi, F., and Zatti, M. Mechanism of the respiratory stimulation in saponine-treated leucocytes. *Biochim. Biophys. Acta 153:* 296–299, 1968.

64. Rubin, R. P., and Laychock, S. G. Prostaglandins and calcium-membrane interactions in secretory glands. *Ann. N.Y. Acad. Sci. 307:* 377–390, 1978.

65. Rubin, R. P., Sink, L. E., Schrey, M. P., Day, A. R., Liao, C. S., and Freer, R. J. Secretagogues for lysosomal enzyme release as stimulants of arachidonyl phosphatidyl inositol turnover in rabbit neutrophils. *Biochem. Biophys. Res. Commun. 90:* 1364–1370, 1979.

66. Rubin, R. P., Sink, L. E., Schrey, M. P., Day, A. R., Liao, C. S., and Freer, R. J. Secretagogues for lysosomal enzyme release as stimulants of arachidonyl phosphatidyl inositol turnover in rabbit neutrophils. *Biochem. Biophys. Res. Commun. 90:* 1364–1370, 1980.

67. Salmon, D. M., and Honeyman, T. W. Proposed mechanism of cholinergic action in smooth muscle. *Nature. 284:* 344–345, 1980.

68. Schrey, M. P. and Rubin, R. P. Characterization of a calcium-mediated activation of arachidonic acid turnover in adrenal phospholipids by corticotropin. *J. Biol. Chem. 254:* 11234–11241, 1979.

69. Seligmann, B. E., and Gallin, J. I. Secretagogue modulation of the response of human neutrophils to chemoattractants: studies with a membrane potential sensitive cyanine dye. *Mol. Immunol. 17:* 191–200, 1980.

70. Serhan, C., Anderson, P., Goodman, E., Dunham, P., and Weissmann, G. Phosphatidate and oxidized fatty acids are calcium ionophores. Studies employing arsenazo III in liposomes. *J. Biol. Chem. 256:* 2736–2741, 1981.

71. Serhan, C., Korchak, H. M., Hoffstein, S. T., and Weissmann, G. PGB_x, a prostaglandin derivative, mimics the action of calcium ionophore A23187 on human neutrophils. *J. Immunol. 125:* 2020–2024, 1980.

72. Shain, W., and Gallin, J. I. Interaction of chemotactic factors with human polymorphonuclear leukocytes: studies using a membrane potential sensitive cyanine dye. *J. Memb. Biol. 52:* 257–272, 1980.

73. Shinitzky, M. *Physical Chemical Aspects of Cell Surface Events in Cellular Regulation.* Edited by DeLisi and Blumenthal, pp. 173–181. Amsterdam, Elsevier, pp. 173–181, 1979.

74. Shohet, S. B. Changes in fatty acid metabolism in human leukemic granulocytes during phagocytosis. *J. Lab. Clin. Med. 75:* 659–671, 1970.

75. Showell, H. J., Naccache, P. H., Sha'afi, R. I., and Becker, E. L. Inhibition of rabbit neutrophil lysosomal enzyme secretion, nonstimulated and chemotactic factor stimulated locomotion by nordihydroguiaretic acid. *Life Sci. 27:* 421–426, 1980.

76. Siegel, M. I., McConnell, R. T., Bonser, R. W., and Cuatrecasas, P. The production of 5-Hete and leukotriene B in rat neutrophils from carrageenan pleural exudates. *Prostaglandins 21:* 123, 1981.

77. Simchowitz, L., Fischbein, L. C., Spilberg, I., and Atkinson, J. P. Induction of a transient elevation in intracellular levels of adenosine-3',5'-cyclic monophosphate by chemotactic factors: an early event in human neutrophil activation. *J. Immunol. 124:* 1482–1491, 1980.

78. Smith, R. J. Modulation of phagocytosis by and Lysosomal enzyme secretion from guinea-pig neutrophils: effect of non-steroid antiinflammatory agents and prostaglandins. *J. Exp. Pharmacol. Ther. 200:* 647, 1976.

79. Smith, R. J., and Iden, SS. Phorbol myristate acetate induced release of granule enzymes from human neutrophils: inhibition by the calcium antagonist 3-(*N,N*-diethylamino)-oxyl 3,4,5-trimethoxy benzoate hydrochloride. *Biochem. Biophys. Res. Commun. 91:* 263–271, 1979.

80. Smolen, J. E., Korchak, H. M., Serhan, C. N., and Weissmann, G. The relative roles of extracellular and intracellular calcium in lysosomal enzyme release and superoxide anion generation by polymorphonuclear leukocytes. *J. Cell Biol. 87:* 303a, 1980.

81. Smolen, J. E., Korchak, H. M., and Weissmann, G. Increased levels of cyclic adenosine-3'5'-monophosphate in human polymorphonuclear leukocytes after surface stimulation. *J. Clin. Invest. 65:* 1077–1085, 1980.

82. Smolen, J. E., and Shohet, S. B. Remodeling of granulocyte membrane fatty acids during phagocytosis. *J. Clin. Invest. 53:* 726–734, 1974.

83. Sostry, P. S., and Hokin, L. E. Studies on the role of phospholipids in phagocytosis. *J. Biol. Chem. 241:* 3354–3361, 1966.

84. Tesch, H., and Konig, W. Phospholipase A₂ and arachidonic acid: a common link in the generation of the eosinophil chemotactic factor (ECF) from human PMN by various stimuli. *Scand. J. Immunol. 11:* 409–418, 1980.

85. Tou, J-S. Modulation of ³²Pi incorporation into phospholipids of polymorphonuclear leukocytes by ionophore A23187. *Biochem. Biophys. Acta 531:* 167–178, 1978.

86. Tou, J-S., and Stjernholm, R. L. Stimulation of the incorporation of ³²Pi and myo [2³H]-inositol into the phosphoinositides in polymorphonuclear leukocytes during phagocytosis. *Arch. Biochem. 160:* 487–494, 1974.

87. Tyson, C. A., Van de Zande, H., and Green, D. E. Phospholipids as ionophores. *J. Biol. Chem. 251:* 1326–1332, 1976.

88. Utsumi, K., Sugiyama, K., Miijahara, M., Naito, M., Awai, M., and Ivove, M. Effect of concanavalin A on membrane potential of polymorphonuclear leukocyte monitored by fluorescent dye. *Cell Struct. Funct. 2:* 203–209, 1977.

89. Volpi, M., Naccache, P. H., and Sha'afi, R. I. Arachidonate metabolite(s) increase the permeability of the plasma membrane of the neutrophils to calcium. *Biochem. Biophys. Res. Commun. 92:* 1231–1237, 1980.

90. Waite, M., DeChatelet, L. R., King, L., and Shirley, P. S. Phagocytosis-induced release of arachidonic acid from human neutrophils. *Biochem. Biophys. Res. Commun. 90:* 984–992, 1979.

91. Walenga, R. W., Showell, H. J., Feinstein, M. B., and Becker, E. L. Parallel inhibition of neutrophil arachidonic acid metabolism and lysosomal enzyme secretion by hordihydroguiaretic acid. *Life Sci. 27:* 1047–1053, 1980.

92. Weiss, S. J. and Putney, J. W., Jr. The relationship of phosphatidyl inositol turnover to receptors and calcium ion channels in rat parotid acinar cells. *Biochem. J. 194:* 463–468, 1981.

93. Weissmann, G., Hoffstein, S., Korchak, H., and Smolen, J. E. The earliest membrane responses to phagocytosis: membrane potential changes and Ca²⁺ loss in human granulocytes. *Trans. Am. Assoc. Phys. 91:* 90–101, 1979.

94. Weissmann, G., Smolen, J. E., and Korchak, H. *Adv. Prostaglandin Thromb. Res. 8:* 1637–1653, 1980.

95. Weissmann, G., Smolen, J. E., and Korchak, H. M. Release of inflammatory mediators from stimulated neutrophils. *N. Engl. J. Med. 303:* 27–34, 1980.

96. Wentzel, B., and Epand, R. M. Stimulation of release of prostaglandins from polymorphonuclear leukocytes by the calcium ionophore A23187. *FEBS Lett. 86:* 255–258, 1978.

97. Whitin, J. C., Chapman, C. E., Simon, E. R., Chovaniec, M. E., and Cohen, H. J. Correlation between membrane potential changes and superoxide production in human granulocytes stimulated by phorbol myristate acetate. *J. Biol. Chem. 255:* 1874–1878, 1980.

98. Zatti, M., and Rossi, F. Relationship between glycolysis and respiration in surfactant-treated leucocytes. *Biochim. Biophys. Acta 148:* 553–555, 1967.

99. Zurier, R. B. Prostaglandin release from human polymorphonuclear leukocytes. *Adv. Prostaglandin Thromb. Res. 2:* 815–818, 1976.

100. Zurier, R. B., and Sayadoff, D. M. Release of prostaglandins from human polymorphonuclear leukocytes. *Inflammation 1:* 93–101, 1975.

101. Zurier, R. B., Weissmann, G., Hoffstein, S., Kammerman, S., and Tai, H. Mechanisms of lysosomal enzyme release from human leukocytes. II. Effects of cAMP and cGMP, autonomic agonists and agents which affect microtubule function. *J. Clin. Invest. 43:* 297–309, 1974.

Chapter 7

The Role of Bacterial Adherence in Infection

GERALD T. KEUSCH

Pathogenic microorganisms are endowed with specific attributes called virulence factors that contribute to their disease-provoking ability (37). This ability can be attributed to four cardinal properties, including the capacity to enter the host, to multiply in or on host tissues, to resist or not stimulate host defenses, and to damage the host (37). In some instances these properties can be ascribed to specific virulence factors, and these often turn out to be surface components of the organism. Microbial and mammalian cell surfaces are currently one of most intensively studied areas in science, and the nature of cell-cell interactions in health and disease is of widespread interest.

In this paper is reviewed one important surface property of pathogenic bacteria, their ability to adhere to and colonize mammalian cell surfaces (2, 11, 23). It is clear that this property is an essential attribute for pathogens not normally found in or on the host animal (15, 37). It also seems to be an important aspect for commensals of the normal flora that are harmless (or even helpful) in their usual habitat (15), but which may become significant agents of disease if and when they establish growth in other habitats. One of the major advances of the past decade has been the definition of specific bacterial determinants as the carrier of this important property (2, 3, 10–16, 23–27, 30, 31, 33, 34, 39–43, 45) and, as a consequence, the initiation of studies to probe the molecular mechanisms involved and the conceptualization of strategies for therapy (28).

BASIC MECHANISMS

RECOGNITION PHENOMENA

Few pathogens of mammals are catholic in taste, with an ability to infect all species of animals, all tissues or organ systems, or all cell types. Rather, there is a clearly expressed preference for one or several, but not all, potential hosts (host adaptation), for one or several, but not all, tissues (site selectivity), and generally for some, but not all, differentiated cell types (cell specificity) (15, 28). What governs this adaptation, selectivity, and specificity?

Current concepts of receptor-ligand interactions in various cellular communication systems, such as drug-response and hormone-response interactions, are useful models to consider (4, 8, 28). In these instances the drug or homone can be considered to be a water-soluble message which must be recognized and received by the appropriate cell type, following which the message must be uncoded and routed within the cell to be translated into the appropriate action. Three functions are thus defined in the stimulus-response model under discussion: a cognitive (receptor) function, an effector (action) function, and a transduction function which serves to link the two (Fig. 7.1) (18). While the receptor is logically placed on the cell surface where it can contact the soluble circulating message, the effector could be at the cell surface, buried within the cell membrane or at its cytoplasmic face, or even within the cytoplasm. Much of contemporary pharmacology and endocrinology has been concerned with these issues.

These concepts have recently been applied to pathogenic microorganisms that secrete soluble virulence factors such as toxins (28). Several bacterial toxins, for example diphtheria or cholera toxins, are the cause of clinical disease and act as enzymes, catalyzing an ADP-ribosylation of the target protein (7, 16, 17) resulting eventually in the "effector response" recognized as the disease. These molecules exhibit specificity for host, organ, and cell as well, and therefore appear to possess the necessary information to both participate in a recognition interaction at the cell surface and to act as the transducing element. Bacterial toxins are, in fact, well designed to carry out these two functions: they are constructed as two-domain molecules (the so-called A-B model) (28), often with separate polypeptide chains held together by disulfide bonds to mediate each distinct function (Fig. 7.2). The B subunit is the binding portion of the molecule that is recognized by

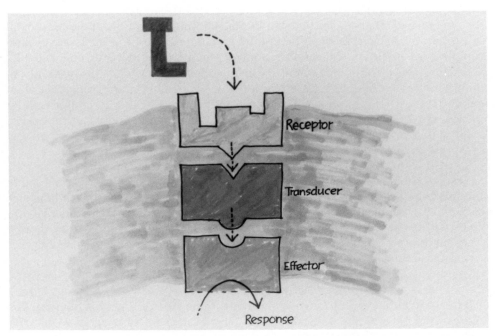

FIG. 7.1. The three functional requirements of a receptor-ligand communiction system. The ligand (*L*) binds to a receptor on the external cell surface which communicates information through a transducing mechanism to the biological effector system somewhere within the plasma membrane.

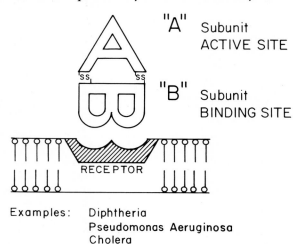

"A" Subunit
ACTIVE SITE

"B" Subunit
BINDING SITE

Examples: Diphtheria
             Pseudomonas Aeruginosa
             Cholera
             Ricin

FIG. 7.2. The general A-B model of toxins. The biologically active A subunit is linked to a distinct B subunit which mediates binding to the cell surface receptor. In many instances, the A and B polypeptides are separate chains, covalently linked together through disulfide bridges.

the cell surface receptor. As in cholera toxin, it may be a multimer of smaller subunit monomers, which provides for multivalency of binding on the cell surface (4, 16), or a single peptide chain, as in diphtheria toxin (7, 16). The A subunit is the biologically active portion of the molecule which transduces the message to the effector (or effected) mechanism in the cell. In the example of cholera toxin, this occurs at the level of the GTP regulatory component of the adenylate cyclase complex, derepressing the catalytic unit of the enzyme and thus operationally activating the effector adenylate cyclase complex (6, 17). In the example of diphtheria toxin, the A subunit enzymatically ADP-ribosylates cytoplasmic elongation factor 2 (EF-2), which serves to inactivate the EF-2 and inhibit cellular protein synthesis (7, 16). One molecule of diphtheria toxin is sufficient to catalytically and irreversibly inactivate all EF-2 and to completely shut off protein synthesis, and the "effected" cell dies (16).

The problem with which we must deal here is the extension of these concepts to two insoluble components (in a cell to cell adhesion interaction), as opposed to the binding of a soluble ligand to an insoluble cellular receptor. Is the language of communication the same? Is there a distinct message and a definable receptor involved? Is there translation of message into a biological response? Is there a transduction or effector mechanism in fact present, or are bacterial adherence reactions simply ecological (28)?

RECEPTOR-LIGAND BINDING

The optimal placement for a receptor to interact with a ligand is obviously on the exterior face of the cell membrane (18). If it is to function in a selective fashion, then the receptor requires "combining site" specificity to permit specific interactions to occur. In fact, if uniqueness is a criterion of receptor function, then nature could be conservative in recognition-response systems such as hormones by using the same or just a few transducer/effector mechanisms (*e.g.*, adenylate cyclase) in different cell types carrying out very different functions (18). A hormone would thus trigger a response only in cells bearing a specific receptor; this process would be mediated through a common intracellular signal (*e.g.* adenylate cyclase), while the ultimate biological effect would be determined by whatever possibilities the process of cellular differentiation has programmed for that particular cell in response to changes in cyclic nucleotide concentration.

Several models have been proposed for this stereospecific ligand binding (Fig. 7.3) (18, 28). The original concept was analogous to a lock and key mechanism, in which a single step binding occurred, the key fitting precisely into the shape of the lock (Fig. 7.3, *1*). However, this imparts extremely strict conformational and orientational requirements to the interaction which might be unrealistically difficult to achieve *in vivo*. Indeed, observations on the binding of drugs to receptors, and particularly structural analogs which have either agonist or antagonist functions, suggest this cannot be the case (8). Many molecules of somewhat differing structure interact productively with individual receptors, albeit with different affinity for binding. Therefore, there must be room for conformational adjustments to occur during a sequential binding process (Fig. 7.3, *middle* and *bottom*), which may occur either in the ligand, the receptor, or both. These models do not introduce any theoretical reasons for alteration of association or equilibrium constants of the interaction, since the final energy state achieved by

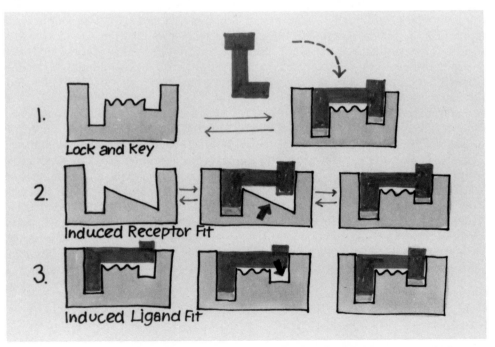

FIG. 7.3. Models for stereospecific receptor-ligand binding. *1*, lock and key model, a single step, conformationally rigid fit of the ligand into the receptor; *2* and *3*, induced receptor or ligand fit, in which conformational changes are induced in either component after the initial binding event to produce a biologically active interaction of ligand with receptor.

lock and key or conformational adjustment models is the same; in all three models the rate-limiting step remains the initial interaction. Importantly, in the latter two more flexible models, the sequential multiple binding interactions that occur are sufficient to provide for the binding specificity requirements. The binding process for soluble ligands is reversible and may be kinetically described by the same mathematical models applied to enzyme-substrate reactions (8, 28). This permits quantitative description of the system in terms of association, dissociation, and equilibrium constants, and comparison of ligands of varying structure. Reversibility also indicates that the binding is noncovalent, but rather a consequence of weak interactions, including van der Waals forces, hydrogen bonding, and ionic or hydrophobic interactions.

A set of criteria can be developed for physiologically relevant receptors, including all of the above physical considerations, as well as tissue or cell distribution consistent with observed *in vivo* events (Table 7.1) (28).

MOLECULAR CONSIDERATIONS

How can these criteria be satisfied at the level of organization of the cell membrane? The first striking characteristic of the lipid bilayer is that hydrophobic determinants are buried within the membrane, whereas hydrophilic determinants are exposed (8, 22). The second striking characteristic of the membrane is that carbohydrate is present only on the external face and not at the cytoplasmic face, whether in glycoprotein or glycolipid (22). In contrast, proteins are found at either surface, within the membrane, partly exposed and partly buried, or even spanning the entire membrane from face to face. The location of the carbohydrates, however, is precisely where the receptor function takes place and on this basis alone could be considered for a role in recognition phenomena. When this insight is combined with the knowledge that great structural diversity of carbohydrates is possible, the sugar sequence at the cell surface becomes of even greater interest. For example, there are 11 stereospecific configurations for a simple glucose disaccharide and 176 for a trisaccharide (22). The number of possible distinct configurations increases still further for mixed oligosaccharides. There are perhaps 4–20 sugar residues in the typical membrane oligosaccharide, composed primarily of six distinct hexoses (glucose, galactose, mannose, fucose, N-acetyl-D-glucosamine, and N-acetyl-D-galactosamine) and sialic acids. It is now well established that these sugars indeed provide the basis for configurational complementarity between many ligands and receptors and in a stereospecific fashion permit a noncovalent, high-affinity, reversible interaction with sensitivity, selectivity, and speed (4, 8, 18, 22, 28). Carbohydrate-specific reception phenomena are, in fact, one of the fundamental mechanisms underlying all of biology.

TABLE 7.1. CRITERIA FOR ASSESSING RECEPTORS

1. High affinity
2. Rapid binding
3. Structural specificity
4. Saturable binding
5. Reversible binding
6. Physiologically relevant tissue distribution
7. Correlation between binding and activity

CELL-CELL INTERACTIONS

Nevertheless, some of these concepts are no longer valid when applied to the interaction between two relatively large, "insoluble" cells involved in cell-to-cell contacts or adherence. First of all, while soluble ligand-receptor interactions may involve multivalency through polymeric binding subunits, in cell-to-cell contacts enormous surface areas are involved so that the appropriate concept is megavalency (Fig. 7.4). This has an important consequence—even if each individual contact is a reversible, noncovalent binding, the sheer number of binding sites involved makes it unlikely that all will become free at the same time to permit the adherent cells to separate, and in practice the attachment becomes irreversible (33). Recent studies on the sugar-dependent attachment of mammalian cells to protein substrates on plastic surfaces demonstrate that this attachment is reversible by sugar haptens only in the first few minutes (5, 35). Once firm attachment has occurred, elution is difficult, even with high concentrations of the hapten inhibitor (35).

Secondly, because of the large size of the cells, surface charge becomes very important. The surface of both eukaryotic and prokaryotic cells has a net negative

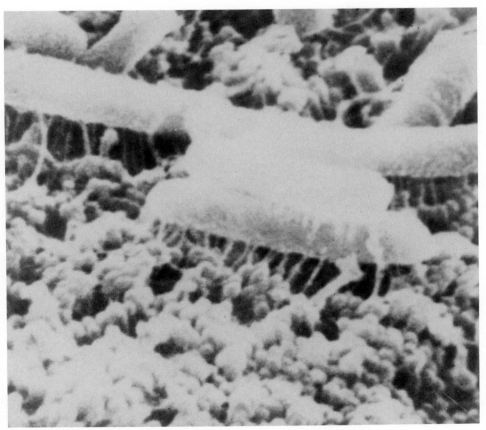

FIG. 7.4. *E. coli* adherent to small bowel mucosa. Of note is the enormous surface areas in contact with each other and the morphological suggestion of multiple adherence sites.

charge due to ionization of various surface groups, especially carboxyls of sialic acid on eukaryotes and teichoic, glucuronic, or hyaluronic acids on prokaryotes (23). Thus, the two apposing surfaces are, electrically speaking, mutually repulsive. It doesn't matter that the net fixed negative surface charges attract a layer of positive ions from the surrounding fluid. Although the positively charged ions for all practical purposes become a part of the membrane as a diffuse double ion layer, even moving together with the cell in electrical fields, the apposing surfaces are still mutually repulsive.

If the above is true, and yet cells still come into close contact and indeed adhere to one another, then there must be attracting forces which overcome the charge effects. These forces do exist and include the same weak interactions involved in receptor-soluble ligand binding, including focal ionic attractions, van der Waals forces and hydrogen bonding, and hydrophobic interactions (2, 11, 23, 33, 40, 43). The magnitude of each of these forces is affected by distance, temperature, and ionic strength of the medium. The resultant force is therefore complex and variable under different conditions of study. For example, increasing ionic strength of the medium will reduce ionic interactions but enhance hydrophobic interactions (40).

Thirdly, the larger the size of the adhering cells, the greater the importance of geometric considerations, for example, the radius of curvature of the surface profiles in attachment (Fig. 7.5). As the radius decreases, the repulsive forces decrease much more than the attractive forces diminish, thus producing a net

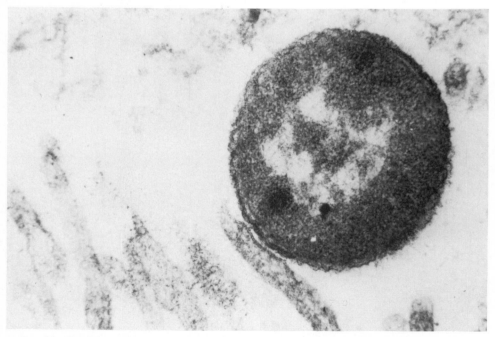

FIG. 7.5. K-88$^+$ *E. coli* adherent to microvillus of porcine proximal small bowel. Note the closeness of the adherence, the relative size of the bacterium and microvillus, and the large radius of contacting cell surface. (Courtesy of Richard Sellwood.)

increase in the attractive forces (23). As the distance between the cells narrows, interactions develop between hydrophobic regions on the two surfaces (for example, stretches of peptides with many apolar amino acids, hydrogen atoms, methyl or methoxy groups on carbohydrates or lipids), and the resulting displacement of water causes a favorable change in free energy and a strong adherence.

In vitro studies in a simplified system designed to examine the extent and specificity of adhesion of mammalian cells to proteins coated onto plastic surfaces have shown that hapten-inhibitable binding to lectins, galactose oxidase (a lectin-like enzyme), and fibronectin is inhibitable by agents such as azide, cytochalasin B, EDTA, diamide (a nontoxic sulfhydryl oxidant), or N-ethyl maleimide (a sulfhydryl blocking agent) only during the first few minutes of interaction (5). Later addition of the drugs or chemical agents is without effect, suggesting that the initial specific recognition is quickly followed by an active, irreversible cell-dependent attachment process. It has been suggested that in this system the primary role of the adhesion surface is in fact to stimulate a cell-dependent attachment process (5).

Given these considerations, one would predict that bacteria wishing to adhere to mammalian cells might do so initially via a long, thin appendage which would have a small radius of curvature at the tip relative to the organism itself, perhaps with a lower net negative charge than the rest of the cell surface or have hydrophobic patches or groups exposed, and would carry determinants for a receptor-ligand recognition to occur in order to provide for selective and specific interactions with certain cell types (23). Indeed, in many instances, this is what nature has chosen to do.

Specific attachment factors are often found in the form of long, thin 6–8 μM filamentous structures of uniform composition called fimbriae (pili),* or as somewhat irregular stringy thinner (2–3 μM) fibrous protein aggregates termed fibrillae (23). These structures have a high content of apolar amino acids and are quite hydrophobic (40, 43). An initial adhesion via fimbriae or fibrillae could be followed by additional cell-dependent (active) or independent (physical) interactions which become possible because of the initial interaction.

MODEL ADHERENCE SYSTEMS

GENERAL CONSIDERATIONS

A number of models have been employed to study the nature of adherence phenomena between bacteria and mammalian cells and their relevance to virulence and pathogenesis of infections. Many factors can influence the results, including the source of the organism in nature, artifacts resulting from conditions of *in vitro* growth of bacteria which induce phenotypic changes, the phase of growth selected for study or effects of laboratory passage, as well as the nature of the mammalian cells or tissue studied, the species of the donor, age of the host, the integrity of the tissue in *in vitro* systems, the immune state of the host, use of primary or established or transformed cell lines, or the presence of exogenous agents (such as viruses or mycoplasma, specific hapten inhibitors, or toxic agents).

---

* It is becoming an accepted custom now to reserve the term pili for structures involved in transfer of genetic material in bacteria.

ENTERIC PATHOGENS—PORCINE COLIBACILLOSIS

A particularly well-studied example which serves as a good model for conceptualizing the nature and role of adherence phenomena in pathogenesis of disease is the neonatal diarrheal disease of infant piglets caused by certain strains of *Escherichia coli* (38). Newborn pigs are naturally and highly susceptible to these orally acquired small bowel infections, developing severe watery diarrhea which results in significant dehydration and high mortality rates (14, 24, 36, 38, 39). This so-called colibacillosis is a major economic factor in swine husbandry.

CLINICAL CONSIDERATIONS

Watery diarrhea is the cardinal manifestation of disease. Various studies have shown that, like many watery diarrheas of bacterial origin, the target organ is the proximal small bowel which is found to be the source of the voluminous intestinal fluid loss (28, 38). Proximal gut is converted from a net fluid-absorbing organ to a net-secreting one by the infecting agent, which is the consequence of polypeptide hormone-like toxins that activate nucleotide cyclases in intestinal epithelial cells to increase intracellular c-AMP or c-GMP (1, 4, 19, 21, 32). The cyclic nucleotides, in turn, alter absorptive or secretory processes to affect net secretion of isotonic fluid (28). Both heat-labile toxins (LT) and heat-stable toxins (ST) are involved in colibacillosis, similar to human toxigenic *E. coli* disease (1, 9, 16, 21). The sequence of events involved has been traced from ingestion of an inoculum of virulent bacteria to colonization of the proximal gut (Table 7.4) and multiplication of the organism to very high numbers (10^8–10^9/ml of gut contents), local production of LT and/or ST, and initiation of the secretory diarrhea; ingestion of preformed toxin is insufficient.

PHENOTYPIC CHARACTERISTICS OF THE ORGANISM

Three properties of the causative organisms attracted attention as possible virulence factors. These included the ability to produce enterotoxin (LT or ST), the presence of a hemolysin, and production of a surface antigen, K-88, found to mediate hemagglutination of certain erythrocytes (for example, guinea pig RBCs) (39). The potential significance of the enterotoxin is obvious. Interest in hemolysins has always been great because the cell lytic process is dramatic, readily studied, and can be envisioned as a mechanism of damage to cell membranes. Hemolysins are, in fact, considered to play a role in the pathogenesis of certain acute infections (*i.e.*, *Clostridium perfringens* sepsis) or even in the pathogenesis of rheumatic fever (cardiotoxic effects of streptolysin-O (SLO)). K-88 was considered to be a potential factor in the initial colonization of the normally relatively sterile proximal gut because of the hemagglutination it induced in the test tube. Isolates from sich animals were often, if not invariably, positive for these phenotypic traits. Study of their role in pathogenesis was facilitated by the finding that each was controlled by nonchromosomal plasmid inheritance in *E. coli* and could thus be manipulated in the laboratory (19, 34, 39). The traits (Ent, enterotoxin; HLy, hemolysin; K-88) could be individually inserted into or removed from single *E. coli* strains to create a series of otherwise isogenic clones for study (39).

In vivo experiments

When these organisms were studied by *in vivo* challenge experiments of susceptible newborn piglets (39), it was found that the presence or absence of HLy affected neither colonization nor disease production (Tables 7.2 and 7.3). Only Ent or K-88 plasmids appeared to have clinical relevance (24). The relationship between these was studied by Smith and Linggood (39), who sequentially inserted the two plasmids into an avirulent Ent$^-$/K-88$^-$ porcine *E. coli* strain (Table 7.4). Neither trait alone was sufficient to confer significant virulence on the organism. The K88$^-$/Ent$^+$ variant could not colonize and therefore had no opportunity to produce toxins, whereas the K88$^+$/Ent$^-$ strain, which could

TABLE 7.2. CORRELATION OF HEMOLYSIN AND/OR K88 ANTIGEN AND PATHOGENICITY IN PORCINE *E. COLI* (0141: K85 ab)

Plasmid Content		No. Bacteria in Proximal Jejunum (Log$_{10}$)	No. Piglets/Total Infected (% Mortality)
Hl$_y^+$	K-88$^+$	High*	10/10 (50%)
Hl$_y^-$	K-88$^+$	9.1	9/10 (56%)
Hl$_y^+$	K-88$^-$	4.0	0/13 (0%)
Hl$_y^+$ K88$^-$/K-88$^+$†		8.3	9/10 (67%)

Adapted from Smith and Linggood (39).

* Data not reported, but from other data available, one should expect levels in excess of 10^8 bacteria.

† Insertion of K-88 plasmid derived from a different *E. Coli* (08: K-87, K-88 ab) into K-88$^-$ 0141: K-85 ab strain.

TABLE 7.3. CORRELATION OF K-88 AND/OR ENTEROTOXIN PRODUCTION AND PATHOGENICITY IN *E. COLI*

E. coli Phenotype	No. of Bacteria in Proximal Jejunum Log$_{10}$	Animals Sick/Total Infected
K88$^-$/Ent$^-$	5.3	0/8
K88$^-$/Ent$^+$	4.4	0/6
K88$^+$/Ent$^-$	8.3	3/11
K88$^+$/Ent$^+$	9.3	12.16

Adapted from H. W. Smith and M. A. Linggood (39).

TABLE 7.4. EFFECT OF PLASMID INSERTION ON VIRULENCE OF PORCINE *E. COLI* (08: K40)

Plasmid Inserted		Colonization	Disease
K-88	Ent		
−	−	±	0
−	+	±	0
+	−	++++	+*
+	+	++++	++++

Adapted from H. W. Smith and M. A. Linggood (39).

* One-third animals with mild diarrhea.

colonize, was unable to activate the secretory process and was therefore relegated to commensal status. Jones and Rutter (24) showed that only K88$^+$ strains attached to the small bowel mucosa (Fig. 7.5). Virulence, the ability to cause disease, required both attributes, each of which was a virulence factor, necessary for but not sufficient to cause disease.

NATURE OF K-88

The antigen is a simple protein, containing neither carbohydrate nor lipid, and it exists as a long, filamentous, irregular, thin appendage radiating out from the surface of the organism (23, 31). At least three antigenic variants have been identified with only minor alterations in amino acid composition, corresponding to variation in molecular weight of the K-88 subunit peptide from 23,500 to 26,000 daltons by SDS-polyacrylamide gel electrophoresis (31). All three variant proteins have the same isoelectric point (pI = 4.2) by isoelectric focusing, and they share a common determinant. K-88 has been shown to bind *in vitro* to brush border epithelial cells from pig intestine, and this is inhibitable by specific antibody (24). The role of K-88 in mediating virulence is further demonstrated by successful passive immunization of colostrum-deprived neonatal pigs or the protective effects of active immunization of sows subsequently allowed to suckle their litter, in contrast to failure of protection in piglets nursed by sham or control immunized sows (23).

Of interest is the recent report by Middledorp and Wilholt (30), who demonstrated that LT$^+$/K-88$^+$ porcine *E. coli* produce small fragments or vesicles of outer membrane (OM) during *in vitro* growth which are found to be greatly enriched for LT. Compared to the K-88 content of the whole organism, these same OM vesicles were 30-fold enriched for K-88. Such OM fragments were shown to bind effectively to brush border membrane preparations from susceptible pigs, but not to OM vesicles prepared from bacteria grown at 18°C, which phenotypically represses K-88 antigen production. The concentration of the two key virulence factors in OM minicells, if an *in vivo* phenomenon as well, would constitute a neat delivery system for toxin to the brush border surface, since the concentration of attachment factors on a smaller bacterial cell fragment should considerably augment binding to the gut cell compared to the relatively enormous intact bacterium.

THE K-88 RECEPTOR

If K-88 is the ligand for attachment, what is the receptor? Although the precise nature of the intestinal receptor is still uncertain, its existence and importance in pathogenesis of disease due to Ent$^+$/K-88$^+$ *E. coli* is certain. Observations on responses of individual litters to infection, selective breeding experiments, and phenotypic characterization of individual animals has led to the identification of receptor positive and negative pig strains (14, 27, 36). The observation that litters might be uniformly susceptible or resistant to K-88$^+$ organisms, or partially susceptible, became of great potential significance when it was found that this pattern was a consistent result of certain pairings of boar and sow, that is, certain mating pairs produced only susceptible or resistant pairs while others always produced both susceptible and resistant animals (14). Phenotypic analysis of the mating pairs and their progeny, accomplished by an *in vitro* adherence assay of

K-88$^+$ organisms to brush border prepared from the proximal gut (Fig. 7.6) (36), permitted genetic analysis of the results (14). The data (Table 7.5) are consistent with simple Mendelian inheritance of a single locus-two allele system, susceptible (receptor$^+$, S) and resistant (receptor$^-$, s), with S being dominant over s. Selective breeding has therefore been used for production of homozygous ss animals which are resistant to disease caused by K-88$^+$/Ent$^+$ *E. coli* because the organism cannot adhere to the gut cell (Fig. 7.6) and therefore is unable to colonize. This has facilitated comparison of the brush border membranes from receptor$^+$ and receptor$^-$ animals and has produced evidence implicating a glycolipid component as the putative receptor (27). These studies are continuing to further characterize the receptor and to elucidate the nature of the interaction with K-88 antigen.

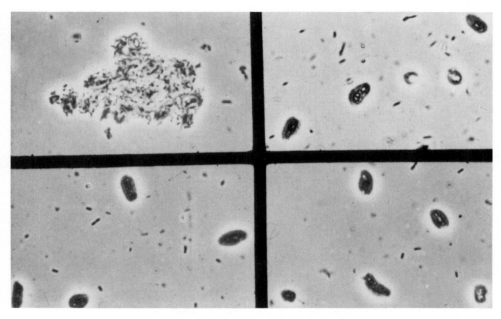

FIG. 7.6. *In vitro* adherence assay for K-88$^+$ *E. coli* and isolated porcine jejunal brush borders. *Top left*, intestinal membrane from receptor$^+$ animal with many adherent, clumped, K-88$^+$. *Top right*, The same brush border preparation has been mixed with organisms grown at 18°C which precludes synthesis of K-88 antigen. No bacterial adherence is seen. *Bottom*, intestinal membrane from receptor$^-$ animal has been mixed with K-88$^+$ bacteria (*left*) or K-88$^-$ bacteria (*right*) as above. The organisms cannot adhere because of the lack of receptors on the gut membrane. (Courtesy of Richard Sellwood.)

TABLE 7.5. K-88 RECEPTOR PHENOTYPES IN PIGLETS FROM MATINGS OF PHENOTYPED PARENTS

Parental Pheno-type	No. of Litters Studied	No. of Animals with Pheno-type*	
		S	s
S* × s	8	36	37
	2	25	0
s × s	9	0	84

Adapted from R. A. Gibbons *et al.* (14).

* S, receptor positive (susceptible); s, receptor negative (resistant).

HYDROPHOBIC INTERACTIONS

Thus it is certain for the K88⁺-porcine *E. coli* system that a receptor-ligand interaction is involved in the recognition. Wadstrom and colleagues (40, 42–44) have proposed that effective adherence following the initial recognition event is attributable to hydrophobic interactions. They have studied K-88 and other similar surface "adhesins" (23) on other toxigenic *E. coli*, including K-99⁺, CFA-I⁺, and CFA-II⁺ strains which affect lambs or cattle (K-99) (10) or humans (CFA-I and CFA-II) (12, 13) for hydrophobicity by adherence to sepharose gels substituted with aliphatic side chains of varying length used for hydrophobic interaction chromatography (40, 43). The binding of bacteria to the gel is in part the consequence of the intrinsic hydrophobicity of the organism, and in part the hydrophobicity of the gel, which can be increased by increasing the degree of substitution and/or length of the fatty acid side chain. With any given combination of an individual organism and a specific gel, the hydrophobic interactions can be enhanced by increasing ionic strength of the buffer. By these means the relative hydrophobicity of the various adhesins has been shown to be CFA-I > CFA-II > K-88 > K-99 (43). Growth of the organisms at 18°C to suppress adhesin production also suppresses hydrophobicity, as does cure of the plasmid coding for the adhesin. Using a binding assay to human adult intestinal epithelial cells (prepared from surgical specimens obtained from patients undergoing bypass surgery for obesity), Wadstrom *et al.*[43] have demonstrated the species selectivity of CFA-I and II and K-88, and the critical role of the adhesin in binding of CFA-I or II positive organisms to the target, presumably the consequence of a specific lectin-like receptor-ligand interaction. Thus at least two types of interaction may be involved in *in vivo* adherence of bacteria to target tissues (Fig. 7.7). In experimental animals Wadstrom *et al.* (44) have also demonstrated the protective effects of hydrophobic gels, which presumably compete with the intestinal cell for attachment of the pathogens and thus effectively inhibit colonization.

CONTROL OF ADHESIN SYNTHESIS

If adherence factors confer selective advantage *in vivo* but are unimportant in other habitats, it would be advantageous to the organisms to repress synthesis until specifically needed. It is not known what might induce adhesin production *in vivo*; however, recent studies with K-99⁺ lamb and bovine strains of *E. coli* suggest some possibilities (10). The information for K-99 antigen, like K-88 antigen of porcine strains, is contained in a 52-megadalton plasmid that associates with certain O antigen types (similar to CFA-I and II), but it has been found that phenotypic expression of K-99 during *in vitro* growth is very dependent on the medium employed. While minimal medium supports K-99 synthesis well, rich or complete media suppress synthesis. De Graaf *et al.* (12) have recently reported that l-alanine partially represses expression of K-99 in minimal medium at relatively low concentrations (0.5 mM) and completely blocks production at 5 mM whereas the product of l-alanine metabolism, pyruvate, is without effect. The plasmid in these studies also codes for a β lactamase controlled by the transposon, Tn 901, and interestingly β-lactamase production is not altered by alanine, thus indicating the specificity of the effect. The authors (10) speculate about possible relevance to *in vivo* responses in which K-99⁺ organisms are

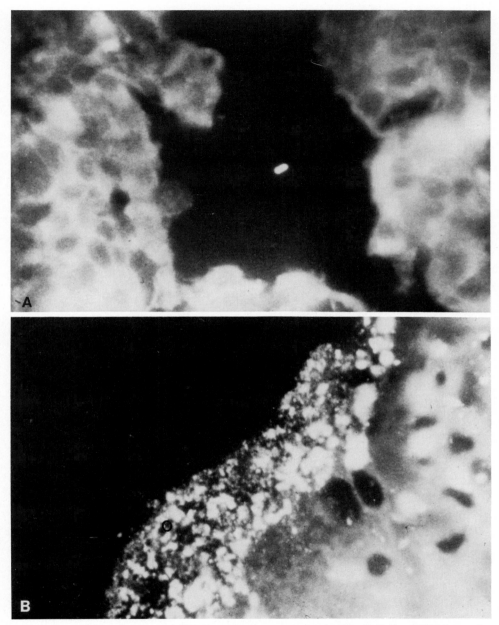

FIG. 7.7. *In vivo* adherence of CFA-I positive human toxigenic *E. coli* (*left*) or CFA-I negative variant 6 hours after infection of infant rabbits. Marked colonization, demonstrated by fluorescent antibody to *E. coli*, is seen with the CFA-I positive organism but not with the strain lacking the factor. (Courtesy of Dolores G. Evans and Doyle J. Evans, Jr.)

naturally pathogenic only for very young animals in the first few days of life. They consider it possible that after birth, protein digestion and the microbial flora may alter the local amino acid concentrations in the gut so that repressive concentrations of alanine are present within days. This would serve to protect the host since failure to produce K-99 would prevent colonization which, in turn, would preclude disease. Whether or not this is true *in vivo* in the example cited is not known; however, the concept that local factors may influence production or function of virulence factors is an important one deserving study as a possible explanation for some particular host-pathogen relationships such as limited age susceptibility and tissue specificity.

Nonintestinal Tract Pathogens

Although the purpose of this paper is to discuss concepts involved in microbial adherence and its relevance to virulence, and not to review each organ system or organism in depth (see recent reviews by Beachey (2), Ellwood *et al.* (11) and Ofek and Beachey (33)), a few additional examples will be discussed to enlarge upon the principles already presented.

Respiratory Tract Pathogens

The specificity of the recognition phenomenon is demonstrated by the adherence of group A beta hemolytic streptococci to upper respiratory (buccal) epithelial cells. Initially, this was thought to be related to the M-protein-containing (M^+) surface fibrillar layers, since M-protein-deficient (M^-) streptococci or trypsinized M^+ strains were denuded of fibrillae and lacked adhesion properties (2, 23, 33). However, in a series of studies Beachey and Ofek (3) have demonstrated that the M-protein content is not of importance in adherence but rather the presence of lipoteichoic acid (LTA) (3). Extraction of LTA always reduces adhesiveness, whereas selective removal of M-protein does not. Consistent with these observations, LTA was also found to be a hapten inhibitor of streptococcal adherence. The surface of the organism, *Streptococcus pyogenes*, is also very hydrophobic, especially the M^+ strains, as shown by hydrophobic interaction chromatography (42). It is not unlikely that M-protein, which clearly acts as a virulence factor because of its antiphagocytic properties, can also contribute to adherence and colonization by virtue of its hydrophobic properties, conferring additional survival value for M^+ strains in the *in vivo* milieu. Adherence of *S. pyogenes* to neonatal cells was found to be much decreased compared to that to adult cells, although the number of LTA receptors determined by studies with purified, labeled LTA was not much different between the two (33). The discrepancy was resolved when it was shown that homogenization or freeze thawing of neonatal cells would restore adherence to near adult levels, apparently by fully exposing partially masked LTA receptors which were unable to interact with native LTA on the bacterial surface.

Another host factor in determination of adherence capacity is suggested by studies of unencapsulated *Pseudomonas aeruginosa* binding to upper respiratory tract (buccal) cells (45). This organism is neither a pathogen nor commensal of the upper airway of normal humans, and it fails to adhere to their buccal epithelial cells. In contrast, it may be an important pathogen of debilitated patients and is a common respiratory organism in patients with cystic fibrosis (CF), and it adheres well to buccal epithelium from CF patients. Normal cells will, in fact, permit a similar degree of attachment of *P. aeruginosa* as CF cells if the epithelium is first trypsinized to remove surface fibronectin, suggesting the presence of a masked determinant (45). When the fibronectin content of buccal epithelium from CF patients was examined, there was an 83% decrease in fibronectin content of the CF cells, associated with an 8.3-fold increase in bacterial adherence. As a possible explanation for diminished cell-associated fibronectin, the proteolytic activity of secretions bathing the buccal epithelium was measured. Protease activity was three times increased in saliva of the CF patients compared to that of normal controls. Whatever the primary defect may be, these data suggest that *in vivo* modification of host cell surfaces may affect adherence of specific microorganisms, and thereby alter colonization and virulence.

URINARY TRACT PATHOGENS

A number of investigations have implicated fimbriae on infecting microorganisms as adhesins for uroepithelial cells. These adherence factors have frequently been studied *in vitro* using hemagglutination assays with specific types of erythrocytes, for the fimbriae are involved in this response as well (20, 23, 25, 26, 41). Many Enterobacteriaceae produce a common pilus (termed Type 1) which causes agglutination of guinea pig cells specifically inhibited by the monosaccharide mannose (mannose-sensitive hemagglutination, MSHA) (23). Because Type 1 pili are found on so many organisms, both pathogens and nonpathogens, it is generally believed that they play no role in virulence, and organisms are therefore frequently screened for potentially significant adherence in the presence of 10–100 mM mannose to select strains causing mannose-resistant hemagglutination (MRHA). This procedure would preclude detection of a mannose-inhibitable factor which was unrelated to Type 1 pili, and therefore is not the optimal strategy to adopt. When *E. coli* isolated from children with urinary tract infections was studied, it was found that the capacity to attach to human urinary tract epithelium was related to the severity of the infection produced by the organism (acute pyelonephritis, acute cystitis, asymptomatic bacteriuria) and paralleled MRHA of human erythrocytes (41). Seventy-seven percent of strains from pyelonephritis patients showed this MRHA, compared to 16% of strains from fecal isolates from health subjects. Kallenius and colleagues (25, 26) have identified the specific carbohydrate determinants of the P blood group antigens on human erythrocytes that are involved in this MRHA. Pyelonephritis strains of *E. coli* were found to bind to P^+ but not P^- cells. There are three glycosphingolipid determinants and five phenotypes involved in the P system (Table 7.6, Fig. 7.8). The pyelonephritis strains adhered equally as well to the most simple phenotype, p^k_2, containing the shortest carbohydrate chain, as they did to more complex P^+ cells, and indeed the isolated, reduced trisaccharide moiety of the trihexosylcer-

TABLE 7.6. PHENOTYPIC VARIANTS OF HUMAN P BLOOD GROUP SYSTEM

Phenotype Designation	P Determinant(s)	Frequency
P_1	P, P_1, p^k	75%
P_2	P, p^k	25%
p^k_2	P_1, p^k	Rare
$\bar{p}$	p^k	Rare
	Nil	Rare

FIG. 7.8. The oligosaccharide structure of the three P blood group determinants showing the common disaccharide group linked to ceramide.

Specificity	Structure
p^k	α-D-Gal$p$-(1-4) ⟍
p_1	α-D-Gal$p$-(1-4)-β-D Gal$p$-(1-4)-β-D-GlcNAcp-(1-3)-β-D-Gal$p$-(1-4)-β-D-Glc$p$-Ceramide
P	β-D-GalNAcp (1-3)-α-D-Gal P (1-4) ⟋

amide of the p^k molecule (present on all P^+ cells) was found to be an effective inhibitor of agglutination of P^+ erythrocytes, whereas monosaccharides (D-galactose, 1-O-α-D-galactopyranoside, N-acetyl-D-galactosamine) or other α-D-galactosyl containing oligosaccharides (stachyose, melibiose) or glycosphingolipids (globoside) were ineffective (26). Subsequently, the authors were able to show that specificity in fact is retained in the nonreducing terminal disaccharide, α-D-Gal$p$-(1-4)-β-D-Gal$p$, common to both p^k and P_1 glycosphingolipids, which thus constitutes the minimum receptor structure for the adhesin on these *E. coli* strains (25). While the receptor on urinary tract epithelium is still unknown, a major glycosphingolipid in normal human kidney is galactobiosyl-ceramide (29), containing exactly the same disaccharide as the p^k and P_1 substances, and this is highly suggestive that P blood group determinants on renal cells may be directly involved in pathogenesis of *E. coli* pyelonephritis.

THERAPEUTIC IMPLICATIONS

Based on the specificity of receptor-ligand interactions, there are four strategies to consider for receptor-based therapy (28). First, to compete with natural receptors for attachment of the pathogen using an artificial receptor complex of great or greater avidity for the ligand or with a sufficiently high concentration to drive the interaction in favor of the artificial receptor (receptor (mega) therapy). Second, the receptor could be blocked with an analogue of the ligand which occupies a sufficient number of all surface receptors to prevent attachment (receptor blockade). This could be a sugar binding lectin, the binding portion of the adhesin, or an antireceptor antibody. Thirdly, the receptor could be structurally altered, for example, enzymatically cleaved from the cell surface or sterically blocked with bulky side groups or addition or removal of monosaccharide units from the carbohydrate portion (receptor modification). Finally, specific soluble hapten inhibitors, whether mono- or oligosaccharides, glycopeptides, or glycolipids, could be employed as competitive inhibitors to reverse the initial binding, before operationally irreversible attachment occurs (elution therapy).

A form of receptor-based therapy has recently been attempted in experimental enteric infections with human CFA-I and *E. coli* in infant rabbits (41). The CFA-I antigen confers hydrophobic properties to the bacterial cell surface, as described earlier in this paper. Therefore, Wadstrom and colleagues (44) elected to administer hydrophobic gels per os as a competitive adherence factor in orally infected animals. Control animals were treated with a hydrophilic gel instead. The results were striking; all animals given hydrophilic gels developed diarrhea, whereas over 90% given hydrophobic gels, even 6 hours after the bacterial inoculum, were protected. Since neither LT or ST *E. coli* enterotoxins interacted with the gel, it presumably had its effect by adherence to the CFA-I positive organisms, thus preventing colonization of the mucosal surface itself.

SUMMARY
The data presented in this review indicate that bacteria have developed mechanisms to facilitate adherence to target mammalian cells, often present in filamentous structures of varying organization at the cell surface, classified together as *adhesins*. These may contain distinctive molecular sequences, often including sugars, which function as ligands for specific interactions with receptors on mammalian cells. Such receptor-ligand interactions determine species, organ, and cell specificity of adherence by individual bacterial strains. In some examples, this adherence phenomenon can be demonstrated to be an essential virulence attributed of pathogens which must adhere in order to colonize and then cause disease. While considerable detailed knowledge has accumulated about certain adhesins (*e.g.*, K-88) or some mammalian cell receptors (*e.g.*, the p^k blood group-related disaccharide on human erythrocytes for pyelonephritis strains of *E. coli*), in no instance do we know the nature of an adhesin *and* its specific receptor to fully define the actual chemistry of the binding, but we undoubtedly will in the near future. Avidity of adherence is attributable to multiple forces, in particular hydrophobic interactions in prokaryote-eukaryote systems. Therapeutic strategies to alter these relationships and thereby to prevent or treat disease are already being applied to model *in vitro* and experimental *in vivo* infections.

REFERENCES

1. Aldorete, J. F., and Robertson, D. C. Purification and chemical characterization of the heat-stable enterotoxin produced by porcine strains of enterotoxigenic *Escherichia coli*. *Infect. Immun.* 19: 1021–1030, 1978.
2. Beachey, E. H. *Bacterial Adherence*. London, Chapman & Hall, Methuen, Inc., 1980.
3. Beachey, E. H., and Ofek, I. Epithelial cell binding of group A streptococci by lipoteichoic acid on fimbriae denuded of M protein. *J. Exp. Med. 143:* 759–771, 1976.
4. Bennett, V., Craig, S., Hollenberg, M.D., O'Keefe, E., Sahyoun, N., and Cuatrecasas, P. Structure and function of cholera toxin and hormone receptors. *J. Supramol. Struct. 4:* 99–120, 1976.
5. Carter, W.G., Rauvala, H., and Hakomori, S.I. Studies on cell adhesion and recognition. II. The kinetics of cell adhesion and cell spreading on surfaces coated with carbohydrate-reactive proteins (glycosidases and lectins) and fibronectin. *J. Cell Biol. 86:* 138–148, 1981.
6. Cassel, D., and Pfeuffer, T. Mechanism of cholera toxin action: covalent modification of the guanyl nucleotide-binding protein of the adenylate cyclase system. *Proc. Natl. Acad. Sci. USA* 75: 2669–2673, 1978.
7. Collier, R. J. Inhibition of protein synthesis by exotoxins from *Corynebacterium diphtheriae* and *Pseudomonas aeruginosa*. In: *Receptors and Recognition. The Specificity and Action of Animal, Bacterial and Plant Toxins.* Series B, Vol 1, edited by P. Cuatrecasas, pp. 67–98. New York, Halsted Press, 1977.
8. Cuatrecasas, P., and Hollenberg, M.D. Membrane receptors and hormone action. *Adv. Protein Chem. 30:* 251–451, 1976.
9. Dallas, W., and Falkow, S. The molecular nature of heat-labile enterotoxin of *Escherichia coli*. *Nature 277:* 406–407, 1979.
10. de Graaf, F. K., Klaasen-Boor, P., and van Hees, J. E. Biosynthesis of the K99 surface antigen is repressed by alanine. *Infect. Immun. 30:* 125–128, 1980.
11. Ellwood, D.C., Melling, J., and Rutter, P. Adhesion of microorganisms to surfaces. London, Academic Press, 1979.
12. Evans, D. G., and Evans, D. J., Jr. New surface-associated heat-labile colonization factor antigen (CFA/II) produced by enterotoxigenic *Escherichia coli* of serogroups 06 and 08. *Infect. Immun. 21:* 638–647, 1978.
13. Evans, D. G., Silver, R. P., Evans, D. J., Jr., and Gorbach, S. L. Plasmid-controlled colonization factor associated with virulence in *Escherichia coli* enterotoxigenic for humans. *Infect. Immun.* 12: 656–667, 1975.

14. Gibbons, R. A., Sellwood, R., Burrows, M., and Hunter, P. A. Inheritance of resistance to neonatal *E. coli* diarrhoea in the pig: examination of the genetic system. *Theor. Appl. Genet. 51:* 65–70, 1977.

15. Gibbons, R. J., Spinell, D. M., and Skobe, Z. Selective adherence as a determinant of the host tropisms of certain indigenous and pathogenic bacteria. *Infect. Immun.* 13:238–246, 1976.

16. Gill, D. M. Seven toxic peptides that cross cell membranes. In: *Bacterial Toxins and Cell Membranes.* Edited by J. Jeljaszewicz, and T. Wadstrom, New York, Academic Press, 1978 pp. 291–332.

17. Gill, D. M., and Meren, R. ADP-ribosylation of membrane proteins catalyzed by cholera toxin: basis of the activation of adenylate cyclase. *Proc. Natl. Acad. Sci. USA 75:* 3050–3054, 1978.

18. Greaves, M.F. Cell surface receptors: a biological perspective. In: *Receptors and Recognition.* Series A, Vol. 1, edited by P. Cuatrecasas and M. F. Greaves, pp. 1–32. London, Chapman Hall, 1976.

19. Gyles, C., So, M., and Falkow, S. The enterotoxin plasmids of *Escherichia coli. J. Infect. Dis.* 130:40–49, 1974.

20. Hagberg, L., Jodal, U., Korhonen, T. K., Lidin-Janson, G., Lindberg, U., and Svanborg Eden, C. Adhesion, hemagglutination, and virulence of *Escherichia coli* causing urinary tract infections. *Infect. Immun. 31:* 564–570, 1981.

21. Hughes, J. M., Murad, F., Chang, B., and Guerrant, R. L. Role of cyclic GMP in the action of heat stable enterotoxin of *Escherichia coli. Nature 271:* 755–756, 1978.

22. Hughes, R. C. The complex carbohydrates of mammalian cell surfaces and their biological roles. *Essays Biochem.* 11:1–36, 1975.

23. Jones, G. W. The attachment of bacteria to the surface of animal cells. In: *Receptors and Recognition. Microbial Interactions,* Series B, Vol. 3, pp. 141–176. London, Chapman & Hall, 1977.

24. Jones, G. W., and Rutter, J. M. Role of the K88 antigen in the pathogenesis of neonatal diarrhoea caused by *Escherichia coli* in piglets. *Infect. Immun. 6:* 918–927, 1972.

25. Kallenius, G., Molby, R., Svenson, S.B., Winberg, J., and Hultberg, H. Identification of a carbohydrate receptor recognized by uropathogenic *Escherichia coli. Infect. Immun. 3:* 288–293, 1980.

26. Kallenius, G., Mollby, R., Svenson, S. B., Winberg, J., Lundblad, A., Svensson, S., and Cedergren, B. The p^k antigen as receptor for the haemagglutinin of pyelonephritic *Escherichia coli. FEMS Microbiol. Lett. 7:* 297–302, 1980.

27. Kearns, M. J., and Gibbons, R. J. The possible nature of the pig intestinal receptor for the K88 antigen of *Escherichia coli. FEMS Microbiol. Lett. 6:* 165–168, 1979.

28. Keusch, G. T. Specific membrane receptors: pathogenetic and therapeutic implications in infectious diseases. *Rev. Infect. Dis. 1:* 517–529, 1979.

29. Martensson, E. Sulfatides of human kidney: isolation, identification and fatty acid composition. *Biochim. Biophys. Acta 116:* 521–531, 1966.

30. Middeldorp, J. M., and Witholt, B. K88 mediated binding of *Escherichia coli* outer membrane fragments to porcine intestinal epithelial cell brush borders. *Infect. Immun. 31:* 42–57, 1981.

31. Mool, F. R., and de Graaf, F. K. Isolation and characterization of K88 antigens. *FEMS Microbiol. Lett. 5:* 17–21, 1979.

32. Newsome, P. M., Burgess, M. N., and Mullan, N. A. Effect of *Escherichia coli* heat-stable enterotoxin on cyclic GMP levels in mouse intestine. *Infect. Immun. 22:* 290–291, 1978.

33. Ofek, I., and Beachey, E. H. Bacterial adherence. In Adv. Int. Med., pp. 503–532. Chicago, Year Book Medical Publishers, 1980.

34. Orskov, I., and Orskov, F. Episome-carried surface antigen K8 of *Escherichia coli.* I. Transmission of the determinant of the K88 antigen and influence on the transfer of chromosomal markers. *J. Bacteriol. 91:* 69–75, 1966.

35. Rauvala, H., Carter, W. G., and Hakomori, S. I. Studies on cell adhesion and recognition. I. Extent and specificity of cell adhesion triggered by carbohydrate-reactive proteins (glycosidases and lectins) and by fibronectin. *Cell. Biol. 86:* 127–137, 1981.

36. Sellwood, R., Gibbons, R. A., Jones, G. W., and Rutter, J. M. Adhesion of enteropathogenic *Escherichia coli* to pig intestinal brush borders: The existence of two pig phenotypes. *J. Med. Microbiol. 8:* 405–411, 1975.

37. Smith, H. Microbial surfaces in relation to pathogenicity. *Bacteriol. Rev. 41:* 475–500, 1977.
38. Smith, H. W., and Jones, J. E. T. Observations on the alimentary tract and its bacterial flora in healthy and diseased pigs. *J. Pathol. Bacteriol. 86:* 387–412, 1963.
39. Smith, H. W., and Linggood, M. A. Observations on the pathogenic properties of the K88, HLY and ENT plasmids of *Escherichia coli* with particular reference to porcine diarrhoea. *J. Med. Microbiol. 4:* 467–485, 1971.
40. Smyth, C. J., Jonsson, P., Olsson, E., Soderlind, O., Rosengren, J., Hjerten, S., and Wadstrom, T. Differences in hydrophobic surface characteristics of porcine enteropathogenic *Escherichia coli* with or without K88 antigen as revealed by hydrophobic interaction chromatography. *Infect. Immun. 22:* 462–472, 1978.
41. Svanborg Eden, C., Jodal, U., Hanson, L. A., Lindberg, U., and Sohl Akerlund, A. Variable adherence to normal urinary tract epithelial cells of *Escherichia coli* strains associated with various forms of urinary tract infection. *Lancet ii:* 490–492, 1976.
42. Tylewska, S., Hjerten, S., and Wadstrom, T. Contribution of M protein to the hydrophobic surface properties of *Streptococcus pyogenes*. *FEMS Microbiol. Lett. 6:* 249–253, 1979.
43. Wadstrom, T., Faris, A., Freer, J., Habte, D., Hallberg, D., and Ljungh, A. Hydrophobic surface properties of enterotoxigenic *E. coli* (ETEC) with different colonization factors (CFA/I, CFA/II, K88 and K99) and attachment to intestinal epithelial cells. *Scand. J. Infect. Dis (Suppl.) 24:* 148–153, 1980.
44. Wadstrom, T., Faris, A., Hjerten, S., Lindahl, M., Lovgren, K., and Agerup, B. Prevention of enterotoxigenic *E. coli* (ETEC) diarrhea by hydrophobic gels. In: *Third International Symposium on Neonatal Diarrhea*. Edited by S. Acres. Saskatoon, Canada, VIDO, 1980.
45. Woods, D. E., Bass, J. A., Johanson, W. G., Jr., and Straus, D. C. Role of adherence in the pathogenesis of *Pseudomonas aeruginosa* lung infection cystic fibrosis patients. *Infect. Immun. 30:* 694–699, 1980.

Chapter 8

Pathophysiological Mechanisms in Pyogenic Infections: Two Examples— Pleural Empyema and Acute Bacterial Meningitis

FRANCIS A. WALDVOGEL

INTRODUCTION

Phagocytosis, the process of "cellular eating," was first observed by Elie Metchnikoff in cells from invertebrates. Only later did it become apparent that leukocytes from higher animals were also engaged in active engulfment of foreign particles, a phenomenon that has stimulated the interest of many clinicians and investigators. Thus, the bactericidal potential of certain mammalian cell populations such as the macrophage system and the granulocyte pool has received a great deal of attention, and their functional properties probably represent advanced steps of a remarkable evolutionary process; macrophages and polymorphonuclear cells (PMN) have become so highly specialized in their phagocytic function that they are considered today by many investigators as the professional phagocytes (2, 10). As a matter of fact, they have many characteristics of true professionals, as we encounter them in various sport competitions on both sides of the Atlantic; they have special metabolic properties and have special food requirements, tailored for their activities. When they are asked to perform, they accomplish their task swiftly and with dedication, provided that the local environmental conditions are suitable. Finally, the tough competition they are submitted to takes its toll, leaving behind at best an exhausted population of fighters who will take time to recuperate; injury is frequent, and phasing out of competition is a common event.

Phagocytic cells have other human characteristics; they possess sensory organs at their surface, *i.e.* membrane receptors, which are triggered by various, highly specific stimuli such as chemotactic factors (5). Other receptors are involved in the anchoring of pathogenic organisms to the cell surface after their interaction with the humoral immune system. This interaction corresponds at a molecular level to the coating of the bacterial cell surface by either a complement component, by immunoglobulins, or by both, and is referred to as *opsonization* (11).

This study was supported in part by a grant from the Swiss National Foundation (Grant 3.836-0.79) and a grant from Beecham Pharmaceuticals Research Laboratories, Berne, Switzerland.

115

Phagocytic cells also have an internal musculoskeletal system made of microfilaments and of contractile proteins. They can therefore ambulate or rather crawl, often at random, occasionally into a well-defined direction determined by chemotactic gradients. They are sensitive to hormonal influences and secrete a variety of mediators (16). Last but not least, they have an insatiable appetite for well-prepared, *i.e.*, opsonized foreign particles, at the risk of all kinds of side effects including poor digestion, regurgitation, and death caused by overindulgence (6, 17).

Let us now consider the process of opsonization, a chain of biochemical and biophysical events leading to the coating of bacteria by two types of serum proteins, resulting in recognition of the bacterium by the phagocytic cells. Unopsonized bacteria are not attractive and are barely recognized by PMNs and macrophages; it follows that any specific or general defect of opsonization means for the host either an enhanced risk or the persistence of pyogenic bacterial infections. Thus, congenital or acquired defects of complement activity (particularly of C3, a key and central component of the cascade) have been repeatedly demonstrated to lead to recurrent infections (1), and the *in vitro* correlate of this clinical observation can be easily demonstrated by a test-tube phagocytic-bactericidal assay. Immunoglobulin deficiencies, which have been known for many years to be associated with a high risk of bacterial infections, will also show defective opsonization when tested in such a phagocytic assay.

So far, the interest of most researchers has concentrated on congenital, generalized defects in opsonization; few studies have dealt with acquired, or local defects. One of the exceptions is a study demonstrating that rheumatoid factor activity, present in up to 50% of patients with subacute bacterial endocarditis, has an inhibitory action on opsonization of the patient's own infecting microorganism (9). Other acquired conditions with deficient opsonization should also be considered; poor diffusion of opsonic factors within the human body, their delayed ingress during inflammation, or their continuous breakdown could also promote infection or favor overwhelming microbial multiplication or persistence of microorganisms. With an appropriate phagocytic bactericidal assay, using as an opsonic source the suspected fluids and as test organisms bacteria requiring either complement or immunoglobulins as sole opsonic factors, such postulates are presently amenable to formal *in vitro* testing. Over the last few years, we have studied several such possibilities. First, empyema formation either during or after bacterial pneumonia can be shown to represent a clinical situation where opsonically active factors are continuously degraded (7, 8). In other studies, we have explored the opsonic activity of normal body fluids particularly prone to bacterial invasion. Thus, normal cerebrospinal fluid (CSF), which is characterized by a very low protein concentration, seems to represent a closed sanctuary with almost undetectable opsonic activity, favoring the rapid ingress and multiplication of encapsulated microorganisms during bacterial meningitis (14, 20).

OPSONIC ACTIVITY IN PLEURAL EFFUSIONS

Pleural empyema—a closed space infection characterized by its chronicity and persistence despite adequate antibiotic therapy—shows by definition on microscopic examination the simultaneous presence of large numbers of PMNs and of pyogenic live bacteria, easily seen on Gram stain. (This means that their concentration must exceed 10^5/ml.) Little is known that explains this biological paradox. The convenient explanation used in the past has been that the PMNs present in an empyema or abscess are dead. Although it is true that certain PMNs undergo lysis in abscesses or empyemas, as demonstrated by the presence of large amounts of nucleoproteins (15), the number of PMNs present in such an encapsulated infectious focus is so high that it must always contain a subgroup of newly attracted, active, functional phagocytes. This has been confirmed experimentally by Ga-labeled PMNs injected into animals with localized subcutaneous abscesses. In a limited study, we have recently been able to analyze various abscesses and pleural empyemas as to their PMN counts, cellular morphology, and functional integrity (Table 7.1). All cell counts in purulent exudates were above 10^7 PMNs/ mm^3, and trypan blue exclusion studies as well as phase contrast microscopy showed more than 50% of them to be viable. PMN integrity was further tested in one single, privileged case of pleural empyema by an *in vitro* phagocytic test, taking peripheral autologous PMNs as a reference. Whereas the fluid phase of the empyema promoted poor opsonization, empyema PMNs showed very active ingestion and bacterial killing, which was as good as that of the control groups. Finally, recent experiments performed on a guinea pig abscess model have confirmed that such PMNs accomplish normal or even enhanced phagocytosis (18). We then examined the opsonic activity of the fluid phase of empyemas, using various types of pleural effusions as opsonic sources and incubating them with peripheral, normal PMNs in a phagocytic bacterial assay. As the biological marker of the assay system, we used *Staphylococcus aureus* strain Wood 46, which grows as single cocci at low concentration and is devoid of protein A, a compound which interacts with immunoglobulin G by coagglutination. Preliminary experiments showed *S. aureus* Wood 46 to require very little, if any, IgG for optimal opsonization, which was almost entirely due to the presence of complement (Table 7.2). When this test was applied to various types of pleural effusions, complement-mediated opsonic activity could be shown to be low or even undetectable in the majority of pleural empyemas, when compared with pleural effusions of other causes, with transudates adjusted for protein concentration, and with the patient's sera (8). Similar results were obtained when complement activity was assayed by a conventional hemolytic method, with both results showing a high correlation coefficient (8).

This low, complement-mediated opsonic activity in pleural empyema, a possible factor contributing to the persistence of bacteria despite the presence of competent PMNs, could be postulated at this stage to be secondary either to decreased

TABLE 8.1. PURULENT EXUDATES: CONCENTRATION OF VIABLE PMNs' AS DETERMINED BY TRYPAN BLUE EXCLUSION

Origin and Microbiology	Total Leukocyte Count	% PMN	% PMN excluding trypan blue
Perianal abscess (*S. aureus*)	10×10^7/ml	95	90
Pleural empyema (mixed anaerobic flora)	4×10^7/ml	95	60
Pleural empyema (mixed anaerobic flora)	15×10^7/ml	95	60

TABLE 8.2. REQUIREMENTS OF TEST STRAIN S. AUREUS WOOD 46[a] FOR OPTIMAL OPSONIZATION

Opsonic Source	Bacterial Killing p̄ 30-min Incubation (%)
Pool serum 10%	95
Individual serum 10%	95
Agammaglobulinemic 10%	90
Pooled serum 10% (56°C for 30 min)	0
Pooled serum 10% (50°C for 20 min)	20
C4 deficient serum, heated 50°C for 40 min	3.5
C4 deficient serum, heated 50°C for 40 min, reconstituted with purified factor B (1 mg/ml)	74

For each assay, 0.05 ml of *S. aureus* Wood 46 (2×10^6) was added to a mixture of 0.4 ml PMNs (3×10^6) in Krebs-Ringer-phosphate medium and 0.05 ml portions of adequately diluted serum. The cell suspensions were incubated at 37°C in a shaking water bath, and samples were taken at 0 and 30 min for plating on Mueller-Hinton medium, after osmotic lysis.

local diffusion/synthesis of complement components necessary for opsonization, or to consumption of some of its components by continuous activation or direct proteolysis. First, evidence for consumption of complement components was sought by different methods, exploiting the fact that some complement factors— such as C3—undergo several cleavage processes during activation or degradation, liberating small byproducts such as C3d. Other components such as factor B of the alternative pathway also undergo cleavage during activation, liberating a small fragment called Ba. Another analysis of 18 empyemas and 18 metapneumonic, sterile effusions confirmed our hypothesis: native C3 and C3d were significantly lower and higher, respectively, in the culture-positive group. Similar results were obtained for factor B and its degradation products (7). We were therefore able to conclude that pleural empyema, a paradigm of a closed, walled-off pyogenic human infection, contained enough functional PMNs for efficient phagocytosis and bacterial killing, but lacked adequate complement-mediated opsonic activity to coat the pathogenic organisms and to promote their efficient ingestion. This low opsonic activity could be correlated with a striking decrease in complement hemolytic activity and in functional factor C3 and factor B levels. On the other hand, high concentrations of the breakdown products of these two factors can be demonstrated in purulent pleural exudates only.

The complement pattern described in these effusions is therefore reminiscent of the well-known, but usually generalized, condition of consumption coagulopathy, wherein biological inefficiency of the clotting system is due to the continuous breakdown of some of its components, accompanied by a simultaneous increase in their breakdown products. Recent evidence suggests that continuous complement activation might also occur in the serum of patients with Gram-negative shock (3).

There are, in our eyes, other analogies between the two systems. Consumption coagulopathy can be induced by continuous triggering of the normal coagulation reaction by certain stimuli, such as bacterial endotoxin; however, it can also be the result of a direct proteolytic cleavage of one or several of its factors, *e.g.*, by proteases secreted by PMNs or their precursors. Could the low complement values measured in pleural empyemas have a similar explanation, *i.e.*, result from their direct, enzymatic proteolysis? To answer this question, we first looked at other opsonic factors, such as immunoglobulins, the quantitation of which showed indeed lower values in culture-positive than in culture-negative effusions (7). Breakdown of IgG in empyema was demonstrated in 11 of 14 empyemas by several techniques, including incubation of culture-positive and culture-negative effusions with ^{125}I-labeled IgG and assessment of cleavage by measuring changes in molecular weight of IgG by sucrose gradients and by ammonium sulfate precipitation; both techniques demonstrated the cleavage of the IgG fraction to occur in culture-positive empyemas only (7). These results indicated that active proteolysis was taking place in a closed space infection and was able to degrade IgG molecules.

Let us now return to complement-mediated opsonization in empyemas. The low complement values found in this condition could be due, as already mentioned, to continuous activation of the cascade along its usual pathways; alternatively, low C3 and high C3d levels could be a consequence of direct, proteolytic cleavage of C3, without involvement of the complement-derived enzymes. Both hypotheses can be easily tested by adequately chosen experimental conditions. Since complement activation is blocked in the absence of divalent cations, any cleavage occurring under such conditions must necessarily be ascribed to other proteolytic enzymes. Thus, Taylor *et al.* have recently shown that in an *in vitro* system, specific cleavage of the alpha chain of C3 can be obtained by the limited digestion of this purified protein by leukocyte elastase, a neutral protease. We therefore devised a simple test for evaluating C3 breakdown in empyema. Human C3 was purified to homogeneity, labeled with ^{125}I, and covalently bound to sepharose beads. This labeled compound was then incubated with several empyema fluids, as well as with sterile pleural fluids of various origins, including neoplastic and post-traumatic effusions. All experiments were carried out in a medium devoid of Ca and Mg ions, in order to inhibit any complement-dependent enzymatic activity. The amount of C3 cleaved was evaluated by measuring supernatant radioactivity after centrifugation of the sepharose beads. Considerable cleavage could be demonstrated for most of the empyemas tested, but for none of the 20 other pleural effusions tested. The proteolytic degradation of purified C3 by empyema fluid was confirmed by the demonstration of the breakdown of the alpha chain of C3, as evidenced by polyacrylamide gel electrophoresis (PAGE). No such breakdown could be demonstrated in the absence of empyema (12). These results are all very consistent with the previously mentioned proteolytic cleavage of C3 by neutrophil elastase in a purified *in vitro* system (13). Present experiments using specific PMN elastase inhibitors and substrates are providing convincing, but indirect, evidence that the majority of the C3-cleaving activity in empyema is related to PMN-elastase activity.

In summary, the data accumulated so far suggest that a hitherto unknown pathophysiological mechanism might favor the persistence of pyogenic organisms in an infected pleural space; the fluid phase of pleural empyema seems to behave like an "immunological no man's land," due to inactivation and cleavage of several opsonic factors by local, not complement-mediated, proteolytic activity.

Neutral protease activity derived from PMN seems to be the best candidate for such a proteolytic activity. Thus, PMNs, the professional phagocytes, can occasionally turn to the enemy's side—another analogy to true professional sportsmen.

OPSONIC ACTIVITY IN CSF

Let us now return to our initial hypothesis suggesting that poor local opsonization might occasionally be a consequence of poor diffusion of opsonic factors into a body fluid. Human CSF represents such a case. Its low protein concentration under normal conditions (<0.5 g/liter) is certainly not compatible with the presence of a high concentration of opsonic factors. Probable absence of opsonic activity under normal conditions is further suggested by the well-known clinical observation of an increased risk of bacterial meningitis when the anatomical barrier separating the nasal cavities or the middle ear and the CSF is breached.

We do not yet know exactly how bacteria gain access to CSF and/or to the bloodstream in bacterial meningitis. Whatever the mechanism of penetration, the disease takes a fulminant course once it has reached the CSF (4). Obviously, first-line defense mechanisms must be poor at the onset of the disease. During the later course of bacterial meningitis, protein concentration in the CSF can reach values close to 5 g/liter, and it would be of interest to know whether, at that stage, inflammatory CSF exhibits measurable complement-mediated opsonic activity. We have tried to answer these questions, using a similar phagocytic-bactericidal assay as described previously. When fresh either diluted or undiluted CSF was assessed in preliminary experiments, no opsonic activity could be demonstrated, despite the fact that our assay was able to demonstrate opsonic activity in corresponding sera diluted to equal protein concentration. In order to sensitize our assay, we concentrated normal CSF obtained under a variety of conditions (spinal anesthesia, myelography, and acute febrile illnesses with photophobia but normal CSF) to 10 times its initial protein concentration by an ultrafiltration device. The results showed that, under the new experimental conditions, normal CSF was able to promote phagocytosis by complement-dependent opsonization, and that the levels of the various complement components were present but too low to be measurable in unconcentrated CSF (19). We then undertook a large study trying to define the response of complement-mediated opsonic activity in various disease states such as viral meningitis, bacterial meningitis, and meningococcemia with positive CSF on culture. No complement-mediated opsonic activity could be measured in CSF samples obtained within 24 hours of onset of the disease from patients suffering from viral meningitis. Quite different was the situation in acute bacterial meningitis, wherein opsonic activity showed great individual variations. Whereas some individuals exhibited no complement-mediated opsonic activity, others showed high levels, which could be titrated up to dilutions of 1:16. These results were of great interest when they were compared with the clinical outcome of the disease. Whereas all patients with a satisfactory evolution (characterized by complete recovery) showed a measurable opsonic activity in their CSF obtained on admission, the patients with a poor evolution (death, or permanent neurological sequelae) were all members of the group with undetectable complement levels in their CSF on admission. There was no difference between the two groups as to age, sex, duration of symptoms before admission, or species of the offending microorganism. However, opsonic titers could be correlated with an interesting microbiological observation: quantitative bacterial counts performed on a limited number of CSF samples showed an inverse correlation with opsonic activity, with low bacterial cell counts being found in patients with high CSF opsonic activity titers. These results suggest that besides early administration of antibiotics, host-derived factors are important in the outcome of bacterial meningitis. Since complement-mediated hemolytic activity and opsonic activity are extremely low in normal CSF, invasion of the subarachnoid space of a susceptible patient lacking type-specific antibodies will lead to a rapid multiplication of the microorganisms on one side and to an inflammatory CSF reaction on the other side, characterized by, among other factors, an increase in CSF protein concentration and CSF PMNs. The degree of the inflammatory reaction seems to be an important determinant of the complement response, which in turn might influence bacterial growth and outcome of the disease. It is of interest to note that infectious disease specialists have insisted for years that meningitis with "normal CSF," *i.e.*, with normal protein concentration and very low cell counts, has a poor prognosis and usually shows a high number of bacteria on CSF Gram stain.

CONCLUSIONS

If the biological mechanisms controlling health and separating it from disease are innumerable, those causing disease are even more intertwined and will lead to a variety of pathological alterations, which in turn will occasionally create new conditions perpetuating the disease. In this setting, friends can turn to foes, and our data on empyema suggest—as also shown by other investigators—that the friendly PMN can do harm to the host under certain conditions. On the other hand, PMN ingress is part of the inflammatory reaction, and a balanced supply of phagocytic cells and opsonic factors certainly helps to fight off infection in closed sanctuaries with no defense mechanisms such as the subarachnoid space. This dual relationship that we entertain with our phagocytic cells is just one of the many ambiguities of our immune system.

ACKNOWLEDGMENTS

This work was performed with the help of the following collaborators: P. H. Lambert, D. Lew, U. Nydegger, S. Suter, P. Vaudaux, and A. Zwahlen. The able technical help of Anneliese Kahr is acknowledged. The secretarial help of Francoise Michaud is gratefully acknowledged.

REFERENCES

1. Agnello, V. Complement deficiency states. *Medicine 57:* 1–23, 1978.
2. Bellanti, J. A., and Dayton, D. H. (eds.). *The Phagocytic Cell in Host Resistance.* New York, Raven Press, 1975.
3. Fearon, D. T., Ruddy, S., Schur, P. H., and McCabe, W. R. Activation of the properdin pathway of complement in patients with gram-negative bacteremia. *N. Engl. J. Med., 292:* 937–940, 1975.
4. Feldman, W. E. Relation of concentrations of bacteria and bacterial antigen in cerebrospinal fluid to prognosis in patients with bacterial meningitis. *N. Engl. J. Med., 296:* 433–435, 1977.

122   *Current Topics in Inflammation and Infection*

5. Gallin, J. I., and Quie, P. G. (eds.). *Leukocyte Chemotaxis: Methods, Physiology, and Clinical Implications.* New York, Raven Press, 1978.
6. Klebanoff, S. J. Oxygen metabolism and the toxic properties of phagocytes. *Ann. Intern. Med., 93:* 480–489, 1980.
7. Lew, P. D., Despont, J-P., Perrin, L. H., Aguado, M-P., Lambert, P. H., and Waldvogel, F. A. Demonstration of a local exhaustion of complement components and of an enzymatic degradation of immunoglobulins in pleural empyema: a possible factor favouring the persistence of local bacterial infections. *Clin. Exp. Immunol., 42:* 506–514, 1980.
8. Lew, P. D., Zubler, R., Vaudaux, P., Farquet, J-J., Waldvogel, F. A., and Lambert, P. H. Decreased heat-labile opsonic activity and complement levels associated with evidence of C3 breakdown products in infected pleural effusions. *J. Clin. Invest., 63:* 326–334, 1979.
9. Quie, P. G., Messner, R. P., and Williams, R. C. Phagocytosis in subacute bacterial endocarditis: localization of the primary opsonic site to Fc fragment. *J. Exp. Med., 128:* 553–570, 1968.
10. Stossel, T. P. Phagocytosis. *N. Engl. J. Med., 290:* 717–723, 774–780, 833–839, 1974.
11. Stossel, T. P. Phagocytosis: recognition and ingestion. *Semin. Hematol., 12:* 83–116, 1975.
12. Suter, S., Nydegger, U., Roux, L., and Waldvogel, F. Decreased complement mediated opsonic activity in pleural empyema: demonstration of enzymatic C3 breakdown by empyema fluid. Abstract 142, Twentieth Interscience Conference on Antimicrobial Agents and Chemotherapy, September 22–24, 1980, New Orleans.
13. Taylor, J. C., Crawford, I. P., and Hugli, T. E. Limited degradation of the third component (C3) of human complement by human leukocyte elastase (HLE): partial characterization of C3 fragments. *Biochemistry, 16:* 3390–3396, 1977.
14. Tofte, R. W., Peterson, P. K., Kim, Y., and Quie, P. G. Opsonic activity of normal human cerebrospinal fluid for selected bacterial species. *Infect. Immun., 26:* 1093–1098, 1979.
15. Vaudaux, P., and Waldvogel, F. A. Gentamicin inactivation in purulent exudates: role of cell lysis. *J. Infect. Dis., 142:* 586–593, 1980.
16. Weissmann, G., Smolen, J. E., and Korchak, H. M. Release of inflammatory mediators from stimulated neutrophils. *N. Engl. J. Med., 303:* 27–34, 1980.
17. Weissmann, G., Zurier, R. B., Spieler, P. J., and Goldstein, I. M. Mechanisms of lysosomal enzyme release from leukocytes exposed to immune complexes and other particles. *J. Exp. Med., 134:* 149–165, 1971.
18. Zimmerli, W., Vaudaux, P., Waldvogel, F. A., and Nydegger, U. E. Foreign body infection: description of an animal model. Submitted for publication, 1982.
19. Zwahlen, A., Nydegger, U., Vaudaux, P., Lambert, P. H., and Waldvogel, F. A. Predictive value of cerebrospinal fluid (CSF) opsonic activity in acute bacterial meningitis (Abstract 141). Twentieth Interscience Conference on Antimicrobial Agents and Chemotherapy, September 22–24, 1980, New Orleans.
20. Zwahlen, A., Nydegger, U., Waldvogel, F. A., and Lambert, P. H. Complement mediated opsonic activity of cerebrospinal fluid in acute meningitis (Abstract 361A). *Clin. Res., 27,* 1979.

Chapter 9

An Update on Legionnaires' Disease and Pneumonias Caused by "New" *Legionella*-like Bacteria

RICHARD L. MYEROWITZ

INTRODUCTION AND HISTORICAL PERSPECTIVE

An outbreak of a febrile respiratory illness in July 1976, affecting almost 200 individuals attending an American Legion convention in Philadelphia (29 of whom died) resulted in the recognition of the first "new pneumonia" (62, 68), Legionnaires' disease (LD). Intensive investigation, predominantly by the Center for Disease Control (26), led to the isolation of an unusual, fastidious gram-negative bacillus which was ultimately dubbed *Legionella pneumophila* (15, 46). The organism failed to grow on routine media but was successfully cultivated by inoculation of embryonated eggs and guinea pigs, techniques generally used for isolation of rickettsia. Following development of a serum indirect fluorescent antibody (IFA) assay using *L. pneumophila* as antigen (75), confirmation of this organism's etiologic role in LD was obtained. Also, other past outbreaks of unexplained pneumonia were quickly shown by serology to have been caused by this organism. Subsequently, sporadic cases of LD have been recognized throughout this and other countries, and current estimates are that LD accounts for about 5% of community-acquired pneumonias (60). *L. pneumophila* has also been shown to be a very significant cause of nosocomial pneumonia, acting as an opportunistic pathogen in immunosuppressed patients (11, 44).

In 1979, investigators at the University of Pittsburgh and the University of Virginia independently noted a cluster of cases of opportunistic pneumonia which were caused by a gram-negative, weakly acid-fast bacillus. The bacilli were easily visualized in lung tissue but failed to grow on routine media, including mycobacterial media (49, 58). The Pittsburgh group successfully cultivated the organism using techniques identical to those used for isolation of *L. pneumophila* (53) and demonstrated seroconversion by the patients to their isolates. They tentatively named the bacterium Pittsburgh Pneumonia Agent for which the name *Legionella micdadei* (32) has subsequently been proposed. "Pittsburgh pneumonia" has subsequently been identified in several areas besides Pittsburgh and Charlottesville but appears to occur exclusively in immunosuppressed patients who have received high doses of corticosteroids.

As part of their environmental studies on the ecology of *L. pneumophila*, investigators at the Center for Disease Control utilized newly developed agar media which support the growth of *L. pneumophila* to look for the organism in environmental water samples. Not only was *L. pneumophila* found, but several strains of fastidious bacteria were isolated which were bacteriologically similar to, yet antigenically distinct from, *L. pneumophila*. This group of bacteria was called *Legionella*-like organisms (LLO) (18) and, using the IFA technique, three serogroups of LLO were defined. Several patients with pneumonia of previously unknown etiology were shown to have serologic rises in antibody titer to at least one of the serogroups of LLO. Also, LLO were isolated from lung tissue of two patients with fatal pneumonia (41, 65). The names *Legionella bozemanii*, *Legionella dumoffii*, and *Legionella gormanii* have been proposed for the three serogroups of LLO (Table 9.1) (8, 9).

Thus a new family of bacteria, the Legionellaceae, has come to be recognized which presently consist of five species (Table 9.1), all of which have unique microbial, serologic, and biochemical properties and most of which have been either proven or implicated as a cause of human pneumonia.

Many years earlier, isolates of fastidious "rickettsia-like" organisms had been reported but had gone largely unnoticed. In 1943, Tatlock (63) isolated an organism from the blood of a young military recruit with "Fort Bragg fever" using guinea pig and egg inoculation. His isolate would not grow on blood agar, and no antibodies were detectable in his patient using a complement fixation assay. The organism was thought to be a pathogen of the guinea pig. In 1947, Jackson *et al.* (36) isolated a similar organism acronymically designated OLDA from the blood of a patient with a febrile respiratory illness. However, he too was unable to demonstrate seroconversion in the patient and, hence, the significance of his isolate was unclear. Some years later Bozeman *et al.* (7) isolated two similar rickettsia-like agents, one from the blood of a patient with pityriasis rosea (designated HEBA) and one from the lung of a skin-diver with fatal pneumonia (designated WIGA). Bozeman's group used cross-protection analysis in guinea

TABLE 9.1. Five Species in the Family Legionellaceae

Original Designation(s)	Author(s) & Ref.	Proposed Genus and Species	Author(s) & Ref.
1. Legionnaires' disease bacillus (LDB)	McDade *et al.* (46)	*Legionella pneumophila*	Brenner *et al.* (9)
OLDA	Jackson *et al.* (36)		
2. Pittsburgh Pneumonia Agent	Pasculle *et al.* (53)	*Legionella micdadei*	Hébert *et al.cfl (32)*
TATLOCK	Tatlock (63)	*Legionella pittsburgensis*	*Pasculle et al. (51)*
HEBA	Bozeman *et al.*		
3. WIGA MI-15, GA-PH	Bozeman *et al.* (7) Cordes *et al.* (18) Thomason *et al.* (65)	*Legionella bozemanii*	Brenner *et al.* (8)
4. NY-23 Tex-KL	Cordes *et al.* (18) Lewallen *et al.* (41)	*Legionella dumoffii*	Brenner *et al.*
5. LS-13	Cordes *et al.* (18)	*Legionella gormanii*	Brenner *et al.* (manuscript in preparation)

pigs to demonstrate that the TATLOCK and HEBA isolates were antigenically similar, that OLDA had antigens which were distinct from the other three, and that WIGA shared some antigenicity with both OLDA and TATLOCK/HEBA. As each of the new pneumonias were discovered, these isolates were restudied. OLDA was found to be *L. pneumophila* (45), TATLOCK/HEBA are both *L. micdadei* (31, 33), and WIGA is a strain of LLO (*Legionella bozemanii*) (65). Thus, although recognition of these three new pneumonias has only been accomplished within the last 5 years, all of the etiologic agents had been isolated two to three decades earlier and had not been recognized as significant because of the lack of modern serologic tools (*e.g.*, IFA) to make the vital connection between isolation of an agent and demonstration of its role as the cause of an infectious disease.

This essay will attempt to summarize and update the rapidly accumulating knowledge about these three new pneumonias, especially with respect to epidemiology, pathogenesis, gross and microscopic pathology, microbiology, immunity, and diagnosis. The clinical, radiographic, and therapeutic (including antibiotic susceptibility) aspects of these new infectious diseases are amply covered in the references cited.

LEGIONNAIRES' DISEASE

LD is an acute febrile respiratory infection which appears to be acquired by the airborne route (26). Other more mild febrile syndromes which do not include pneumonia, such as Pontiac fever, also have been described. There is still no evidence of man-to-man transmission, *i.e.*, contagion, yet clusters of LD cases occur both in hospitals and in other settings. Some of the more recent outbreaks have been clearly related to contamination of environmental water, *e.g.*, cooling tower water with presumed transmission via aerosolization through air-conditioners (20) or potable water with transmission via aerosolization from shower taps (59, 66). Animal models of LD have been developed in guinea pigs in which infection occurs either by inhalation of infected aerosols (4) or by direct intratracheal inoculation (73). In both instances the disease that results bears much of a similarity to human LD. Thus, LD can presumably be acquired via the inhalation of infected droplets from the environment. However, the hypothesis that LD may also result from reactivation of a latent previous infection has not been ruled out. This hypothesis appears especially relevant to cases in immunosuppressed patients. Intact cell-mediated immune mechanisms appear to be an important aspect of host defense against *L. pneumophila* (see below), and suppression of cell-mediated immunity could reactivate latent infection analogous to other intracellular pathogens such as cytomegalovirus or *Toxoplasma gondii*.

The gross and histopathologic changes in LD have been well described (5, 6, 37, 74). Macroscopically, LD is a nodular consolidative bronchopneumonia frequently associated with fibrinous or fibrinopurulent pleuritis. A pattern of lobar pneumonia can also occur. Frank abscess formation with cavitation has been described, especially in nosocomial cases occurring in compromised hosts (42). Microscopically, cases of LD in an early stage of evolution studied by open lung biopsy demonstrate a fibrinopurulent intraalveolar exudate. Numerous bacilli are present within this exudate and, therefore, within respiratory secretions and, occasionally, pleural fluid. *L. pneumophila* is a thin, faintly staining, gram-negative bacillus which may, therefore, be difficult or impossible to visualize in sections stained with tissue gram stains such as the Brown and Brenn or Brown and Hopps technique. Imprint smears stained with the routine gram procedure will usually allow visualization of the bacilli. The Dieterle silver impregnation stain, which was the first technique successfully used to demonstrate *L. pneumophila* in tissue sections (15), is difficult to perform and is nonspecific, *i.e.*, it will stain any bacterium, since such LD cases often demonstrate numerous bacilli with the Dieterle technique. It is important to remember though that the Dieterle stain is *not specific* for *L. pneumophila* and only suggests the diagnosis of LD when gram stains are negative. Most recently, immunochemical staining of tissue sections using direct fluorescent antibody (DFA) techniques (16) or immunoperoxidase techniques (61) has been described. In autopsy cases, the inflammatory cell component of the alveolar exudate often shows a predominance of alveolar macrophages, many of which are laden with large numbers of intracellular bacilli. The polymorphonuclear leukocytes may show pronounced leukocytoclasis. Alveolar septal necrosis, often with septic vasculitis, is also common and probably represents the early stages of frank abscess formation which occurs in a minority of cases.

Extrapulmonary alterations in LD have been sought to explain the high frequency of extrapulmonary clinical signs and symptoms, *e.g.*, obtundation, diarrhea, abnormal liver function tests, hematuria, azotemia, and hypophosphatemia. However, markedly little pathology has been found which is ascribable to *L. pneumophila*. The organism has been isolated from blood (21) and has been visualized by DFA in intravascular sites within the kidney (70) and by DFA and electron microscopy in the sinusoidal lining cells of the spleen and liver (67). One case of myocarditis (70) and one of pericarditis (Pasculle *et al.*, 52) due to *L. pneumophila* have been described in which the organism was identified by DFA and culture. Most recently, Weisenburger *et al.* (69) have described a previously healthy patient who succumbed to LD and had focal necrosis of pulmonary hilar lymph nodes, bacilli within glomerular capillaries, and clusters of histiocytes with intracellular bacilli in the nodes, spleen, and bone marrow. The latter finding is especially interesting since it is similar to findings in animals experimentally infected with Pittsburgh pneumonia agent (PPA) (see below). The paucity of anatomic findings has led to the suggestion that *L. pneumophila* may elaborate exotoxins which act on human tissues. Some experimental evidence exists to support this notion (2, 27).

Bacteriologically, the Legionellaceae are unique in several ways. All species fail to grow on routine agar or broth media but are cultivatable in the yolk sacs of embryonated eggs. Recently, agar media have been developed which support their growth. These media contain two key nutrients which are essential for successful cultivation of all Legionellaceae, *i.e.*, iron (usually in the form of ferric pyrophosphate) and cysteine. The pH must be carefully adjusted to precisely 6.9, and a buffer may be added. At present, the best agar medium is charcoal yeast extract (CYE) agar (24) or buffered charcoal yeast extract (BCYE) agar (51). Broth media such as yeast extract broth have also been devised (56). At present neither agar nor broth media are selective. A second unique feature of the

Legionellaceae is their high content of branched-chain cell wall fatty acids (47). These fatty acids can be separated by gas-liquid chromatography, and the chromatographic pattern can be useful in specific identification of an isolate.

The ultrastructure of *L. pneumophila* has been extensively studied (13, 14, 28, 39, 50, 57). The organism is 2–4 μm long and 0.5–1.0 μ wide. Filamentous forms occur frequently. A single subpolar flagellum is present (64). The organism has the general structure of a bacterium with an ill-defined nucleoid, cytoplasmic ribosomes, and no mitochondria. Cytoplasmic vacuoles containing lipid have also been noted. The cell wall is typical of other gram-negative bacilli, consisting of an outer trilaminar membrane and an inner trilaminar cell membrane separated by an electron lucent periplasmic space. Cell division occurs by nonseptate pinching fission. When studied in infected human tissues, the organisms are predominantly intracellular, often occurring in large clusters sequestered in the cytoplasm of phagocytes within a well-defined membranous sac (phagosome).

Host immunity to *L. pneumophila* has only begun to be investigated. It is clear that *L. pneumophila* has a complex antigenic structure. Six different serotypes are now recognized with serotype 1 (the type which occurred in the Philadelphia epidemic) still recognized as most common. Common antigens do exist among all strains of *L. pneumophila*, including the flagellar antigen (76). Patients with LD make a brisk humoral immune response to these antigens. Yet, it is unclear as to what, if any, significance this response has with respect to recovery from the disease and protection against recurrent infection. Conflicting reports exist concerning the susceptibility of *L. pneumophila* to complement-mediated serum bactericidal activity (1, 35). Antibody and complement have been shown to be required *in vitro* for attachment and ingestion of *L. pneumophila* by human polymorphonuclear leukocytes and monocytes. However, intracellular killing by either phagocytic cell is poor despite the presence of excess antibody and complement (35). These *in vitro* data may explain why inflammatory cells in the lungs of patients with LD are often laden with intracytoplasmic bacilli. These data also suggest that humoral immunity may not be effective against *L. pneumophila*. Much precedent exists for this phenomenon with other intracellular bacteria, *e.g.*, *Salmonella* and *Listeria*. Acquired resistance to infection with *L. pneumophila* can be produced in experimental animals by immunization with the whole bacterium (7) or a crude soluble antigen (34). It is likely that this resistance is mediated predominantly by cellular immune mechanisms, although no direct evidence for this hypothesis is presently available. *L. pneumophila* is also able to parasitize and multiply in cells other than leukocytes using cell-culture systems (76).

The diagnosis of LD can now be made in several ways. The most rapid technique involves use of the DFA technique for demonstration of bacilli in specimens such as sputum, transtracheal aspirates, fine needle aspirates of lung, imprints of lung tissue obtained by biopsy, or pleural fluid (10). Studies to date indicate a rather high degree of specificity and predictive value of a positive result in respiratory secretions and pleural fluid (72). However, the sensitivity of the test is not great, indicating that a negative result does not rule out the diagnosis (22). One problem is the serotypic heterogeneity of *L. pneumophila* requiring that polyvalent antisera be available. However, cross-reactions with other medically important bacteria have thus far been infrequent so that false positives are rare. A similar approach to rapid diagnosis has been the development of an antigen detection test using urine as the sample and either an enzyme-linked immunosorbent (ELISA) assay (3) or radioimmunoassay (40). Preliminary results appear promising.

Cultivation of *L. pneumophila* from specimens such as sputum, transtracheal aspirates, pleural fluid, or lung tissue can not be accomplished using BCYE agar. The yield from sputum in confirmed cases is not great, possibly because of inhibition of *L. pneumophila* growth by contaminating indigenous pharyngeal bacteria (25). The development of selective media should improve the frequency of isolation of *L. pneumophila* from mixed cultures. Specimens from sites not generally contaminated, *e.g.*, pleural fluid or transtracheal aspirates have a high culture yield in patients with LD.

Serodiagnosis of LD using the IFA test provides a method of retrospective case confirmation (75). The current diagnostic criteria include a fourfold or greater rise in titer to a level ≥1/128 or a single standing titer ≥1/256. There seems to be no advantage to measuring Ig subclass specific titers (*e.g.*, IgM) since titer rises and falls occur in all immunoglobulin classes simultaneously. Other serodiagnostic assays, such as ELISA, are being developed. Sera must be tested against all six serotypes of *L. pneumophila* and, in general, titers will be highest against the serotype of the infecting strain. However, some sera show equivalent titers against multiple serotypes. Thus, a diagnostic titer against a single serotype of LD does not prove that the infection was due to that serotype.

"PITTSBURGH" PNEUMONIA

Pneumonia due to *L. micdadei* is an acute febrile illness which occurs almost exclusively as a nosocomial infection in immunosuppressed patients and has a high case fatality ratio. The original isolates designated TATLOCK and HEBA came from noncompromised patients with illnesses very different from Pittsburgh pneumonia, raising the possibility that *L. micdadei*, like *L. pneumophila*, may ultimately be shown to cause other febrile syndromes. Case clustering of Pittsburgh pneumonia has occurred in two locations (49, 58) but sporadic cases have been seen in Boston, Massachusetts (12), Derby, Connecticut (17, 49), and San Francisco, California. The source or reservoir of *L. micdadei* has not been adequately defined. However, *L. micdadei* has been isolated from water in a hospital ultrasonic nebulizer (29), as well as in a cooling tower (Cordes *et al.*, manuscript in preparation). As with LD, disease acquisition by inhalation appears to be the most likely pathogenesis. Since *L. micdadei* occurs in patients treated with corticosteroids, the possibility of reactivation of latent infection also seems plausible.

Macroscopically, *L. micdadei* pneumonia is a nodular bronchopneumonia which is frequently bilateral and often cavitary (Fig. 9.1). Fibrinopurulent pleuritis is common due to the often peripheral location of consolidated foci. These latter features account for the usual radiographic finding of peripheral nodular infiltrates (Pazin *et al.*, unpublished data) and frequent occurrence of pleuritic pain as a presenting symptom. Microscopically, the changes are virtually identical to those seen in LD, *i.e.*, biopsies generally show an acute fibrinopurulent alveolar

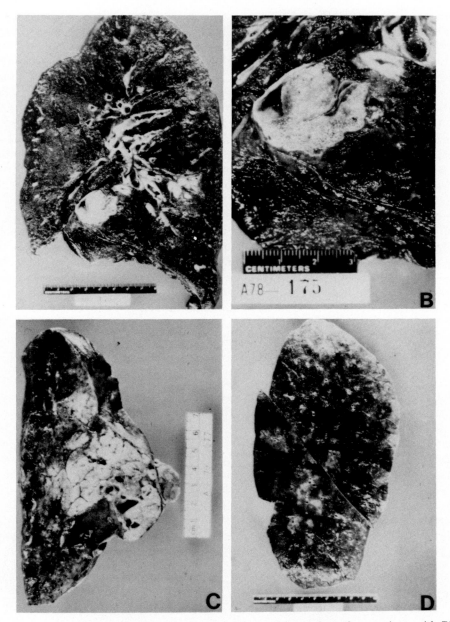

FIG. 9.1. Composite photograph of postmortem lung specimens from three patients with Pittsburgh pneumonia. (*A*) Left lung shows two areas of abscess in the lower lobe. (*B*) Closer view of the larger abscess shown in *A*. The abscess is cavitary, measures 2.8 cm in maximum diameter, and is subpleural, causing a localized fibrinous pleuritis. (*C*) Left lower lobe from a second patient showing extensive consolidation, cavity formation, and diffuse fibrinopurulent pleuritis. (*D*) Left lung slice from a third patient demonstrating a pattern of patchy consolidation involving both upper and lower lobes. The intervening nonconsolidated parenchyma is intensely congested.

exudate with preservation of lung architecture, whereas autopsies usually show a greater component of alveolar macrophages in the inflammatory infiltrate and a high frequency of alveolar septal necrosis progressing to cavitary abscess. Imprint smears of consolidated lung usually show large numbers of intracellular, thin, faintly staining, gram-negative bacilli identical in morphology to *L. pneumophila*. This appearance is characteristic or sufficiently distinctive to allow morphologic separation from other common gram-negative lung pathogens, including enteric bacteria, *Pseudomonas aeruginosa*, and *Haemophilus influenzae*. However, the faint staining and thin diameter make the organism easy to overlook in smears. The most distinctive histochemical feature of *L. micdadei*, as compared with other Legionellaceae, is its property of weak acid-fastness. In smears, the organisms will not retain carbol fuchsin using a standard Ziehl-Neelsen stain. However, using a weaker decolorizer (1% aqueous sulfuric acid) for a shorter period (the "modified" Z-N stain, usually used to identify *Nocardia* species), *L. micdadei* is partially acid-fast, *i.e.*, about 10–25% of the bacilli stain red whereas the rest are stained with the methylene blue counterstain. Using tissue stains, the same phenomenon applies, *i.e.*, the acid-fastness of the bacilli is best demonstrated with the Putt (54) or Fite (43) stains whereas the Z-N or Kinyoun techniques may decolorize the bacilli.

An animal model of *L. micdadei* pneumonia has been developed (52) in which guinea pigs are inoculated intratracheally with agar-grown PPA. The animals develop fever, leukocytosis, and profound weight loss. They ultimately succumb to a confluent bronchopneumonia (Figs. 9.2 and 9.3) which resembles the human

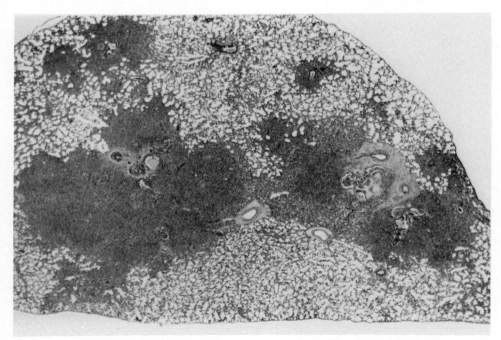

Fig. 9.2. Low magnification photomicrograph of lung from a guinea pig inoculated intratracheally with 10^8 cfu of agar-grown *L. micdadei*. The animal was sacrificed 2 days after inoculation. There is a patchy peribronchial alveolar consolidation, *i.e.*, nodular bronchopneumonia (H & E, ×9).

Brown and Brenn technique, LLO appear as bacilli which are blue (gram-positive) (23). The blue color is less intense than that usually seen with other gram-positive bacilli, *e.g.*, *Clostridia*, but is quite distinctive from the gram reaction of *L. pneumophila* and *L. micdadei*.

LLO are fastidious bacteria which will grow on CYE and BCYE agar and in yeast extract broth. The major phenotypic distinction of LLO from *L. pneumophila* and *L. micdadei* is the production of a fluorescent pigment which causes colonies to be brightly fluorescent when examined under a Wood lamp and which allows rapid presumptive identification. The chromatographic pattern of the cell wall branched-chain fatty acids in the various LLOs is distinctive, for each LLO, as well as for *L. pneumophila*. As mentioned above, *L. bozemanii* shares some cell wall antigens with *L. pneumophila*, but the cell wall antigens of *L. dumoffii* and *L. gormanii* do not cross-react with each other, other LLO, or *L. pneumophila*.

Diagnosis of future cases of pneumonia due to LLO will be made by DFA, culture, or serodiagnosis using the same techniques described above. Insufficient experience does not allow estimation of the sensitivity of specificity of these methods for these particular pathogens.

SUMMARY

Since the recognition of Legionnaires' disease in the summer of 1976, a great deal has been learned about the epidemiology, pathogenesis, gross and microscopic pathology, bacteriology, host immunity, and diagnosis of this "new" disease and its etiologic agent, *L. pneumophila*. We have also come to recognize a group of *Legionella*-like organisms which include *L. micdadei* and three other species, all of which share certain special bacteriologic characteristics with *L. pneumophila* and two of which (*L. micdadei* and *L. bozemanii*) appear to be important causes of human pneumonia. Because they are phenotypically similar but sufficiently genetically distinct, as determined by DNA homology studies (8, 33, 65), *L. pneumophila*, *L. micdadei*, and LLO such as *L. bozemanii* have been placed in the same family (Legionellaceae) and genus (*Legionella*) but in separate species. The phenotypic similarities and differences between *L. pneumophila*, *L. micdadei*, and *L. bozemanii* are summarized in Table 9.2.

TABLE 9.2. Phenotypic Properties of Bacteria in the Family Legionellaceae

	L. pneumophila	LLO*	*L. micdadei*
Requires iron and cysteine	+	+	+
Primary growth on charcoal yeast extract agar	+	+	+
Primary growth of F-G agar	⊞	−	−
Weakly acid-fast in tissues	−	−	⊞
Brown pigment	+	+	+
Blue fluorescence	−	⊞	−
Catalase	+	+	+
Gelatinase	+	+	+
Oxidase	+	⊟	+
B-lactamase	+	±	⊟
Motility (single subpolar flagellum)	+	+	+

* *Legionella*-like organisms (*e.g. L. bozemanii*).

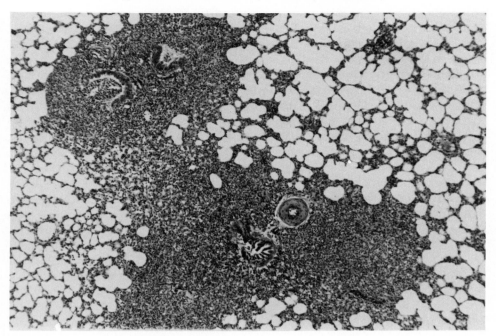

FIG. 9.3. Higher magnification of lung from a similarly challenged guinea pig. Note the purulent exudate in the bronchial lumen and in the peribronchial alveoli (H & E, ×96).

disease. Interestingly, extrapulmonary pathology in the form of nodular aggregates of macrophages with intracellular bacilli are regularly seen in the spleen and liver. These changes are similar to those recently seen in a patient with LD (69). However, no such changes have been described in the autopsies of human patients with *L. micdadei* pneumonia. Nevertheless, the possibility that human PPA pneumonia, like LD, is frequently complicated by bacteremia, is raised by the animal model data.

L. micdadei has been cultivated on CYE (33) and BCYE agars (51). The organism is even more fastidious than *L. pneumophila* and will not grow in primary isolation on supplemented Mueller-Hinton agar or Feeley-Gorman agar. *L. micdadei* will grow in yeast extract broth (56). *L. micdadei* loses its property of acid-fastness after cultivation on artificial medium. Also, serial agar subculture leads to a change in colonial morphology (type 2) from the prototype colony type (type 1). Type 2 colonies grow faster than type 1 (25) and are less virulent for chick embryos and guinea pigs (52). Like *L. pneumophila*, PPA also has a high content of cell wall branched-chain fatty acids, but its chromatographic pattern is distinct from *L. pneumophila* and the other three species of LLO (31). The ultrastructure of *L. micdadei* differs from that of *L. pneumophila* by virtue of the presence of a 70–75 nm electron-dense band in the periplasmic space of *L. micdadei* (48). This band, presumably a mucopeptide layer, is lost after subculture on agar and appears only after several days of intracellular growth in a monkey kidney (Vero) cell culture system (55). The relationship of this structure to acid-fastness and to virulence remains to be elucidated.

Host immunity to *L. micdadei* appears to be similar to that of *L. pneumophila*.

The cell wall antigens of *L. micadadei* are distinctive from other Legionellaceae, with the exception of *L. bozemanii*, with which PPA has some cross-reactivity. The flagella of *L. micdadei* are probably antigenically identical to those of *L. pneumophila* and other LLO. Using an IFA procedure, a brisk humoral immune response in both infected human patients and infected guinea pigs has been demonstrated. However, in at least one patient, recrudescence of clinical disease occurred in the face of high titers of serum *L. micdadei* antibodies. These data, plus the intracellular location of *L. micdadei* and the occurrence of disease exclusively in steroid-treated patients, strongly suggest that cell-mediated immunity is the major arm of host defense against *L. micdadei*. Direct support for this hypothesis has been provided by successful demonstration of adoptive transfer of acquired resistance to *L. micdadei* from guinea pigs previously sublethally infected with *L. micdadei* to otherwise susceptible guinea pigs using spleen cells (48). Passive transfer of hyperimmune serum may also have some protective activity, but it is much weaker than that provided by cell transfer.

The diagnosis of *L. micdadei* pneumonia can be made on the same specimens described for LD by DFA using specific antiserum (17, 33) by culture using CYE or BCYE agars. Serodiagnosis using the IFA technique can also be accomplished (49). Experience with the latter technique is small, but preliminary analysis indicates that the criteria used for serodiagnosis of LD are also applicable to *L. micdadei* pneumonia.

PNEUMONIA DUE TO OTHER LEGIONELLA-LIKE ORGANISMS

To date, only five patients have been described in whom a diagnosis of pneumonia due to LLO has been made by cultivation of the organism from lung tissue or by DFA analysis of lung tissue. These include a skin diver who died of pneumonia due to *L. bozemanii* (7), a patient with chronic lymphocytic leukemia in remission who died of *L. bozemanii* pneumonia shortly after exposure to brackish pond water (18, 65), two immunosuppressed renal transplant recipients who died of nosocomial *L. bozemanii* pneumonia (J. Keller, J. Goldstein, *et al.*, unpublished data), and a patient with oat cell carcinoma receiving cytotoxic chemotherapy who died of pneumonia due to *L. dumoffii* (41). Ten other patients, about whom limited clinical information was given, had pneumonia of unknown etiology but seroconverted to *L. bozemanii* antigen by IFA analysis (18).

From this limited experience one can only make very preliminary hypotheses concerning epidemiology and pathogenesis. However, it appears likely that pneumonias due to LLO other than *L. micdadei* will be predominantly caused by *L. bozemanii*. As with LD and *L. micdadei* pneumonia, contact with water and inhalation of infected aerosols may be important. As mentioned before, LLO were initially discovered as environmental isolates from aqueous samples. Pneumonia due to *L. micdadei* also appears to occur in both community-acquired and nosocomial settings, the latter predominantly in immunosuppressed patients.

The pathologic changes in *L. micdadei* pneumonia, as seen in the five autopsy cases described above, are very similar to those described for *L. micdadei* pneumonia. Leukocytoclasis of alveolar inflammatory cells has been an especially prominent feature. The major distinction from LD and *L. micdadei* pneumonia involves the histochemical properties of the bacilli in tissue sections. Using the

The discovery of these "new pneumonias" was the direct result of thorough epidemiologic study backed up by equally thorough laboratory study, including the application of unusual isolation techniques (*e.g.*, inoculation of embryonated eggs and guinea pigs) to the diagnosis of bacterial pneumonia and the application of modern serodiagnostic tools, such as the IFA and DFA techniques. Information concerning these new pneumonias is accumulating at a furious pace which will undoubtedly continue for some time. Some major areas that need to be addressed in the near future are: (a) elucidation of the complete clinical spectrum of disease caused by these agents; (b) investigation of the possibility that control of these diseases can be accomplished through alteration of the environment, *e.g.*, treatment of environmental water; (*c*) improvements in our diagnostic armamentarium, *e.g.*, selective media or more sensitive immunologic tools; and (*d*) a more complete understanding of host immunity to these agents leading to new diagnostic and, possibly, disease prevention methods. The years to come promise to be as exciting in this field as the years which have passed since the summer of 1976.

REFERENCES

1. Arko, J., Wong, K. H., and Feeley, J. C. Immunologic factors affecting the in-vitro survival of LDB. *Ann. Intern. Med. 90:* 680–683, 1979.
2. Baine, W. B., Rasheed, J. K., Mackel, D. R., *et al.* Exotoxin activity associated with Legionnaires' disease bacterium. *J. Clin. Microbiol. 9:* 453–459, 1979.
3. Berdal, B. P., Farshy, C. E., and Feeley, J. C. Detection of *Legionella pneumophila* antigen in urine by enzyme-linked immunospecific assay. *J. Clin. Microbiol. 9:* 575–578, 1979.
4. Berendt, R. F., Young, H. W., Allen, R. G., *et al.* Dose-response of guinea pigs experimentally infected with aerosols of *Legionella pneumophila. J. Infect. Dis. 141:* 186–192, 1980.
5. Blackmon, J. A., Chandler, F. W., and Hicklin, M. D. Legionnaires' disease: a review for pathologists. *Pathol. Annu., Part 2:* 303–404, 1979.
6. Blackmon, J. A., Hicklin, M. D., Chandler, F. W., *et al.* Legionnaires' disease. Pathological and historical aspects of a 'new' disease. *Arch. Pathol. Lab. Med. 102:* 337–343, 1978.
7. Bozeman, F. M., Humphries, J. W., and Campbell, J. M. A new group of rickettsia-like agents recovered from guinea pigs. *Acta Virol. 12:* 87–93, 1968.
8. Brenner, D. J., Steigerwalt, A. G., Gorman, G. W., *et al. Legionella bozemanii* (sp. nova) and *Legionella dumoffii* (sp. nova): classification of two additional species of *Legionella* associated with human pneumonia. *Curr. Microbiol.,* 4: 111–116, 1980.
9. Brenner, D. J., Steigerwalt, A. G., and McDade, J. E.: Classification of the Legionnaires' disease bacterium: *Legionella pneumophila,* genus novum, species nova, of the family Legionellaceae, familia nova. *Ann. Intern. Med. 90:* 656–658, 1979.
10. Broome, C. V., Cherry, W. B., Winn, W. C., Jr., *et al.* Rapid diagnosis of Legionnaires' disease by direct immunofluorescent staining. *Ann. Intern. Med. 90:* 1–4, 1979.
11. Broome, C. V., Goings, S. A. J., Thacker, S. B., *et al.* The Vermont epidemic of Legionnaires' disease. *Ann. Intern. Med. 90:* 573–576, 1979.
12. Case Records of the Massachusetts General Hospital, 42-1978. *N. Engl. J. Med. 299:* 939–946, 1978.
13. Chandler, F. W., Blackmon, J. A., Hicklin, M. D., *et al.* Ultrastructure of the agent of Legionnaires' disease in the human lung. *Am. J. Clin. Pathol. 71:* 43–50, 1979.
14. Chandler, F. W., Cole, R. M., Hicklin, M. D., *et al.* Ultrastructure of the Legionnaires' disease bacterium. A study using transmission electron microscopy. *Ann. Intern. Med. 90:* 642–647, 1979.
15. Chandler, F. W., Hicklin, M. D., and Blackmon, J. A. Demonstration of the agent of Legionnaires' disease in tissue. *N. Engl. J. Med. 297:* 1218–1220, 1977.
16. Cherry, W. B., Pittman, B., Harris, P. P., *et al.* Detection of Legionnaires disease bacteria by direct immunofluorescent staining. *J. Clin. Microbiol. 8:* 329–338, 1978.

17. Cordes, L. G., Myerowitz, R. L., Pasculle, A. W., *et al. Legionella micdadei* (Pittsburgh pneumonia agent): Direct fluorescent antibody examination of infected human lung tissue and characterization of clinical isolates, *J. Clin. Microbiol. 13:* 720–722, 1981.

18. Cordes, L. G., Wilkinson, H. W., Gorman, G. W., *et al.* Atypical *Legionella*-like organisms: Fastidious water-associated bacteria pathogenic for man. *Lancet ii:* 927–931, 1979.

19. D. J. Brenner, unpublished data.

20. Dondero, T. J., Jr., Rendtorff, R. C., Mallison, G. F., *et al.* An outbreak of Legionnaires' disease associated with a contaminated air-conditioning cooling tower. *N. Engl. J. Med. 302:* 365–370, 1980.

21. Edelstein, P. H., Meyer, R. D., and Finegold, S. M. Isolation of *Legionella pneumophila* from blood. *Lancet i:* 750–751, 1979.

22. Edelstein, P. H., Meyer, R. D., and Finegold, S. M. Laboratory diagnosis of Legionnaires' disease. *Am. Rev. Resp. Dis. 121:* 317–327, 1980.

23. Ewing, E. P., Chandler, F. W., Hicklin, M. D., *et al.* Histopathology of pneumonia due to bacteria resembling *Legionella pneumophila*: presumptive differentiation from Legionnaires' disease using special stains (abstract). *Lab. Invest. 42:* 114, 1980.

24. Feeley, J. C., Gibson, R. J., Gorman, G. W., *et al.* Charcoal-yeast extract agar: primary isolation medium for *Legionella pneumophila. J. Clin. Microbiol. 10:* 437–441, 1979.

25. Flesher, A. R., Kasper, D. L., and Modern, P. A. Growth inhibition of *Legionella pneumophila* by indigenous pharyngeal flora. Abstract 504, 20th Interscience Conference on Antimicrobial Agents and Chemotherapy, New Orleans, La., 1980.

26. Fraser, D. W., Tsai, T. R., Orenstein, W., *et al.* Legionnaires' disease. Description of an epidemic of pneumonia. *N. Engl. J. Med. 297:* 1189–1196, 1977.

27. Friedman, R. L., Iglewski, B. H., and Miller, R. D. Identification of a cytotoxin produced by *Legionella pneumophila. Infect. Immun. 29:* 271–274, 1980.

28. Glavin, F. L., Winn, W. C., Jr., and Craighead, J. E. Ultrastructure of lung in Legionnaires' disease. Observations of three biopsies done during the Vermont epidemic. *Ann. Intern. Med. 90:* 555–558, 1979.

29. Gorman, G. W., Yu, V. L., Brown, A., *et al.* Isolation of Pittsburgh pneumonia agent from nebulizers used in respiratory therapy. *Ann. Intern. Med. 92:* 572–573, 1980.

30. Gress, F. M., Myerowitz, R. L., Pasculle, A. W., *et al.* Ultrastructural morphology of "Pittsburgh pneumonia agent." *Am. J. Pathol. 101:* 63–78, 1980

31. Hébert, G. A., Moss, C. W., McDougal, L. K., *et al.* The rickettsia-like organisms TATLOCK (1943) and HEBA (1959): bacteria phenotypically similar to but genetically distinct from *Legionella pneumophila* and the WIGA bacterium. *Ann. Intern. Med. 92:* 45–52, 1980.

32. Hébert, G. A., Steigerwalt, A. G., and Brenner, D. J. *Legionella micdadei* species nova: Classification of a third species of *Legionella* associated with human pneumonia. *Curr. Microbiol. 3:* 255–257, 1980.

33. Hébert, G. A., Thomason, B. M., Harris, P. P., *et al.* "Pittsburgh pneumonia agent": a bacterium phenotypically similar to *Legionella pneumophila* and identical to the TATLOCK bacterium. *Ann. Intern. Med. 92:* 53–54, 1980.

34. Hedlund, K. W., McGann, V. G., Copeland, D. S., *et al.* Immunologic protection against the Legionnaires' disease bacterium in the AKR/J mouse. *Ann. Intern. Med. 90:* 676–679, 1979.

35. Horwitz, M. A., and Silverstein, S. C. The Legionnaires' disease bacterium resists killing by human phagocytes, antibody, and complement. Abstract 350, 20th Interscience Conference on Antimicrobial Agents and Chemotherapy, New Orleans, La., 1980.

36. Jackson, E. B., Crocker, T. T., and Smadel, J. E. Studies on two rickettsia-like agents probably isolated from guinea pigs. *Bacteriol. Proc.:* 119, 1952.

37. Kariman, K., Shelburne, J. D., Gough, W., *et al.* Pathologic findings and long-term sequelae in Legionnaires' disease. *Chest 75:* 736–739, 1979.

38. Katz, S. M., Brodsky, I., and Kahn, S. B. Legionnaires' disease. Ultrastructural appearance of the agent in a lung biopsy specimen. *Arch. Pathol. Lab. Med. 103:* 261–264, 1979.

39. Keel, J. A., Finnerty, W. R., and Feeley, J. C. Fine structure of the Legionnaires' disease bacterium. *In vitro* and *in vivo* studies of four isolates. *Ann. Intern. Med. 90:* 652–655, 1979.

40. Kohler, R. B., Zimmerman, S., Allen, S., *et al.* Detection and partial characterization of an antigen in the urine of patients with Legionnaires' disease. Abstract 503, 20th Interscience Conference on Antimicrobial Agents and Chemotherapy, New Orleans, La., 1980.

41. Lewallen, K. R., McKinney, R. M., Brenner, D. J., *et al.* A newly identified bacterium phenotypically resembling but genetically distinct from *Legionella pneumophila*: An isolate in a case of pneumonia. *Ann. Intern. Med. 91:* 831–834, 1979.
42. Lewin, S., Brettman, L. R., Goldstein, E. J. C., *et al.* Legionnaires' disease. A cause of severe abscess-forming pneumonia. *Am. J. Med. 67:* 339–342, 1979.
43. Luna, L. G. *Manual of histologic staining methods of the Armed Forces Institute of Pathology*, Ed. 3. pp. 217–219, 222–223. New York, McGraw-Hill, 1968.
44. Marks, J. S., Tsai, T. F., Martone, W. J., *et al.* Nosocomial Legionnaires' disease in Columbus, Ohio. *Ann. Intern. Med. 90:* 565–568, 1979.
45. McDade, J. E., Brenner, D. J., and Bozeman, F. M. Legionnaires' disease bacterium isolated in 1947. *Ann. Intern. Med. 90:* 659–661, 1979.
46. McDade, J. E., Shepard, C. C., Fraser, D. W., *et al.* Legionnaires' disease. Isolation of a bacterium and demonstration of its role in other respiratory disease. *N. Engl. J. Med. 297:* 1197–1203, 1977.
47. Moss, C. W., and Dees, S. B. Further studies of the cellular fatty acid composition of Legionnaires' disease bacteria. *J. Clin. Microbiol. 9:* 648–649, 1979.
48. Myerowitz, R. L., Dowling, J. N., and Pasculle, A. W. Immunity to Pittsburgh pneumonia agent in guinea pigs. Abstract 497, 20th Interscience Conference on Antimicrobial Agents and Chemotherapy, New Orleans, La., 1980.
49. Myerowitz, R. L., Pasculle, A. W., Dowling, J. N., *et al.* Opportunistic lung infection due to Pittsburgh pneumonia agent. *N. Engl. J. Med. 301:* 953–958, 1979.
50. Neblett, T. R., Riddle, J. M., and Dumoff, M. Surface topography and fine structure of the Legionnaires' disease bacterium. A study of six isolates in hospitalized patients. *Ann. Intern. Med. 90:* 648–651, 1979.
51. Pasculle, A. W., Feeley, J. C., Gibson, R. J., *et al.* Pittsburgh pneumonia agent: direct isolation from human lung tissue. *J. Infect. Dis. 141:* 727–732, 1980.
52. Pasculle, A. W. Experimental studies with Pittsburgh pneumonia agent. In *Microbiology—1981*, edited by D. W. Schlesinger, American Society for Microbiology, pp. 169–172.
53. Pasculle, A. W., Myerowitz, R. L., Rinaldo, C. R. New bacterial agent of pneumonia isolated from renal transplant recipients. *Lancet ii:* 58–61, 1979.
54. Putt, F. A. A modified Ziehl-Neelsen stain: for demonstration of leprosy bacilli and other acid-fast organisms. *Am. J. Clin. Pathol. 21:* 92, 1951.
55. Rinaldo, C. R., Jr., Pasculle, A. W., Myerowitz, R. L., *et al.* Growth of the Pittsburgh pneumonia agent in animal cell cultures. Abstract 499, 20th Interscience Conference on Antimicrobial Agents and Chemotherapy, New Orleans, La., 1980.
56. Ristroph, J. D., Hedlund, K. W., and Allen, R. G. Liquid medium for growth of *Legionella pneumophila. J. Clin. Microbiol. 11:* 19–21, 1980.
57. Rodgers, F. G., Macrae, A. D., and Lewis, M. J. Electron microscopy of the organism of Legionnaires' disease. *Nature 272:* 825–826, 1978.
58. Rogers, B. H., Donowitz, G. R., Walker, G. K., *et al.* Opportunistic pneumonia: A clinicopathologic study of five cases caused by an unidentified acid-fast bacterium. *N. Engl. J. Med. 301:* 959–961, 1979.
59. Shands, K. N., Ho, J. L., Meyer, R. D., *et al.* Potable water: possible role in epidemic Legionnaires' disease (LD). Abstract 501, 20th Interscience Conference on Antimicrobial Agents and Chemotherapy, New Orleans, La., 1980.
60. Storch, G., Baine, W. B., Fraser, D. W., *et al.* Sporadic community-acquired Legionnaires' disease in the United States. A case-control study. *Ann. Intern. Med. 90:* 596–600, 1979.
61. Suffin, S. C., Kaufmann, A. F., Whitaker, B., *et al. Legionella pneumophila.* Identification in tissue sections by a new immunoenzymatic procedure. *Arch. Pathol. Lab. Med. 104:* 283–286, 1980.
62. Swartz, M. N. Another new pneumonia: Pandora's box reopened? *N. Engl. J. Med. 301:* 995–996, 1979.
63. Tatlock, H. A rickettsia-like organisms recovered from guinea pigs. *Proc. Soc. Exp. Biol. Med. 57:* 95–99, 1944.
64. Thomason, B. M., Chandler, F. W., and Hollis, D. G. Flagella on Legionnaires' disease bacteria: an interim report. *Ann. Intern. Med. 91:* 224–228, 1979.

65. Thomason, B. M., Harris, P. P., Hicklin, M. D., *et al.* A *Legionella*-like bacterium related to WIGA in a fatal case of pneumonia. *Ann. Intern. Med. 91:* 673–676, 1979.

66. Tobin, J. O'H., Beare, J., Dunnhill, M. S., *et al.* Legionnaires' disease in a transplant unit: isolation of the causative agent from shower baths. *Lancet ii:* 118–121, 1980.

67. Watts, J. C., Hicklin, M. D., Thomason, B. M., *et al.* Fatal pneumonia caused by *Legionella pneumophila*, serogroup 3: demonstration of the bacilli in extrathoracic organs. *Ann. Intern. Med. 92:* 186–188, 1980.

68. Weinstein, L. The "new" pneumonias: the doctor's dilemma. *Ann. Intern. Med. 92:* 559–562, 1980.

69. Weisenburger, D. D., Rappaport, H., Ahluwalia, M. S., *et al.* Legionnaires' disease. *Am. J. Med. 69:* 476–482, 1980.

70. White, H. J., Felton, W. W., and Sun, C. N. Extrapulmonary histopathologic manifestations of Legionnaires' disease. Evidence for myocarditis and bacteremia. *Arch. Pathol. Lab. Med. 104:* 287–289, 1980.

71. White, H. J., Sun, C. N., and Hui, A. N. An ultrastructural demonstration of the agent of Legionnaires' disease in the human lung. *Hum. Pathol. 10:* 96–99, 1979.

72. Winn, W. C., Jr., Cherry, W. B., Frank, R. O., *et al.* Direct immunofluorescent detection of *Legionella pneumophila* in respiratory specimens. *J. Clin. Microbiol. 11:* 59–64, 1980.

73. Winn, W. C., Jr., Davis, G. S., Gump, W., *et al.* Legionnaires' pneumonia after intratracheal inoculation of guinea pigs. Abstract 505, 20th Interscience Conference on Antimicrobial Agents and Chemotherapy, New Orleans, La., 1980.

74. Winn, W. C., Jr., Glavin, F. L., Perl, D. P., *et al.* The pathology of Legionnaires' disease. Fourteen fatal cases from the 1977 outbreak in Vermont. *Arch. Pathol. Lab. Med. 102:* 344–350, 1978.

75. Wilkinson, H. W., Fikes, B. J., and Cruce, D. D. Indirect immunofluorescence test for serodiagnosis of Legionnaires disease: evidence for serogroup diversity of Legionnaires disease bacterial antigens and for multiple specificity of human antibodies. *J. Clin. Microbiol. 9:* 379–383, 1979.

76. Wong, M. C., Ewing, E. P., Jr., Callaway, C. S., *et al.* Intracellular multiplication of *Legionella pneumophila* in cultured human embryonic lung fibroblasts. *Infect. Immun. 28:* 1014–1018, 1980.

Chapter 10

Persistent Viral Infections of Man

JOHN E. CRAIGHEAD

It is customary to think of virus infections as acute, sometimes fulminating events having a short incubation period and a clinical illness of relatively brief duration. As a result we tend to overlook the fact that many common agents exhibit both an acute and a more protracted phase of residence in tissue. Chronicity proves to be a characteristic feature of viral infections, rather than an exceptional and unusual event.

During the past several decades we have become aware of a number of diseases that fail to fit the stereotype of an infection, although an etiologic agent can be transmitted. Virologists now arbitrarily classify these conditions under the rubric of persistent infections, even though they are caused by a variety of viruses having differing biological and clinical patterns of expression. Some of these processes are caused by common viruses occurring under unusual circumstances whereas others are attributable to exotic agents, the characteristics of which are incompletely understood. Yet, all of the so-called persistent viruses have in common an extended, but highly variable, period of apparent dormancy in tissues and a diversity of clinical expressions.

In this review I will neither catalogue nor fully document the large numbers of persistent virus infections of man and lower animals that are now recognized. Rather, I will provide an overview and consider examples of several different clinically important human infections in the perspective of their biologic commonalities.

MODELS OF PERSISTENCE—INTERACTIONS OF VIRUS WITH THE HOST

Table 10.1 categorizes the basic mechanisms of virus persistence as the biology of these infections currently is understood. The features are briefly summarized below.

INTEGRATION OF VIRAL INFORMATION IN HOST CELLS

The RNA retroviruses and members of the DNA containing herpesviruses provide the best examples of infectious agents that persist as integrated messages in the cell. Recent evidence indicates, however, that the genetic material of several additional persistent viruses may also integrate into host DNA. During the past decade the molecular biology of these complex states has been examined

TABLE 10.1. Mechanisms of Viral Persistence in Man

Integrated Infection
  Viral RNA transcribed into DNA or viral DNA-integrated host genome or transmitted to progeny
  cells as independent episome. Infectious progeny are produced sporadically or not at all.
Latent Infection
  Viral expression as gene product and/or a morphologically distinguishable viral component.
  Assembly of infectious virus is variable.
Slow Infection
  Protracted subclinical infection terminating in overt disease in "target" organ.
Chronic Infection
  Chronic disease accompanied by an active but protracted infection.

thoroughly, in part because the phenomena provide insight into mechanisms whereby new genetic information can be transmitted from generation to generation. In addition, this is at least one important means whereby oncogenic genes are conveyed horizontally among populations and vertically to progeny.

Cells infected with retroviruses acquire both an RNA message and an RNA transcriptase from the virus. The enzyme serves as a tool for recording the viral message as a DNA replica into the chromosomal material of the infected cells (Fig. 10.1) (3). Once this event is accomplished, evidence of infection may no longer be apparent since the new genetic information in the host cell is not expressed phenotypically. Activation of the message resulting in either virus production or malignant transformation of the cell (or both) is a poorly understood event, although often it is regulated by genetic and immunologic influences intrinsic to the host. On the one hand, viral information can lie dormant indefinitely; on the other hand, it can be activated either through the mechanism of a concomitant superinfection with another retrovirus or an environmental insult such as cell injury caused by a toxic chemical. So far retroviruses have not been shown to be responsible for disease in man, although some evidence of inapparent human infections has accumulated (38), and cultured mammalian cells can be infected *in vitro* with agents from lower species (6). It is surprising that man has not been shown to be infected with retroviruses since these agents are found in the tissues of a wide variety of lower animals, including a number of subhuman primates. It may be only a matter of time before human retrovirus infections are documented.

The DNA-containing herpesviruses also interact with the host genetic material and are integrated. Viral DNA either bonds covalently with the DNA of the chromatin or becomes established as an independent "provirus" in the cell (Fig. 10.2) (7, 17). In these forms the viral genetic material may serve to redirect cell function, although it often lies dormant indefinitely and is transmitted to progeny cells. Members of the herpesvirus group commonly interact with human cells by this mechanism.

LATENT INFECTIONS

A second, equally complex form of virus-cell interaction is termed latency. Unfortunately, this term means different things to different people. In the latent state, transcription of the viral message is incomplete, and the cell fails to fabricate infectious viral particles. The block in the viral replicative sequence

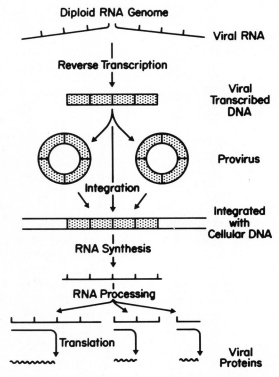

FIG. 10.1. Schema depicting a hypothetical mechanism for integration of a retrovirus RNA message into the DNA genetic material of the cell. (Modified from J. M. Bishop (3)).

may be relatively early, for example, at a stage when only a few viral proteins have been synthesized. Alternatively, it can occur during a late stage of virus assembly. Whereas in the first case it is possible to detect evidence of infection using either immunological or biochemical techniques, in the second the incompletely assembled virus might be demonstrable by ultrastructure.

In subacute sclerosing panencephalitis, caused by either measles or a measles-like virus, evidence of viral replication in cells of the central nervous system can be detected by the above approaches, yet the brain tissue of children with the disease fails to yield infectious virus when cultured by traditional approaches (Fig. 10.3) (24, 35). In the chronic carrier state of type B hepatitis (HBV), the coat antigenic protein (HB_sAg) of the virus often is synthesized in luxuriant quantities (Fig. 10.4). It can be detected by immunohistochemistry and ultrastructure in the cytoplasm of the cell (Fig. 10.5) (2, 23). The outcome of this latent infection is variable. Whereas some cases have a subclinical infection over a lifetime, others evolve into chronic hepatitis and possibly hepatocellular carcinoma.

SLOW VIRUSES

The designation slow virus was coined by Sigurdsson during his studies of the endemic sheep diseases of Iceland: maedi (a chronic pneumonitis), visna (a progressive demyelinating central nervous disorder) and scrapies (a spongiform

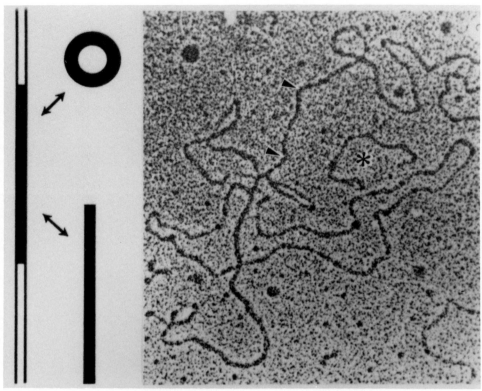

FIG. 10.2. Schema depicting forms of integrated and nonintegrated viral DNA in genetic material of the cell. Note the presumptive insertion site in the cellular DNA strand (*arrowheads*) in the electron micrographs, and the "open-ended" "episome" or "provirus" (*).

encephalopathy) (1, 44, 45). Characteristic of this group of transmissible agents is the persistence of a productive infection in tissues of the host for years *before* the development of disease in the "target" organ. For example, one can recover the agent responsible for scrapies from tissues outside the central nervous system for periods of several years before debilitating neurological disease develops in the animal (16). Similar observations have been made in subhuman primates experimentally infected with the human agents of spongiform encephalopathy (29). "Slow" is a relative term, and thus the criteria for inclusion of virus into the group is somewhat arbitrary. For example, rabiesvirus infections in man and lower animals often are quiescent for protracted periods of time before they are expressed in the form of neurological disease (31, 35). Since our technological capability to detect subtle infection still is limited, it is likely that additional cryptic "slow" viruses will be associated with disease in man.

Chronic Viral Infections

Man is afflicted with a number of chronic viral disease in which the virus actively multiplies for extended periods in tissue exhibiting the characteristic features of disease. For example, in verruca vulgaris, the common wart, papovavirus particles are found in intranuclear inclusions, and the virus can be trans-

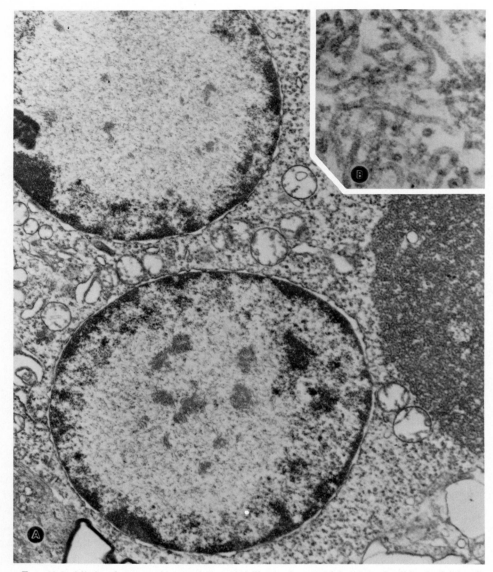

Fɪɢ. 10.3. (A) An electron micrograph (×1,220) illustrating a multinucleated cell in the brain of a hamster infected experimentally with measles virus. Note the nucleocapsid material in the nucleus (B, ×23,100) and the array of intracytoplasmic virions (A). These viral components also are readily demonstrable by fluorescence microscopy. (Courtesy of Cedric S. Raine, Ph.D., and Williams & Wilkins).

mitted to susceptible subjects using homogenates of the lesions (18, 41). Similar papovavirus particles are found in condyloma acuminata and laryngeal papillomata. Characteristically, either normal immune mechanisms fail to control intracellular replication and intercellular spread of the virus or the immunologic response of the host is attenuated. Thus, the lesion and its associated virus persists for extended periods of time.

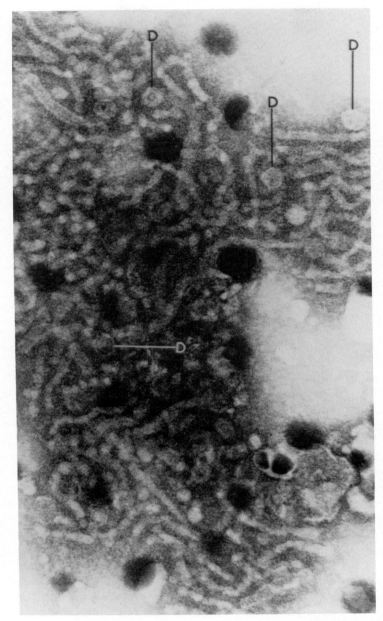

Fig. 10.4. A negatively stained electron micrograph of a homogenate of HBV-infected liver tissue that was treated with HB$_s$Ab to aggregate the coat protein of the virus. Note the abundance of this material in relation to the scarce viral (Dane) particles (*D*). (Courtesy of S. N. Huang and V. Groh (23) and Williams & Wilkins.)

RELATIONSHIP OF ALTERED IMMUNE STATES TO VIRAL PERSISTENCE

It would be difficult to catalogue the wide variety of virus infections that are facilitated, or exacerbated, in the immunologically modified host. I will record

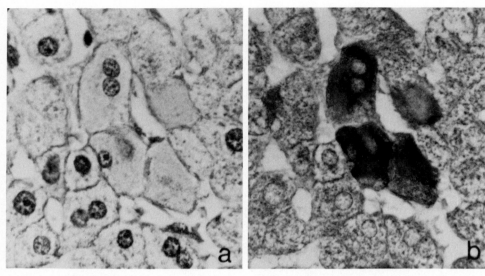

FIG. 10.5. Photomicrograph of paraffin-embedded histologic section of the liver (×385) from a patient with persistent viral hepatitis. The tissue is stained by the immunoperoxidase method (*b*) to reveal HB$_s$Ag and with hematoxylin and eosin to illustrate the characteristic "ground glass" appearance (*a*) of the cytoplasm. (Courtesy of A. P. Afroudakis *et al.* (2)).

here several selected examples to provide insight into the biological mechanisms involved.

Infections with picornaviruses (such as polio, Coxsackie, and ECHO viruses) customarily are systemic during the acute stages and evolve into a chronic intestinal stage with the passage of time. Many of these infections are silent, although occasionally they are of sufficient severity to cause important lesions in "target" organs. Resolution of the infection normally is accompanied by a brisk immunological response that involves both cellular and humoral elements (46, 47). Whereas the latter mechanism provides future protection against infection, the former contributes actively to the resolution of the infection in the cell.

Rarely, persistent picornavirus infections develop in persons with immunological deficiency disorders involving either cellular or humoral immune mechanisms (or both). Although this customarily occurs as an outgrowth of natural exposure, it also has been observed in infants who inadvertently are administered live, attenuated poliovirus vaccine (12, 58). Typically, the process is characterized by chronic tissue infection that initially is clinically inapparent. After a protracted period of weeks or months, the central nervous system is involved, and the child succumbs with encephalomyelitis (Fig. 10.6) (53, 56).

The papovavirus that causes progressive multifocal leukoencephalopathy establishes a dramatically different relationship with the host. This virus, known by the designation JC, customarily infects most of us during the early years of life (36). This event would appear to be asymptomatic (since an association with acute illness has not been established), although the virus might be responsible for one of the nondescript illnesses children invariably experience.

Although JC virus infections would appear to be established and persist in a

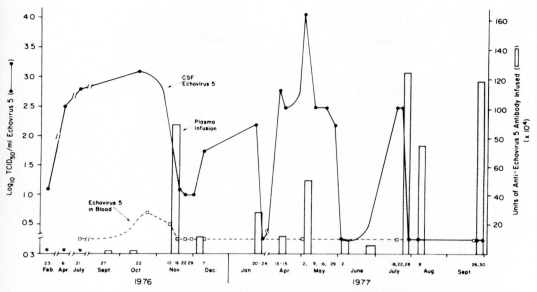

FIG. 10.6. Amounts of echovirus type 5 in the cerebral spinal fluid (●) and blood (□) of a young child with hypogammaglobulinemia. The *bars* indicate therapeutic attempts using intravenous specific antibody. (Courtesy of L. S. Weiner *et al.* (53) and the University of Chicago Press.)

dormant form in most of us, the virus is readily activated by therapeutic interventions which alter cell-mediated immune responses such as the immuno-suppression employed in organ transplantation. For example, virological studies have shown that 20–25% of kidney graft recipients excrete this virus, or a related papovavirus, BK, in the urine, and we and others, have found changing serum concentrations of JC viral antibody during periods of immunosuppression. (11, 37). Although treatment regimens employed in transplantation appear to activate JC virus, progressive multifocal leukoencephalopathy proves to be a rare complication of therapeutic immunosuppression.

Numerous case reports attest to the common association of progressive multi-focal leukoencephalopathy with advanced leukemia and lymphoma, particularly Hodgkin's disease (40, 52). Because of the rarity of this nervous system disease, it is uncertain whether or not the unique altered immune state that accompanies Hodgkin's disease predisposes to activation of JC virus. Of interest is a recent report which documents the presence of both JC and the related BK virus in the urine of a substantial number of healthy women during pregnancy (9). Currently, it is not known why the gestational state predisposes to viral activation.

Recently, an altered state of immune control was proposed by Chisari et al. (8) to account for the sporadic occurrence of chronic hepatitis in persons infected with HBV. These workers suggest that both the production and breakdown of immunoregulatory substances (proteins, lipoproteins) in the liver are altered because of the hepatic disease. This selective immunological abnormality results in an attenuated viral antibody response which would predispose to chronicity of the infection. Additional support for an immunological contribution to the virus

"carrier" state relates to the apparent increase in susceptibility of renal allotrans-
plant recipients to HBV (42).

POSTNATAL INFECTION AFTER *IN UTERO* OR PERINATAL EXPOSURE

Exposure to virus early in life initiates a unique virus-host relationship that
occasionally is followed by a persistent infection in the neonatal period. The basis
for the chronicity of the process has not been defined, but it does not appear to
be attributable to altered immunological protective mechanisms. Although the
outcome can be either severe disability or death, many infants survive without
apparent stigmata of disease despite the persistence of the infection.

Cytomegalovirus by far is the most common infection of the perinatal period.
The conceptus customarily contracts the virus late in pregnancy either via the
placenta (30) or at parturition from an infected cervix uteri (48, 55). Regardless
of the route, a systemic infection of the neonate is established and persists for
varying periods of time thereafter. Studies in newborn nurseries have shown that
0.5–2% of infants yield cytomegalovirus when either the saliva or urine are tested
during the first few days of life (22, 49).

Persistent neonatal cytomegalovirus infection only rarely results in significant
organ abnormalities, and by far most children recover without evidence of central
nervous system disease (22, 27) and overt cytomegalic inclusion disease is uncommon (19, 22, 27, 39). There are no observations in man to suggest that the
outcome is influenced by an altered immunological responsivity of the child,
although evidence in experimental models suggests that cytomegalovirus has a
unique immunosuppressive effect in the acutely infected host (4, 28).

As is well known, rubellavirus infection of the fetus often, but not invariably,
results in embryopathies, and a postnatal chronic infection (Fig. 10.7) (20). When
the infection is severe the infant with congenital rubella succumbs and the viscera
yield enormous amounts of virus. Alternatively, a persistent infection of lesser
severity can smolder for extended periods of time after birth (Fig. 10.8). Although
virus excretion in the saliva has been documented for as long as 2 years in a few
children, there is evidence to indicate that the virus persists cryptically in tissues
for more extended periods of time. Recently, an unusual subacute progressive

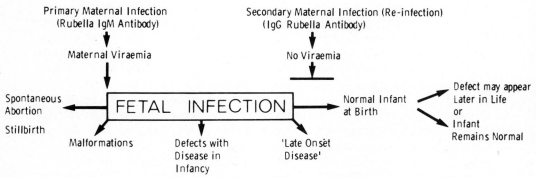

Fig. 10.7. Diverse outcomes of maternal infection with rubellavirus. (Courtesy of J. B. Hanshaw
and J. A. Dudgeon (20), as well as W. B. Saunders.)

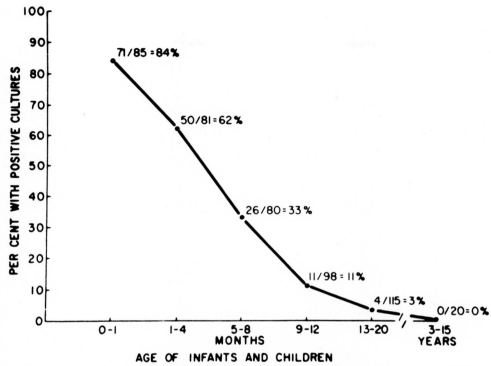

FIG. 10.8. Incidence of virus excretion by age by children congenitally infected with rubellavirus. (Courtesy of J. B. Hanshaw and J. A. Dudgeon (20), as well as W. B. Saunders.)

panencephalopathy has been documented as a late sequela of congenital rubella infection. The evidence suggest that this syndrome is consequent to persistence of the virus into the second decade of life (51, 57).

INFECTIONS OF SENSORY NERVE CELLS

A persistent infection with herpes simplex (herpesvirus hominis, type 1) is established in sensory ganglia of the central nervous system after an initial exposure to this virus (34, 50). The primary infection may be either subclinical or a transient vesicular and inflammatory eruption of the oropharyngeal mucosa or external eye. Apparently herpes simplex virus is transmitted through the sensory axon to the nucleus of a trigeminal ganglion cell where it localizes. The cellular site of the virus and viral genetic information during periods of dormancy in the ganglion is uncertain, and our knowledge of the mechanism of reactivation is scant. Both cellular and humoral immune mechanisms play a role in the control of the persistent infection and prevent reinfection with new "wild" strains of virus (7, 34). As is well known, a variety of nonspecific stimuli activate the viral message in the nucleus of the sensory ganglion, resulting in a productive infectious process and recurrent episodes of herpes labialis and ophthalmitis.

Repeated attempts by virologists to isolate herpes simplex from the trigeminal ganglion during an inactive clinical phase failed until cells from ganglia were cultured *in vitro*. It was then possible to recover the virus by growing susceptible cells with the nerve cells, a technique known as cocultivation. A sizeable body of evidence suggests that viral genetic material is either integrated into the DNA of the host cell or persists as an isolated DNA episome during dormant periods. However, the virus could be present in an elementary form that is not detectable by traditional virological and morphological approaches.

Herpes simplex (type 2) customarily is a genital infection acquired in a venereal fashion (25, 33). The biology of this virus in man has not been studied extensively, and it is not known whether it localizes in the ganglia of the neuraxis after infection of the genitalia. Regardless, both persistent clinically inapparent, and recurrent vesicular-ulcerative processes of the genital organs occur after an initial exposure. Infections of the regional ganglia have been demonstrated in animals after inoculation directly into the cervix.

Varicella virus also persists in tissues in an inapparent form, although the site of localization has not been established (21). Compelling clinical and epidemiological evidence indicates that chickenpox usually is the initial experience with varicella. One might assume by analogy with herpes simplex that sensory ganglia serve as a residence for either the virus or viral genetic information after the subsidence of this systemic infection, but evidence to support this conclusion is limited. During clinical episodes of herpes zoster, sensory neurons in the ganglia exhibit necrosis and inflammation. Morphological evidence of infection is also found in the form of antigens demonstrable by immunofluorescence and virions found by electron microscopy (32). As with herpes simplex, immunological factors influence expression of the virus, but nonspecific insults such as physical trauma often appear to initiate clinical expression as "shingles" in persons with seemingly intact immune systems.

COMPLEX SYNDROMES OF VIRAL PERSISTENCE AND ACTIVATION

Having now considered the spectrum of circumstances under which disease is associated with viral persistence, I will provide in this section a perspective to the diverse clinical features of the infections which accompany three agents of contemporary interest.

Epstein-Barr Virus (EBV) (7, 14, 43)

Knowledge of this virus began with the studies of Sir Dennis Burkitt on the clinical epidemiology of the lymphoma that bears his name. The EB virus was isolated in the late 1950s by Drs. Epstein and Barr from tumor cells cultured from cases in East Africa. Since that time a vast body of fundamental virological information has accumulated on this agent and its interactions with cells. In addition, we have learned a great deal about its epidemiology and the several diseases with which it is associated.

Figure 10.9 summarizes in outline form our current knowledge. EBV appears to be ubiquitous for it has a worldwide distribution. Primary infection occurs by intimate contact among susceptibles and most probably as a consequence of respiratory-droplet transmission. In lower socioeconomic groups the virus is acquired at a relatively early age, and infection is either subclinical or accompanied by a nonspecific illness. In population groups of higher socioeconomic status,

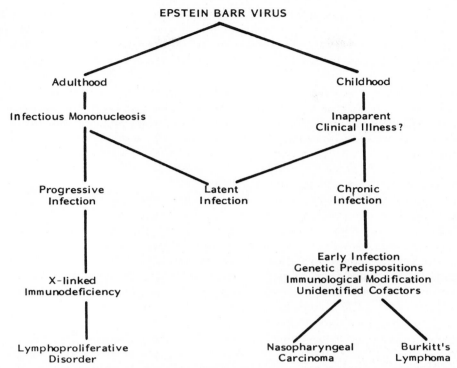

EPSTEIN BARR VIRUS

Adulthood

Infectious Mononucleosis

Progressive Infection

Latent Infection

X-linked Immunodeficiency

Lymphoproliferative Disorder

Childhood

Inapparent Clinical Illness?

Chronic Infection

Early Infection
Genetic Predispositions
Immunological Modification
Unidentified Cofactors

Nasopharyngeal Carcinoma

Burkitt's Lymphoma

FIG. 10.9. Schema depicting the various forms of disease associated with infection by Epstein Barr virus.

infections are experienced later in life and often take the form of infectious mononucleosis.

A persistent infection develops after an initial experience with this virus in persons of all age groups. The biologic features of the associated cellular events are complex and incompletely defined, but viral DNA is incorporated into host cell DNA and it may remain integrated indefinitely. Lymphocytes of the B type are specifically susceptible, and most, if not all, persons suffering from acute infection are carriers of B cells with EB viral genetic material integrated into the DNA of the chromatin. The extent and type of epithelial cell involvement (if it occurs), is obscure, but it is likely that mucosal cells of the oropharynx and salivary glands are involved since carriers of EB virus release small amounts of infectious virus into the oropharyngeal secretions. In addition, virus in B cells of lymphoid organs may be activated so that the cells express either early or late viral antigens. Apparently some of the lymphoid cells support the replication of fully assembled infectious virus and undergo cytolysis. Thus the infection is in a dynamic state of equilibrium. On the one hand, viral genetic information is integrated into host DNA; on the other, it is expressed as an active infection. These events are only partially under the control of immunologic influences.

Infectious mononucleosis is the usual form of disease associated with an initial exposure to EB virus in young adults residing in economically advanced countries. Although the clinical features (pharyngitis, lymphadenopathy, hepatosplenomegaly) appear to reflect the infiltration and proliferative response of T cells to the virus-associated antigens in B cells, the details of this immunologically mediated event are not fully defined. The abnormal antibody responses that occur during the acute illness appear to reflect the stimulation of B cells consequent to infection.

Most patients experience an uneventful recovery although a subclinical infection persists. The factors that influence the subsidence of the acute episode are not known. Many recuperative patients sporadically yield small amounts of virus in the oropharyngeal secretions, and the circulating lymphocytes exhibit viral antigens and have the capacity to proliferate indefinitely when studied *in vitro*. This latter feature is unique to lymphoid cells infected with EB virus. It may be a reflection of the oncogenic potential of this agent.

A lymphoproliferative syndrome having diverse manifestations occurs in male members of certain rare kinships as a consequence of EB virus infection. It appears to be due to an X chromosome-linked, genetically transmitted deficiency which results in defective modulation of the infection. Although a progressive, ultimately fatal infectious mononucleosis is the most common outcome, the manifestations range from lymphoma to dysgammaglobulinemia. Persistence of EB virus in B cells appears to be a key element in this obscure complex of conditions, and a defective response of cytolytic and suppressor T cells accounts for unrestricted B cell proliferation.

Burkitt's lymphoma in tropical Africa and anaplastic nasopharyngeal carcinoma in South China and Southeast Asia also are almost invariably associated with persistent EB virus infection. In children with the lymphoma the immunosuppression that accompanies hyperendemic malaria is believed to play a role, but genetic and other environmental influences may also be important. The pathogenesis of the nasopharyngeal carcinoma is equally obscure. Although one cannot state dogmatically that EB virus is the etiological agent responsible for these rare tumors, it is evident that the genetic material and various expression of its presence (*i.e.*, viral antigens, virions) invariably are demonstrable in tumor cells. The possibility that tumor cells serve as carriers for the virus has not been excluded.

Cytomegalovirus (CMV) (10, 54)

The diverse clinical expressions of cytomegalovirus have been the subject of hundreds of publications during the past two decades. It is now apparent that this ubiquitous virus has the potential to cause human disease in virtually every organ system, yet in most of us it persists either in a dormant state or is expressed as an active, but subclinical infection (Fig. 10.10).

As noted earlier in this chapter, cytomegalovirus commonly is acquired during the perinatal period. In the majority of the population, however, exposure usually occurs later in life. Respiratory droplets and saliva probably are the means of transmission among most children whereas primary infection of adults who lack serum antibody has been documented frequently in recipients of fresh blood transfusions and kidney transplants. Regardless of the means of transmission, a persistent infection is established, and virus is excreted in the oropharyngeal secretions and urine for varying periods of time.

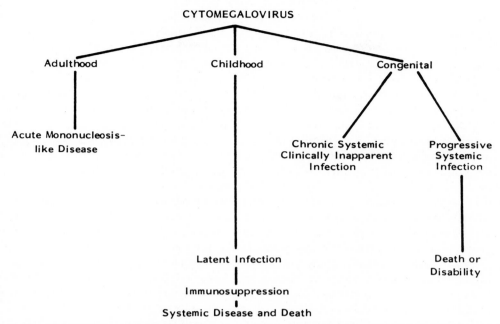

FIG. 10.10. Schema depicting the various forms of disease and central role of the viral persistent state in diseases caused by cytomegalovirus.

Our knowledge of the biological mechanism of persistence of cytomegalovirus is scant, but infection of both lymphoid elements and epithelial cells during clinical dormancy is likely. Although viral genetic material may be integrated with cellular DNA it is often possible to recover the virus from tissues of persons who lack evidence of infection if appropriate virological techniques are employed. Immunological modulation of viral activity seems apparent, but the means by which this is accomplished is obscure. For example, it is not known why generalized cytomegalic inclusion disease occurs in only an occasional infant, even though infection at the time of birth is a relatively common event. Occurrence of disseminated disease in adults also has its anachronistic features. In the older age group, overt infections develop either because a dormant infection is activated or a virus is introduced by a blood transfusion or organ graft. Thus, cytomegalovirus infections almost invariably occur in recipients of the immunosuppressive regimens employed in organ and bone marrow transplantation and are common in terminal Hodgkin's disease and other hematopoietic malignancies. Yet, they usually do not prove to be as imposing a clinical problem in patients receiving chemotherapy for solid tumors and in persons with a variety of heritable syndromes affecting both cellular and humoral mechanisms of immunity.

HEPATITIS B VIRUS, HEPATITIS, AND HEPATOCELLULAR CARCINOMA (5, 28)

Our understanding of the pathobiology of viral hepatitis has been in a state of rapid evolution during the past decade. We have now identified two viruses (HVA, HVB) that play an important etiologic role in the causation of the disease. In addition, one or more additional agents (nonA, nonB) also are believed to have an etiological importance. HVA, which appears to be a picornavirus, causes a relatively mild disease of limited duration. Persistent HVA infections are not known to occur. The second virus (HVB) falls into a new class of agents having genetic material comprised of DNA. It produces a disease of varying degrees of severity and often initiates a persistent state which may result in one or more of the following complications: (a) a chronic "carrier" state; (b) chronic hepatitis; and (c) postnecrotic cirrhosis. In addition, recent evidence strongly argues for a role of this agent in the pathogenesis of hepatocellular carcinoma.

A number of years ago, Blumberg and his colleagues (5) undertook studies of a "new" antigen in the blood serum of inhabitants of Oceania and Southeast Asia. This substance, later termed Australian antigen, proved to be the coat protein of HBV. Later work indicated that the HBV carrier state was commonly associated with a chronic infection of the liver. Although virus persistence is usually subclinical, members of population groups with a high rate of infection often experience chronic aggressive hepatitis and postnecrotic cirrhosis. In these same geographic areas, hepatocellular carcinoma is endemic.

During the past decade, numerous studies have been undertaken to assess the possible role of HBV in the pathogenesis of hepatoma. A strong association of the carrier state with the development of the disease is found both in hyperendemic areas of the world and in countries where the infection is sporadic. In addition, viral antigen has been identified frequently in liver tumors and in cells cultured from these lesions *in vitro*. Recent work has demonstrated the DNA genetic material of HVB integrated into the genome of hepatic tumor cells, an observation which argues for a possible role of the virus in neoplastic transformation.

There are many questions that remain to be resolved in this rapidly evolving story. At present it is not known why certain population groups are unusually predisposed to the infection, although environmental and genetic influences appear to affect the distribution of the virus and individual host susceptibility. The factors influencing the progression of the carrier state to chronic aggressive hepatitis with cellular destruction and cirrhosis also are incompletely defined. Recent studies referred to elsewhere in this chapter strongly suggest that the immunologic control mechanisms of the infected host are modulated by certain proteins elaborated by, and catabolized in, the liver. Thus, the fate of the chronically infected liver may be determined by some subtle but incompletely defined immunologic mechanism. Finally, it remains to be determined whether or not environmental factors other than infection contribute to the development of hepatocellular carcinoma in individuals with chronic HBV infections.

CONCLUDING REMARKS

During the course of a lifetime, man is infected with a wide variety of viruses. Some of these agents persist in tissues in a seemingly dormant state during convalescence, and indefinitely thereafter. Although the factors influencing the persistence of the infection have been the subject of intense clinical and laboratory investigation, we understand only in part the biologic influences that play a role in the development of the virus "carrier" state.

This short paper provides an overview of our knowledge regarding a number of important human diseases resulting from persistent infections. I have stressed the role of the host in viral dormancy and expression and have emphasized the contribution of immunologic factors which appear to modulate these conditions. In this review I have not considered the role of the host's genetic makeup and its effect on viral susceptibility. Regrettably, our understanding of these heritable factors in man is limited. Thus far little attention has been directed to an analysis of the pathogenetic characteristics of the etiologic agents and their unique properties. Although the biologic peculiarities of these so-called persistent viruses are of critical significance, our knowledge is limited almost exclusively to observations in animals and cell culture systems.

Scientists have available to them extraordinary tools to decipher the many biological secrets of the persistent viruses andtrthcoming in future years understanding at present is limited by our imagination and our ability to apply these tools to resolvable problems. Answers should be forthcoming in future years which will provide insight into the mysteries of these intriguing agents (13).

ACKNOWLEDGMENTS

This work was supported in part by USPHS Grant HL 22555. The author would like to express his gratitude to Sophie Hurst for typing this manuscript and to Dr. Linda M. McManus for her helpful comments.

REFERENCES

1. Adornato, B., and Lampert, P. Status spongiosus of nervous tissue: Electron microscopic studies. *Acta Neuropathol. 19:* 271–289, 1971.
2. Afroudakis, A. P., Liew, C. T., and Peters, R. L. An immunoperoxidase technique for the demonstration of hepatitis B surface antigen in human liver. *Am. J. Clin. Pathol. 65:* 533–540, 1976.
3. Bishop, J. M. The molecular biology of RNA tumor viruses: a physician's guide. *New Engl. J. Med. 303:* 675–681, 1980.
4. Bixler, G., and Booss, J. Establishment of immunologic memory concurrent with suppression of the primary immune response during acute cytomegalovirus infection of mice. *J. Immunol. 125:* 893–896, 1980.
5. Blumberg, S. S., and London, W. T. Hepatitis B virus and the prevalence of primary hepatocellular carcinoma. *New Engl. J. Med. 304:* 782–784, 1981.
6. Boettiger, D. Activation and repression of virus expression in mammalian cells infected by Rous sarcoma virus. *Symp. Quant. Biol.* 1169–1172, 1975.
7. Centiganto-Fitzgerald, Y. M., and Kaufman, H. E. Avirulent herpesvirus strains and ocular disease (abstract). *Fed. Proc. 40:* 777, 1981.
8. Chisari, F., Routenberg, J., Anderson, D., and Edgington, T. Cellular immune reactivity. In *JBV-induced Liver Disease in Viral Hepatitis.* Edited by G. Vyas, S. Cohen, and R. Schmid, pp. 245–266. Philadelphia, Franklin, 1978.
9. Coleman, D. V., Wolfendale, M. R., Daniel, R. A., Dhanjal, N. K., Gardner, S. D., Gibson, P. E., and Field, A. M. Infectious diseases: a prospective study of human polymavirus infection in pregnancy. *J. Infect. Dis. 142:* 1–8, 1980.
10. Craighead, J. E. Cytomegalovirus pulmonary disease. *Pathobiol. Ann. 5:* 197–220, 1975.
11. Craighead, J. E., Padgett, B. L., and Walker, D. L., unpublished data.
12. Davis, L. E., Bodian, D., Price, D., Butler, I. J., and Vickers, J. H. Chronic progressive poliomyelitis secondary to vaccination of an immunodeficient child. *New Engl. J. Med. 297:* 241–245, 1977.
13. U. S. Department of Health, Education and Welfare, *Persistent Viral Infections in Virology,* NIAID Task Force Report, Vol. III, Publication No. 79-1833.
14. de-The, G. Role of Epstein-Barr virus in human diseases: infectious mononucleosis, Burkitt's lymphoma, and Nasopharyngeal carcinoma. In *Viral Oncology.* edited by G. Klein, pp. 769–797. New York, Raven Press, 1980.

15. Dierks, R. E. Rabies pathogenesis and diagnosis. *J. Lab. Clin. Med. 94:* 1–4, 1979.
16. Eklund, C. M., Hadlow, W. J., and Kennedy, R. C. Some properties of the scrapie agent and its behavior in mice. *Proc. Soc. Exp. Biol. Med. 112:* 974–979, 1963.
17. Epstein, M. A., and Achong, B. G. The *Epstein-Barr Virus*. Edited by M. A. Epstein, and B. G. Achong. Heidelberg, Springer-Verlag, 1979.
18. Gordon, R. S. From the NIH: human wart virus found in many papillomas. *JAMA, 244:* 2041, 1980.
19. Hanshaw, J. B., and Dudgeon, J. A. Congenital cytomegalovirus. In *Viral Diseases of the Fetus and Newborn*. Edited by A. J. Schaffer, and M. Markowitz, pp. 97–152. Philadelphia, W. B. Saunders, 1978.
20. Hanshaw, J. B., and Dudgeon, J. A. Evidence for the viral etiology of congenital defects. In *Viral Diseases of the Fetus and Newborn*. Edited by A. J. Schaffer and M. Markowitz, pp. 10–96. Philadelphia, W. B. Saunders, 1978.
21. Hanshaw, J. B., and Dudgeon, J. A. Varicella-zoster infections. In *Viral Diseases of the Fetus and Newborn*. Edited by A. J. Schaffer and M. Markowitz, pp. 192–207. Philadelphia, W. B. Saunders, 1978.
22. Huang, E-S., Alford, C. A., Reynolds, D. W., Stagno, S., and Pass, R. F. Molecular epidemiology of cytomegalovirus infections in women and the infants. *New Engl. J. Med. 303:* 958–962, 1980.
23. Huang, S. N., and Groh, V. Immunoagglutination electron microscopic study on virus-like particles on Australian antigen in liver tissue. *Lab. Invest. 29:* 353–366, 1973.
24. Jenis, E. H. *et al.* Subacute sclerosing panencephalitis: immunoultrastructural localization of measles-virus antigen. *Arch. Pathol. 95:* 81–89, 1973.
25. Juel-Jensen, B. E., and MacCallum, F. O. Herpes simplex. In *Herpes Simplex, Varicella and Zoster*, Chap. 2, pp. 6–31. Philadelphia, J. B. Lippincott, 1972.
26. Kew, M. C. Hepatoma and the HBV. In *Viral Hepatitis*. Edited by G. N. Vyas, S. N. Cohen, and R. Schmid, pp. 439–450. Philadelphia, The Franklin Institute Press, 1978.
27. Larke, B. R. P., Wheatley, E., Saigal, S., and Chernesky, M. Congenital cytomegalovirus infection in an urban Canadian community. *J. Infect. Dis. 142:* 647–652, 1980.
28. Loh, L., and Hudson, J. B. Immunosuppressive effect of murine cytomegalovirus. *Infect. Immunol. 27*(1): 54–60, 1980.
29. Masters, C. L., Gajdusek, D. C. and Gibbs, Jr., C. J. The spongiform encephalopathies: the natural history of Creutzfeldt-Jakob disease and its relationship to kuru and scrapie. In *Search for the Cause of Multiple Sclerosis and Other Chronic Diseases of the Central Nervous System*. Proceedings of the First International Symposium of the Hertie Foundation. Edited by A. Boese, Frankfurt/Main, Verlag Chemie, Weinheim, September 1979, 1980.
30. Monif, G. R., and Dische, R. M. Viral placentitis in congenital cytomegalovirus infection. *Am. J. Clin Pathol. 58:* 445–449, 1972.
31. Murphy, F. A. Rabies pathogenesis: brief review. *Arch. Virol. 54:* 279–297, 1977.
32. Nagashima, K., Nakazawa, M., Endo, H., Kurata, T., and Aoyama, Y. Pathology of the human spinal ganglia in varicella-zoster virus infection. *Acta Neuropathol. 33:* 106–117, 1975.
33. Nahmias, A. J., and Josey, W. E. Epidemiology of Herpes Simplex Viruses 1 and 2. In *Viral Infections of Humans: Epidemiology and Control*. Edited by A. S. Evans, pp. 253–272. New York, Plenum Publishing Corporation, 1976.
34. Openshaw, H., Puga, A., and Notkins, A. L. Herpes simplex virus infection in sensory ganglia: immune control, latency, and reactivation. *Fed. Proc. 38:* 2660–2664, 1979.
35. Oyanagi, S., terMeulen, V., Muller, D., Katz, M., and Koprowski, H. Electron microscopic observations in subacute sclerosing panencephalitis brain cell cultures: their correlation with cytochemical and immunocytological findings. *J. Virol. 6:* 370–379, 1970.
36. Padgett, B. L., and Walker, D. L. Natural history of human polyomavirus infections. In *Persistent Viruses*. Edited by J. Stevens, G. Todaro, and C. F. Fox, pp. 751–757. New York, Academic Press, 1978.
37. Padgett, B. L., Walker, D. L., ZuRhein, G. M., Hodach, A. E., and Chou, S. M. J. C. papovavirus in progressive multifocal leukoencephalopathy. *J. Infect. Dis. 133:* 686–690, 1976.
38. Panem, S., and Reynolds, J. Retrovirus expression in normal and pathogenic processes of man. *Fed. Proc. 38:* 2674–2680, 1979.
39. Pass, R. F. *et al.* Outcome of symptomatic congenital cytomegalovirus infection: results of long-term longitudinal follow-up. *Pediatrics 66:* 758–762, 1980.

40. Richardson, E. P., Jr. Progressive multifocal leukoencephalopathy. *N. Engl. J. Med. 265:* 815–823, 1961.
41. Rowson, K. E., and Mahy, B. W. Human papova (wart) virus. *Bacteriol. Rev. 31:* 110–131, 1967.
42. Scullard, G. H., Robinson, W. S., Merigan, T. C., and Gregory, P. B. The effect of immunosuppressive therapy on hepatitis B viral infection in patients with chronic hepatitis. *Gastroenterology 77:* 40, 1978.
43. Seemayer, T. A., Oligny, L. L., and Gardner, J. The Epstein-Barr virus. In *Perspectives in Pediatric Pathology*, Vol. 6, edited by H. S. Rosenberg and J. Bernstein, pp. 1–48. New York, Masson Publishing, 1981.
44. Sigurdsson, B. Maedi, a slow progressive pneumonia of sheep: an epizoological and a pathological study. *Br. Vet. J. 110:* 255–271, 1954.
45. Sigurdsson, B., Palsson, P. A., and Grimson, H. Visna, a demyelinating transmissable disease of sheep. *J. Neuropathol. Exp. Neurol. 16:* 389–403, 1957.
46. Sissons, J. G., and Oldstone, M. B. Killing of virus-infected cells: the role of antiviral antibody and complement in limiting virus infection. *J. Infect. Dis. 142:* 442–448, 1980.
47. Sissons, J. G. P., and Oldstone, M. B. Killing of virus-infected cells by cytotoxic lymphocytes. *J. Infect. Dis. 142:* 114–119, 1980.
48. Stagno, S., Reynolds, D., Tsiantos, A., Fuccillo, D. A., Smith, R., Tiller, M., and Alford, C. A. Cervical cytomegalovirus excretion in pregnant and non-pregnant women: suppression in early gestation. *J. Infect. Dis. 131:* 522–527, 1975.
49. Stern, H., and Tucker, S. M. Prospective study of cytomegalovirus infection in pregnancy. *Br. Med. J. 2:* 269–270, 1973.
50. Stevens, J. G. Latent herpes simplex and the nervous system. *Curr. Top. Microbiol. Immunol. 70:* 31–48, 1975.
51. Townsend, J. J. *et al.* Progressive rubella panencephalitis: late onset after congenital rubella. *N. Engl. J. Med. 292:* 990–998, 1975.
52. Walker, D. L. Progressive multifocal keukoencephalopathy: an opportunistic viral infection of the central nervous system. In *Handbook of Clinical Neurology*, Vol. 34, Part II, Chap. 16, edited by P. J. Vinken and G. W. Bruyn, pp. 307–329. New York, North Holland, 1978.
53. Weiner, L. S., Howell, J. T., Langford, M. P., Stanton, G. J., Baron, S., Goldblum, R. M., Lord, R. A., and Goldman, A. S. Effect of specific antibodies on chronic echovirus type 5 encephalitis in a patient with hypogammaglobulinemia. *J. Infect. Dis. 140:* 858–863, 1979.
54. Weller, T. H., and Hanshaw, J. B. Virologic and clinical observations on cytomegalic inclusion disease. *N. Engl. J. Med. 266:* 1233–1244, 1962.
55. Wenckebach, G. F., and Curry, B. Cytomegalovirus infection of the female genital tract: histologic findings in three cases and review of the literature. *Arch Pathol. Lab. Med. 100:* 609–612, 1976.
56. Wilfert, C. M., Buckley, R. H., Mohanakumar, T., Griffith, J. F., Katz, S. L., Whisnant, J. K., Eggleston, P. A., Moore, M., Treadwell, E., Oxman, M. N. and Rosen, F. S. Persistent and fatal central nervous-system echovirus infections in patients with agammaglobulinemia. *N. Engl. J. Med. 296:* 1485–1490, 1977.
57. Wolinsky, J. S., Berg, B. O., and Meitland, C. J. Progressive rubella panencephalitis. *Arch. Neurol. 33:* 722–723, 1976.
58. Wyatt, H. V. Poliomyelitis in hypogammaglobulinemics. *J. Infect. Dis. 128:* 802–806, 1973.

Chapter 11

The Biology of Viral Hepatitis*, †

EVGENYA ZHKARINSKY AND EMANUEL RUBIN

During the last three centuries, infectious disease of the liver has been alluded to by terms such as epidemic jaundice, infectious jaundice, benign jaundice, catarrhal jaundice. The description of epidemic jaundice in the Hippocratic writings (*De Internis Affectionibus*) was pointed out by Cockayne (40) in 1912. According to Sherlock (263) the earliest record in Western Europe is in a letter by Pope Zacharias to St. Boniface (751 A.D.). It is worth noting that several other infections associated with jaundice, *e.g.*, Weil's disease (leptospirosis), yellow fever, sepsis, and relapsing fever due to infection with *Borrelia recurrentis* could have been included under the umbrella of infectious jaundice. Virchow coined the term "catarrhal jaundice" to designate any jaundice not explained by mechanical obstruction of the bile duct. The views of Bamberger and of Virchow in 1865, ascribing jaundice to catarrh of the duodenum and common bile duct, suggested mechanical obstruction as the cause of jaundice (307). In the 19th and early 20th centuries, this concept was challenged by some investigators who suggested that epidemic and sporadic jaundice were caused by an infectious hepatotropic agent. Although a viral etiology was suggested as early as 1908 (198), the concept of catarrhal jaundice persisted at least until 1940.

Clinical observations had previously suggested at least two types of hepatitis which were morphologically indistinguishable. One was recognized to have a short incubation period, a high rate of contagion, and a fecal-oral route of transmission. By contrast, another type of hepatitis, having a longer incubation period and being less contagious, was reported as early as 1885 among shipyard workers who had been inoculated with smallpox vaccine prepared from glycerinated human lymph (177). This so-called serum hepatitis, postvaccinal hepatitis, or transfusion jaundice was thought to be transmitted only parenterally, *e.g.*, by blood transfusion or contaminated needles.

The greatest incidence of long incubation hepatitis occurred among patients who were treated for venereal diseases (134, 160, 208), diabetes (100, 305),

---

* This work was supported in part by Grant AA 3442.

† The following abbreviations are used in this review: HB, hepatitis B; HA, hepatitis A; NANB hepatitis, non-A, non-B hepatitis; HBV, hepatitis B virus; HAV, hepatitis A virus; HBsAg, hepatitis B surface antigen; HBcAg, hepatitis B core antigen; HBeAg, hepatitis B "e" antigen; HAAg, hepatitis A antigen; anti-HBs, hepatitis B surface antibody; anti-HBc, hepatitis B core antibody; anti-HBe, hepatitis B "e" antibody; anti-HA, hepatitis A antibody; PHC, primary hepatocellular carcinoma.

tuberculosis, and rheumatoid arthritis (109). After the introduction of new vaccines, postvaccinal jaundice was noted to increase among those vaccinated against yellow fever (80, 83) and sand-fly fever (270). The use of convalescent serum for treatment or prevention of infectious diseases culminated in the occurrence of epidemics among military personnel. It occurred with prior administration of pooled measles (237) and mumps (18) convalescent serums. Almost half of American soldiers who received mumps convalescent serum developed icterus (18). In 1945, 23% of all cases of viral hepatitis in USA army hospitals were plasma-associated (261). Outbreaks of serum hepatitis also occurred among children inoculated with measles or mumps convalescent serum. In 1946, Nefe and coworkers (212) proposed the names "infectious" and "serum" hepatitis, terms which remained in general use until a decade ago.

Many of the initial studies relating to the etiology of hepatitis were stimulated by the fact that hepatitis was an important military problem. The repeated failures to propagate specific viruses led to human transmission studies from the 1940s to the early 1960s (110, 178, 212, 225). In 1947 Mac Callum proposed that the terms "infectious hepatitis virus" and "serum hepatitis virus" be replaced by "hepatitis virus A" and "hepatitis virus B" (76, 178). However, it was not until the discovery of the Australia antigen by Blumberg and his colleagues (23) in the early 1960s that the virus of hepatitis B (HB) was identified. This antigen, discovered in the serum of an Australian aborigine during an unrelated study on genetically determined protein polymorphism, reacted with antibody from a multiply transfused patient with hemophilia. The antigen, which was also demonstrated in patients with Down's syndrome and viral hepatitis, was later associated exclusively with type B hepatitis (223, 234).

At about the same time, Krugman *et al.* (152) demonstrated two types of infectious hepatitis by inoculating serum from infected individuals into institutionalized mentally retarded children, who almost invariably contracted the disease spontaneously. The short incubation type, designated MS-1, proved to be hepatitis A (HA), and the long incubation variety, MS-2, was later shown to be HB (92).

The availability of sera infective for HA and HB provided the opportunity to demonstrate that HB could be spread not only by direct parenteral exposure but also from person to person through intimate contact, *e.g.*, oral or venereal ((153). Since the inactivated MS-2 serum was antigenic but noninfectious, it was a potential source of antigen for the development of an inactivated HB vaccine (154, 155).

Despite the advances in understanding HB, there was a consistent failure to visualize the virus responsible for HA, a malady documented only by the demonstration of infectivity of sera from patients with HA in marmosets (119, 152, 239). In 1973, this virus was demonstrated by immune electron microscopy following incubation of stool filtrates from patients with HA convalescent serum (63, 77). In 1975 a simple method to detect anti-HA was developed, namely, the immune adherence hemagglutination test, using HAV antigen derived from liver homogenates of infected marmosets (240) or human stool (204). Subsequently, a microtiter assay for HAV antigen (245) and the enzyme-linked immunoabsorbent assay (ELISA) became widely used (310). These techniques are based on modifications of similar radioimmunoassays for the detection of hepatitis B surface antigen (HBsAG) and hepatitis B central core antigen (HBcAg). Currently a highly specific competitive inhibition radioimmunoassay test kit and a sandwich solid-phase radioimmunoassaay for IgM anti-HAV are commercially available (186).

Despite the ability to detect HBsAG in blood used for transfusions, the incidence of transfusion-associated hepatitis was reduced only 25–30% (1). Hepatitis B virus (HBV) now accounts for less than 10% of transfusion-related hepatitis (96). Of the 3 million Americans who receive transfusions each year, 0.7% still develop hepatitis. About 90% of these new cases of hepatitis are negative for markers of HA or HB viruses, or other viruses that occasionally produce liver disease. This third major cause of viral hepatitis, diagnosed by serological exclusion, has been designated non-A,non-B (NANB) hepatitis.

There are other viruses capable of causing liver disease. Some are hepatotropic, *e.g.*, yellow fever virus and Epstein-Barr virus. Others, such as herpesvirus, cytomegalovirus, and rubella virus may be associated with hepatitis, in congenital as well as in postnatal forms. This review will be limited to HB, HA, and NANB hepatitis.

HEPATITIS B

Although it is generally accepted that the incubation period of HB is 60–180 days, this interval depends on the dose of viral inoculum and the route of exposure. For instance, in one study it varied from 29 to 43 days after parenteral inoculation and from 68 to 81 days after oral exposure (153). The larger the dose of the virus, the shorter the incubation period and the time of appearance of HBsAG in serum (15). Krugman *et al.* (158) demonstrated HBsAG as early as 6 days after parenteral exposure to HBV.

Jaundice may or may not herald the onset of clinical HB. Studies of Krugman and Giles (155) indicate that anicteric mild infection occurs more frequently among children. They usually have mild or inapparent symptoms and exhibit only slight elevation of the serum transaminase activity. In icteric hepatitis, symptoms usually gradually diminish after jaundice appears. There is a correlation between the depth of jaundice (in most cases, the maximum concentration of bilirubin is less than 10 mg/dl) (290) and the severity of symptoms. The serum transaminase activity may reach 2000 IU/ml in the first week following the appearance of symptoms. The liver displays lobular inflammatory, degenerative, and regenerative changes, all of which seem to be present simultaneously. Degenerative changes most commonly are represented by swelling and ballooning of the cytoplasm of hepatocytes, and hepatocytolysis, which eventually leads to the drop-out necrosis of liver cells (180). Acidophilic bodies, *i.e.*, round, refractile, and eosinophilic structures, are remnants of necrotic hepatocytes extruded into the sinusoidal spaces (142). These "Councilman-like" bodies are not absolutely specific for viral hepatitis, but when severe, suggest this diagnosis (35). The presence of mitotic figures and bi- and trinucleated liver cells indicates regeneration. The severity of cholestasis, which is variable, is usually mild and is most prominent in the perivenular area (zone 3 of Rappaport) (249). Because degeneration and regeneration in the liver are concomitant, the architecture of the liver remains unchanged. The inflammatory infiltrate is composed predominantly of lymphocytes, with a few segmented leukocytes and plasma cells. The presence of plasma cells should not be misinterpreted as evidence of chronic hepatitis (265). Universal triaditis, with a tendency to extension into the adjacent parenchyma, is characteristic.

Occasionally, the predominant manifestations of HB are cholestatic, that is, they mimic extrahepatic biliary obstruction. The moorphologic features include extensive bile retention in the cytoplasm of hepatocytes and Kupffer cells, and bile plugs in dilated canaliculi.

In most cases of HB, the disease begins to subside within 3–4 weeks. In this stage of resolving or subsiding hepatitis, inflammatory cells tend to disappear from the lobules and are confined to the portal tracts, which show a well-defined limiting plate (54). Clumps of macrophages and Kupffer cells with prominent phagocytic activity in sinusoids, variation in liver cell size, and acidophilic bodies may persist for some time (227). Complete clinical recoveery occurs in 80% of cases of HB in 3–4 months, and in an additional 10–15% of patients in 6 months (139).

Acute hepatitis with bridging necrosis (subacute hepatic necrosis, subacute hepatitis, impaired regeneration syndrome, submassive necrosis, bridging necrosis) (228) is a more severe form of acute viral hepatitis, in which the typical initial symptoms and findings are prolonged and in which the malady becomes progressively debilitating. The names "subacute hepatitis" or "hepatic necrosis" are confusing because they are often applied to changes in chronic active hepatitis (28, 283) and may have prognostic implications in this condition. Since the definitive diagnostic procedure is a liver biopsy, it seems preferable to use the term "acute hepatitis with bridging necrosis."

In this variant of HB, extensive confluent necrosis involves the central and midzones (zones 3 and 2 of Rappaport (249)). Collapse and condensation of the reticulin framework result in thin septa or bridges. Areas of necrosis connect vascular structures, producing central-central and central-portal bridging (28, 146, 266). In one study, death occurred in 19%, and cirrhosis developed in 37% (28).

Rarely, patients with acute viral hepatitis develop a fulminant course (251); HBV has been reported to account for 40–50% of such patients (84, 190). In such cases, 1 or 2 weeks after the onset of symptoms, acute hepatic failure develops, manifested by deep jaundice, encephalopathy, and coma. Few patients survive fulminant hepatitis, the mortality being reported as 65–80%. The liver typically displays confluent necrosis affecting all zones of the lobules. Lobular collapse, with prominence or reticulum framework, is common. Spaces of Disse and sinusoids contain necrotic debris, scavenger cells, and red blood cells. Mild to moderate inflammatory reaction is present. Scattered small groups of regenerating cells, frequently arranged in duct-like structures adjacent to the portal areas, are observed. In addition proliferated ductules, or "neocholangioles" (229), are often prominent. Those patients who survive fulminant hepatitis (128, 141) may display a "postnecrotic" (multilobular, irregular) cirrhosis, but others regain a normal liver (42).

One of the characteristics of HB, as opposed to HA, is the occasional progression to chronic disease. Approximately 10% of patients develop chronic viral hepatitis (213, 252), of which two types are distinguished, clinically and morphologically. These are chronic persistent hepatitis, a condition with a generally good prognosis, and chronic active hepatitis, the more severe disorder, which occurs 2–3 times less often than the former (252). Chronic active hepatitis should be considered after about 6 months of continuing symptoms and should not be overdiagnosed within a few months of the onset of acute hepatitis.

Progression from acute to chronic hepatitis is likely in patients whose biopsies show combined features of acute and chronic active hepatitis (20, 180, 264). Histologically, the principal diagnostic feature of chronic active hepatitis is a portal inflammatory reaction involving the periportal parenchyma (20, 232). The limiting plate is irregular as a result of the loss of periportal hepatocytes and their replacement by lymphocytes and plasma cells (51, 232). In severe forms bridging necrosis also occurs (27), and portal-to-central bridging may insidiously progress to cirrhosis (20), a process which may require 2–5 years. Membrane-associated HBsAG in the cytoplasm and HBcAG in the nucleus of hepatocytes have been particularly related to the development of chronic hepatitis B (22, 102, 250, 315). Because the activity of serum transaminase and other laboratory values does not necessarily correlate with the progression of chronic active hepatitis (202), liver biopsy remains the best procedure to evaluate the nature and extent of the liver disease. These two conditions must be distinguished from the chronic viral carrier state and are defined as primary inflammatory diseases of the liver with a prolonged clinical course, usually persisting for more than 6 months, and with laboratory and/or histologic evidence of hepatocellular damage (20, 41, 262). Chronic hepatitis may be a sequel to other diseases such as NANB viral hepatitis, alcohol- and drug-induced hepatitis, Wilson's disease, and autoimmune hepatitis (95, 180, 181, 284).

In contrast to chronic active hepatitis, chronic persistent hepatitis is generally self limited. The portal tracts exhibit chronic inflammation and expansion, but the lobular architecture is preserved, the limiting plate is sharp, and the liver parenchyma, normal. Restoration of normal structure and function is the rule.

HEPATITIS B VIRUS

The highly species-specific hepatitis B virus belongs to a group of enveloped DNA viruses which exhibit a unique antigenic structure and genetically heterogeneous DNA capable of producing liver disease in man, chimpanzees, woodchucks, and a few other species. No cell culture in which hepatitis B virus can be propagated is presently known.

Morphologic Structure

HBV, as visualized by electron microscopy, is a 42-nm (48) double-coated particle, which is a complete infective virion (8), and was originally named the Dane particle. Of the two smaller particles, the most numerous are spherical, with diameters ranging from 16 to 25 nm. Elongated filamentous forms, with a diameter of 22 nm and a length ranging up to several hundred nm, are also seen. The latter two forms represent the incomplete viral coat, presumably a result of overproduction of coat proteins by the infected cell.

The complete virus consists of an outer lipoprotein coat and an inner 27-nm core particle. The core contains hepatitis B virus-specific DNA polymerase (257) and circular, predominantly double-stranded DNA, with a molecular weight of 1.6×10^6 daltons (123, 256). One strand is approximately 3200 nucleotide bases in length, and its 3′ and 5′ ends are not covalently bound. The other DNA strand is incomplete for a variable portion of its length (1700 to 2800 nucleotides (258, 287). This single-stranded region in the circular DNA molecule accounts for about one-fourth of its length (129). The DNA polymerase appears to use the short strand as a primer to fill the single-stranded gap. This reaction is probably necessary to initiate replication of the virus and may relate to possible integration of the viral DNA into host DNA (114).

The antigenic determinants of HBV appear to be specified by the hepatitis viral genome. The complete virion contains two main antigens, the hepatitis B surface antigen (HBsAg), also known as Australia antigen, expressed on the outer lipoprotein coat of the Dane particles, and the central core antigen (HBcAg), which is expressed on the internal core particle and can be released from the virion by treatment with detergents.

The three forms of HBsAg share common group-specific determinants, designated "a," on their surfaces (8). HBsAg also shares subtype-specific determinations, designated HBsAg/adr, HBsAg/ayr, HBsAg/adw, and HBsAg/ayw (14). HBsAg contains lipid (145), carbohydrates (276), and proteins (255). Seven polypeptides ranging from 23,000 to 97,000 daltons were observed in purified prepartions of HBsAg (272). The isolated polypeptides stimulated both group-specific and subtype-specific antibodies to HBsAg, suggesting that they contain viral-specific determinants (68, 271).

The major polypeptide of HBcAg is approximately 17,000 (31) to 19,000 (130) molecular weight. The combined weights of the polypeptides from HBsAg and HBcAg exceed the coding capacity of the small HBV genome, and the amount of virus-specified unique gene product in these structures may be limited.

Two other HBV-related antigens have been described. The "e" antigen (HBeAg), first described in 1972 by Magnius and Espmark (182), now appears to have several antigenic determinants, HBe_1Ag, HBe_2Ag, and HBe_3Ag (312). The true nature of the antigen and the structural relationship with the hepatitis B virus are unclear. Four major polypeptides with molecular weights of 23,000, 27,000, 50,000, and 70,000 daltons were identified in HBeAg. This soluble antigen is found only in serum that also contains HBsAg (182). It is not detectable either on the surface or the core of the Dane particle, but some evidence exists to support the concept that there is, at least, partial viral specification of HBeAg (302). HBeAg has been related to HBsAg, albumin (166), an albumin-binding component, and lactic dehydrogenase isoenzyme, LDH-5ex (309). A relationship of HBeAg to the forementioned substances may be indirect, as in the case of an additional isoenzyme, LDH-5ex, detected in HBeAg-positive sera. Although there is a strong correlation between HBeAg and LDH-5ex, the latter is identical neither with HBeAg nor the HB virus. HBeAg may act as a ligand in serum, attaching to several normal serum proteins (309). Recent data suggest that HBeAg may be a metabolic breakdown product of the HBV core (319).

Another recently described antigen associated with hepatitis B is the delta antigen, demonstrated by immunofluorescence in the nuclei of hepatocytes in biopsies of patients with HBsAg-positive chronic hepatitis. However, HBcAg and HBsAg were not found on electron microscopy in this case (54, 253). The significance of these findings are not yet clear.

HEPATITIS B SEROLOGIC EVENTS

The sequence of the appearance and disappearance of various antigens and antibodies in the serum of patients infected with HBV has come from experimental infections of volunteers (116, 209) and individuals with high risks of hepatitis (158). Approximately 30–40% of infected adults develop acute clinically apparent disease. In this type of HB, HBsAg appears in the serum during the late incubation period, about 1–4 weeks after exposure to HBV, well before the onset of serum biochemical changes, symptoms, and jaundice. The antigen persists for 3–6 months, but generally peaks in titer simultaneously with the peak of biochemical and clinical manifestations of disease; it disappears with recovery. Antibody to HBsAg (anti-HBs) appears during convalescence (161). There may be a gap of 1–2 months, during which time neither HBsAg nor anti-HBs is detected. In a small percentage of cases, anti-HBs never develops, and the patient remains a carrier of HBV. Anti-HBs is considered a serologic marker of recovery and immunity. Antibody to HBcAg (anti-HBc) appears and rises quickly in titer at the onset of disease, usually 2–4 weeks after the appearance of HBsAg. It is detectable in all patients with acute HB (124, 158). Both anti-HBs and anti-HBc may persist indefinitely. During the gap between the disappearance of HBsAg and the detectability of anti-HBs, the only serologic marker of the disease may be the presence of anti-HBc. As detected by radioimmunoassay, HBeAg appears at the same time or shortly after HBsAg, but disappears well before appearance of HBsAg. After a variable period, from a few days to a few months, anti-HBe is found and may persist up to several years.

The majority (50–60%) of those exposed to HBV have asymptomatic subclinical infection. These patients have HBsAg in the serum for a brief period (approximately 2 weeks). The development of high and sustained titers of anti-HBs and low and sometimes transient titers of anti-HBc follows quickly (124, 158, 161). Biochemical changes of hepatitis are minimal or absent, and lasting immunity results; 5–10% of adults who manifest HB develop a chronic carrier state for HBsAg. Strictly speaking, the term "carrier" has been reserved for individuals who have neither symptoms nor significant liver disease. Because of natural history, clinical course, and serology of the chronic HBsAg carrier state, two main types are distinguished; one is the asymptomatic serological carrier with HBsAg in the blood, normal liver function tests (127, 277), and essentially normal liver biopsy (with the exception of the presence of "ground-glass" hepatocytes containing HBsAg). The second type comprises asymptomatic and symptomatic patients with altered liver function tests and histological alterations of chronic persistent or chronic active hepatitis. The histopathologic feature common to both types of chronic HBsAg carriers is the presence of "ground-glass" hepatocytes (180, 277), *i.e.*, cells which contain HBsAg (108). Ground glass hepatocytes are larger than normal and have smooth, uniform, pale eosinophilic cytoplasm and nuclei frequently displaced toward the periphery. In chronic asymptomatic carriers, ground-glass cells are present in clusters, whereas in patients with chronic hepatitis and cirrhosis, the distribution is irregular (87).

In the persistent HBsAg carrier, shortly after exposure to HBV, HBsAg appears in the serum, rises to high titers, and persists. HBeAg accompanies HBsAg, typically in high titer (158, 214). Anti-HBc is detected early and persists in high and sustained titer (124). The persistance of high titers of anti-HBc is a characteristic feature of chronic infection with HBV. In some instances, HBV carriers also contain large amounts of HBcAg; this is more frequent in carriers with chronic active or chronic persistent hepatitis (297). In such cases, anti-HBs is not detected. This does not imply that anti-HBs is not produced, but if it is, it is in the form of immune complexes. At any rate, the antibody response is not sufficient to clear the virus. This period of chronic hepatitis can last less than a year to a decade or more. The asymptomatic "healthy" carrier state coincides with the disappearance of serum HBeAg and the appearance of anti-HBe. Other markers of the virus, such as DNA-polymerase activity, HBV DNA, and serum Dane particles, decrease in amount, or disappear. In acute cases, the presence of HBeAg indicates early and active infection and correlates well with infectivity of the blood (207, 222), while the seroconversion to anti-HBe is a sign of the beginning of the disease resolution and protection against infection with HBV (222).

In chronic HBsAg-positive states, the presence of HBeAg or anti-HBe has important clinical and serologic correlations. The presence of anti-HBe indicates a low level of infectivity (12, 17, 182, 222, 226,, 273). HBsAg carriers positive for HBeAg tend to be young, to have had a recent onset of the carrier state, to have elevated transaminasees, and to have active liver disease. Carriers with anti-HBe are usually older, have been carriers for a long time, and have normal liver function tests and inactive liver disease (120, 214, 300). Chronic HBsAg and HBcAg-positive mothers transmit type B hepatitis to their newborns. By contrast, anti-HBe-positive mothers rarely transmit the disease (17, 222). Serum levels of HBeAg and anti-HBe closely correlate with those of the HBV-specific DNA polymerase, increased activity of which indicates that viral replication continues. Currently, the HBeAg and anti-HBe tests are recommended for all individuals positive for HBsAg. This includes individuals with HB who may transmit the disease to sexual partners, dialysis patients, infected health care personnel, pregnant women, and others in potentially infectious environments.

INTERPRETATION OF SEROLOGIC MARKERS

Various combinations of HBV markers in the serum are helpful in the diagnosis of the state of the disease. The most common is the combination of serum HBsAg and anti-HBc, which occurs in acute HB and in the chronic HBsAg carrier state. Serologic markers alone do not differentiate acute from chronic HB. Although it has been suggested that determination of anti-HBc titer, which should be low or moderate in early HB and high in the chronic carrier state (17, 121), is useful, this differentiation usually requires clinical and biochemical or histologic evaluation (34, 90). HBsAg uncommonly may be present alone. This may occur in the early presymptomatic period of acute HB. The combination of anti-HBs and anti-HBc indicates full recovery and immunity to HB. Patients with that combination cannot transmit HBV. The interpretation of the presence of anti-HBc alone, without HBsAg and anti-HBs, depends on the titer of anti-HBc in the serum. Low titers of IgG anti-HBc are found in individuals who had remote HBV infections. High titers of anti-HBc usually are found in persons who have recently had either acute HB and are in the immediate convalescence period (the "gap"), or are in the resolution of the chronic HBsAg carrier state. In later cases, infection with the virus persists, but production of HBsAg is at undetectable levels. Patients with high titers of anti-HBc alone are potentially infectious for HB (122). Rare patients may have anti-HBs in the absence of anti-HBc. The interpretation of this pattern is also dual. It occurs in individuals who have had subclinical HB long before the antibodies were found and in people who have been immunized with HBsAg (125, 158) or have become immunized as a result of environmental exposure (67) and thus have never been infected with HBV (112, 113, 157, 193, 244).

TISSUE MARKERS OF HBV

HBsAg and HBcAg have been demonstrated in hepatocytes using specific fluoresceinated antibodies, by the peroxidase-antiperoxidase method in frozen or formalin-fixed tissues (88, 130, 256), and by electron microscopy. HBsAg gives positive fluorescence of the cytoplasm of hepatocytes, particularly in ground glass liver cells, plasma membranes (88, 132, 256), and sometimes Kupffer cells (33). The same pattern of distribution of HBsAg is seen using simple histochemical stains such as the Shikata (orcein), Gomori's aldehyde fuchsin, aldehyde thionine (149), and a modified trichrome (101). However, discrete linear membrane localization of HBsAg, demonstrated by immunofluorescence and by the peroxidase-antiperoxidase method (130), cannot be seen with current histochemical procedures. Hepatocytes containing HBsAg are often found in chronic carriers without significant hepatocellular damage (34, 101, 317) and in immunosuppressed patients with mild chronic persistent hepatitis (218, 230). There seems to be an inverse correlation between the number of HBsAg-bearing hepatocytes and the severity of hepatocellular injury (15, 34, 230, 250, 284).

HBcAg is found in the nuclei of hepatocytes. Small amounts of HBcAg have been identified in the perinuclear cytoplasm and diffusely in the cytoplasm, sparing the nuclei (250), but the significance of the latter pattern is unclear. Excessive accumulation of HBcAg in the nuclei can be appreciated in routine H&E stains as eosinophilic inclusions, which do not stain with orcein, PAS, and Feulgen stains (20). The only reliable method for detection of the HBcAg is the immunohistochemical technique, which gives a mild granular nuclear and cytoplasmic pattern by specific immunofluorescence.

ELECTRON MICROSCOPY

HBV has been extensively studied by ordinary transmission (11, 86, 132) and immune electron microscopy (131–133). In tissue sections HBsAg consists of 20–30 nm diameter filamentous structures of various lengths, which are in the cisternae of the endoplasmic reticulum. In cross-section, these filaments measure 20–35 nm in diameter and display electron-dense centers (88). Particles of HBcAg, located primarily in the nuclei of the hepatocytes, are spherules composed of capsomeres and 7–10 nm spikes, organized in an icosahedral symmetry (115).

Clusters of uncoated particles of core antigen are also seen along the nuclear membranes or associated with the rough endoplasmic reticulum.

IMMUNE THEORIES OF HB

In HB, the cells harboring the virus show little evidence of cell damage. This suggests that host-determined genetic and immunologic factors may be responsible for elimination of the virus and that infected cells or immunologic reactions may be the cause of the liver cell damage (72). There is no convincing evidence to support the role of genetic factors in the pathogenesis of HB, but there is an abundance of studies demonstrating a variety of alterations involving immunologic reactions in association with HB. Because of absence of methods for propagation of HBV and, therefore, of the possibility to study the infected cells *in vitro*, definitive evidence that cellular immunity is involved in the pathogenesis of viral hepatitis is lacking. Since the data are derived from patients studied after the onset of symptoms, it is difficult to be certain whether the immune response causes or results from HB.

There is a striking decrease in T lymphocytes in the peripheral blood in acute HB (38, 55, 203) and in HBsAg-positive chronic active hepatitis (40a, 260). However, a similar decrease in circulating T lymphocytes has been found in chronic active hepatitis unrelated to HB and in alcoholic hepatitis (6, 40a, 203, 260).

Little or no change in the number of circulating B lymphocytes has been reported in most studies. On the other hand, the appearance of an increased number of "null" cells, which do not display markers of T or B lymphocytes, occurs in the majority of cases, a finding which correlates with the decrease in circulating T cells. A normal number of circulating T lymphocytes in acute and chronic HB was demonstrated with neuraminidase-treated sheep red blood cells (38). Therefore, the reduced number of E rosette-forming T lymphocytes in HB may reflect a functional alteration of T cell metabolism.

Two distinct mechanisms for defective rosette formation in HB have been implicated. An "extrinsic" reversible mechanism, in which serum from patients with HB inhibits rosette function of normal T cells by means of a rosette inhibitory factor (RIF) (36), and an "intrinsic" defect in the capacity of T cells from patients with HB to stimulate rosette formation (72). It has been claimed that the persistence of RIF is associated with chronic active hepatitis caused by HBV (37, 38). However, the same findings are reported in HA and NANB hepatitis (38).

Diminished responsiveness of stimulation of cellular DNA synthesis by phytohemagglutinin (PHA) is observed in viral (217), neoplastic (97), and hepatic diseases, including acute and chronic HB (4). In acute cases PHA reactivity is reduced, but returns to normal after the first 2 weeks of disease (94, 318). It is normal in the healthy carrier state, but is persistently suppressed in patients with chronic active HB.

Specific cellular immune reactivity to HBsAg, shown by leukocyte migration inhibition and lymphocyte transformation techniques, correlates with sensitization of lymphocytes to antigens of HBV (71, 75, 135–137, 164, 165, 299). A high incidence of cellular sensitization to HBsAg has been demonstrated in acute and recovered HB, and in chronic active hepatitis. The incidence of cellular immune responses is negligible in cases of chronic persistent hepatitis, in asymptomatic carriers of HBV, and in controls. It should be noted that cellular immune responses have also been reported in 58% of patients with chronic active hepatitis whose serum is negative for HBsAg (164).

The pathogenetic significance of cellular sensitization to HBsAg is not yet clear. Studies of lymphocyte reactivity *in vitro* give limited information, since only sensitization to a specific antigen can be recognized. The high incidence of sensitization among healthy convalescents suggests that cellular reactivity to HBsAg may not be sufficient by itself to induce hepatocellular damage. There is no coexistence of cellular reactivity to HBsAg with the expression of HBsAg at the surface membrane of the hepatocytes in HBsAg-positive chronic hepatitis (127). It was recently suggested that the antibody response to HBsAg may suppress the surface expression and synthesis of HBV (72). Suppression of surface expression of HBsAg would then affect hepatocellular susceptibility to HBsAg-specific cellular attack systems. Suppression of viral synthesis would determine the development of the chronic carrier state. Thus, the humoral immune response may play an important but indirect role in the termination of hepatocellular injury and viral synthesis in viral hepatitis.

LIVER-SPECIFIC ANTIGENS

A liver-specific hepatocyte surface membrane lipoprotein (LSP) has been suggested as the target antigen in viral hepatitis (126, 201). In these studies, immunization of rabbits with LSP led to the synthesis of immunoglobulins directed against hepatocyte membranes, stimulation of humoral antibodies against hepatocyte membranes, a cellular immune response to LSP, and histologic lesions consistent with chronic active hepatitis. Sensitization to LSP is detectable in 50% of the patients with acute HB but is not detectable upon recovery (165, 205). Sensitization persists in 71% of untreated patients with chronic active hepatitis, either positive or negative for HBsAg.

The loss of sensitization to LSP with the clinical recovery from HB, and the equal frequency of sensitization in patients with chronic active hepatitis who are positive or negative for HBsAg, better correlates with hepatocellular injury than sensitization to HBsAg and may have pathogenetic significance.

The presence of anti-LSP antibodies in the serum of patients with HBsAg-negative chronic active hepatitis was demonstrated by Hopf *et al.* (126, 127). In these patients, anti-LSP antibodies were associated with linear staining for IgG on the surface of their own hepatocytes (126, 127). By contrast, in patients with HBsAg-positive chronic hepatitis, serum LSP antibodies were not found, but granular deposits of IgG were present on surface of hepatocytes, suggesting binding of immune complexes. At least in chronic active hepatitis, the activation of the humoral immune response was suggested.

Circulating lymphocytes from patients with acute viral hepatitis, whether positive or negative for HBsAg, exhibit cytotoxic effector cell activity toward hepatocytes. This cytotoxic reactivity disappears with the resolution of the disease, but persists in chronic active hepatitis (39, 85, 224, 311). Cytotoxicity of circulating lymphocytes toward hepatocytes was also found in other hepatic disorders not associated with viruses, *e.g.*, neonatal hepatitis (281), hepatitis owing to alpha₁-antitrypsin deficiency (281), and alcoholic hepatitis (140). Because purified LSP blocks cytotoxicity, it has been argued that the cytotoxic reaction is specific for this surface antigen of hepatocyte (39). With the respect to LSP, the cellular immune response appears to be intact in viral hepatitis.

As suggested above, there seem to be defects of some nonspecific indicators of cellular immunity (4, 37, 38, 55, 71, 94, 318). The function of primary antigen reactive cells may be normal, while antigen-nonspecific immunoregulatory systems display varying degrees of dysfunction.

A role for immune responses in the pathogenesis of hepatic injury is not conclusively proved. Nevertheless, the data, such as the consistency of humoral and cellular immune responses, the presence of abnormal plasma immunoregulatory lipoproteins (RIF) (36–38), decreased suppressor cell activity, and the presence within the liver itself of potent immunosuppressive molecules are compatible with explanations for (a) acute and chronic injury, (b) recovery, and (c) the carrier state.

In patients who recover from HB without complications, anti-HBV antibody leads to clearance of the virus from the blood and the liver. The resulting absence of HBsAg prevents a possible attack by immune systems. At the same time, removal of the virus allows normal regulation of cellular immunity, and suppressor cells may prevent a cellular immune reaction.

Patients with chronic HB do not develop adequate antibody responses to HB viral antigens and thus do not clear the virus. The persistence of HBV genome may result in faulty regulation of cellular immunity, with a progressive cellular attack on hepatocyte autoantigens and perhaps viral antigens. The end result would be chronic active hepatitis.

Asymptomatic carriers of HBV presumably have an impaired antibody response to the virus and, as in the case of patients with chronic hepatitis, do not clear the virus from the blood or the liver. However, the normal function of suppressor cells is preserved, leading to suppression of antiviral and antihepatocyte attack systems.

VIRUSES SIMILAR TO HBV

Early studies of HBV were hindered by the lack of a suitable animal model. Initially, the sequence of events in the epidemiology and pathogenesis of HB was elucidated by experimental infection in man (152, 209). Sera of about 30 different species were surveyed to find animals which might harbor HBV, but HBsAg was not found in any (173). While HBV causes acute hepatitis in chimpanzees (113, 195, 244), this species does not develop chronic active hepatitis, cirrhosis, or hepatocellular carcinoma. The discovery that woodchucks are commonly afflicted with chronic hepatitis and cancer of the liver led in these animals to the identification of a hepatotropic virus similar to HBV. The serum of infected woodchucks contains particles morphologically and chemically similar to HBsAg particles. However, the viruses are not identical, and only 0.1–1% of the surface antigens are shared. There is greater cross-reactivity between the core antigens of HBV and the woodchuck virus, with about 5–10% of antigenic sites being mutal. The fact that a major cause of death in woodchucks is primary hepatocel-

lular carcinoma (25% of the animals studied by Snyder (282)) provides an
opportunity to study the pathogenesis of hepatocellular carcinoma associated
with HB. Similar, but not identical, DNA viruses have now been found in other
species, including ground squirrels (89, 183) and ducks (185). In the latter, the
virus has been found in embryos removed 15 days after the eggs were laid (220),
indicating the possible importance of maternal infection.

RELATION OF HB TO PRIMARY HEPATOCELLULAR
CARCINOMA (PHC)

PHC, although relatively uncommon in the Western world, is one of the major
malignant diseases in Southeast Asia, parts of Africa, Japan, Oceania, Greece,
and Italy (268, 269). In these areas, 5–20% of the population may be carriers of
HBV. Moreover, in these endemic areas, 90% or more of patients with PHC have
HBsAg or high titers of anti-HBc in their blood (192, 210, 294). Even in areas in
which the incidence of hepatocellular carcinoma is low, serologic evidence of
persistent infection with HBV is more common in patients with PHC than in the
general population (25). In many areas, the frequency of anti-HBs is higher in the
population than in cases of PHC (163, 215).

The statistical association between chronic HBV infection and PHC, based on
serologic studies, is supported by the common occurrence of HBV markers in
liver tissue obtained at autopsy. HBsAg and HBcAg are undetectable or present
in very small quantities in the neoplastic cells but are usually present in nonma-
lignant hepatocytes (143, 210, 211, 303, 304). HBV is more common in well-
differentiated than in poorly differentiated tumors (143, 159, 210, 211), a finding
which suggests that viral replication is better maintained by normal hepatocytes
or by neoplastic cells which display only minimal deviation. In a prospective
study in Japan, chronic carriers of HBsAg with cirrhosis had about a 25%
incidence of PHC 3 years later; tumor did not develop in patients with cirrhosis
and anti-HBs and was eventually found in only 1 of 43 cirrhotic patients with no
evidence of previous infection with HBV (219). In a study in Taiwan (16), 49
cases of PHC occurred in a 2- to 4-year period among 3500 asymptomatic carriers
of HBsAg, compared to one in 18,000 HBsAg-negative individuals. The relative
risk of PHC among HBV carriers was thus estimated as 250 times greater than
in noncarriers.

Since the carrier state for the HB virus usually precedes hepatocellular carcinoma by 15 or 20 years, it is likely that transmission from mother to infant is
important in endemic areas (221, 308), particularly when the mothers have a high
titer of HBsAg and display HBeAg (222). Children of mothers who are chronic
carriers are themselves likely to become carriers of HBsAg.

In most cases, PHC arises in a liver that exhibits evidence of chronic injury. It
is most commonly associated with cirrhosis and less commonly with chronic
hepatitis; in about one-tenth of cases of PHC, usually in children, the liver
appears histologically normal (73, 74, 233).

True oncogenic DNA viruses are integrated into the host cell DNA to induce
malignant transformation. At least one, and perhaps as many as six, copies of the
complete DNA sequence of HBV were reported to be integrated into the genome
of a cell line derived from a PHC (179, 184). RNA transcripts for the HBsAg gene

were also isolated from the same cell line (99). Integration of HBV-DNA into cells of PHC has now been reported in three West African patients (30). Further evidence for a role of HBV in PHC is the finding that DNA from the woodchuck hepatitis virus hybridized to the cellular DNA in five woodchuck livers with PHC, but did not hybridize to the DNA in 9 livers without tumor (288, 289). Integration of one or two genomes of the virus into the tumor cells was demonstrated in two woodchucks (288, 289). However, conclusive evidence for the oncogenicity of the virus requires further proof, such as induction of malignant transformation, either of normal liver cells in culture or of hepatocytes in experimental animals. There is some experimental evidence for a synergism between HBV and various chemicals. Chimpanzees with HB, who were treated with the carcinogen diethylnitrosamine, developed mild hepatitis, postnecrotic cirrhosis, and multifocal hepatocellular carcinoma (107). In addition, marmosets with low-grade hepatitis are susceptible to the development of PHC when exposed to aflatoxin (167).

RELATION OF HB TO GENDER

Several studies have indicated an unusual correlation between HB and male gender. The prevalence of the chronic carrier state is at least twice as great in men as in women, even though male and female children are equally exposed to HBV carrier mothers and siblings (26, 70, 174, 293); among individuals found to have persistent infection, females are more likely than males to clear the infection (32, 70, 98, 278). Finally, the complications of chronic active hepatitis cirrhosis and PHC are about five times more common in men than in women (24, 162, 298, 308). The ratio of males to females at birth is increased among the children of HBsAg carrier women (70, 111, 197, 254), while the presence of anti-HBs in mothers has the opposite effect (70). In patients subjected to renal dialysis, the probability of remaining HBsAg-positive is about twice as great for men as for women (174). Chronic carriers of HbsAg or patients who have never been infected with HB show much better survival of a transplanted kidney than recipients who exhibit anti-HBs (175). The decreased survival of the renal graft in recipients with anti-HBs is restricted to transplants from male donors (69).

These data suggest an association between HBsAg and the male sex correlate with the hypothesis that there is cross-reactivity between HBsAg and a male-associated antigen (70). According to this concept, females are more likely to develop an antibody response to HBsAg, while males would be more likely to be tolerant of the antigen and, therefore, have a greater tendency to become carriers. The persistence of HBsAg in the serum of pregnant women may promote cross-tolerance to a male-associated antigen, leading to an enhanced survival of the male fetus. By contrast anti-HBs may cross-react with a male-associated antigen in the conceptus, thus decreasing survival of the male fetus. Finally, anti-HBs in the recipient of a male kidney graft might interact with a male-associated antigen, thus leading to rejection of the kidney.

HEPATITIS A

EPIDEMIOLOGY

Outbreaks of HA have been attributed to contaminated food, milk, water, and shellfish and have occurred among institutionalized persons, within families, and among contacts of infected nonhuman primates (58, 59, 243). This implies almost exclusively the fecal-oral route of transmission, a mode of spread enhanced by poor personal and environmental hygiene, crowding, and poor sanitation.

Although HA can be transmitted experimentally by percutaneous inoculation, HAV plays no role in transfusion-associated hepatitis (63, 78).

Exposure to HAV is not increased among hemodialysis patients and staff (291), health care personnel (194), multiply transfused persons (194, 285), or drug addicts (104). No observations of easy vertical transmission of HAV infection from mother to fetus have been made (301).

HA accounts for 20–40% of sporadic hepatitis cases (62). An enhanced risk of acquiring HA was noticed among homosexual males, particularly among those attending venereal disease clinics (43, 199). This appears to result from oral-anal contact. Spread of HAV was noticed among children in day care centers (286, 313). Children in such centers are often not toilet trained, and infection in young children is usually asymptomatic; this combination permits the transmission of the infection to their families, center personnel and, through them, to the community.

Recent seroepidemiologic studies show that 40–50% of urban adults in the USA display anti-HAV. The prevalence of exposure to HAV increases with increasing age and decreasing socioeconomic status (65). Higher prevalences of anti-HAV among older persons in modern urban populations reflect almost universal exposure of this population at a younger age. The overall decrease in the incidence of HA currently (206) reflects a falling prevalence of HAV exposure in modern urban societies (103).

CLINICAL AND PATHOLOGIC FEATURES

It is generally agreed that HA is, in the vast majority of cases, an entirely benign disease (292). The incubation period for HA, whether transmitted orally or percutaneously, is usually between 2 and 4 weeks (153). In rare instances, HAV infection may be complicated by the development of acute fulminant hepatitis (247). Three of 188 cases of acute fulminant hepatitis were caused by HAV (3). Despite the fact that HAV infection, in rare instances, may cause fulminant hepatitis, HA is self-limited (168, 188, 247, 259), does not cause chronic hepatitis or cirrhosis, and is not associated with a chronic carrier state. No instances of neonatal hepatitis or biliary atresia caused by HAV are known (5, 13).

The histopathological presentation of HAV infection is similar to that of acute HB. Relative mildness of morphologic features and sparing of centrolobular zones has been noticed, findings which coincide with those observed in chimpanzees (56, 61, 231). By contrast, in marmosets with experimental HAV infection, areas of focal necrosis involved the entire lobule and extended to the centrolobular zones (52, 119, 231).

ANIMAL MODELS

An animal model for HA, namely, the marmoset, was discovered almost a decade before the virus itself was identified (176, 241). In addition to marmosets, it is now recognized that chimpanzees are also infected with HAV (56, 196). The availability of experimental animal models allowed successful cultivation of HAV *in vitro*. The inoculum consisted of a liver suspension from a marmoset infected with HAV (239). Several tissue culture systems exist, including Vero cells (172), African Green Monkey kidney cells (49), and fetal rhesus monkey kidney cell lines (82). HAV appears to be cell-associated, is not secreted into the culture medium, and is not cytopathic (172).

STRUCTURE OF HAV

Following the recognition that marmoset monkeys are susceptible to infection with HAV (119, 239), the virus itself was visualized by immune electron microscopy in the stools of inviduals infected with HAV as a 27-nm nonenveloped particle with cubic capsid symmetry. Complete and incomplete virions are both visualized.

HAV contains four polypeptides, with a molecular weight similar to that of the poliovirus (44, 45). The genome of HAV consists of a single-stranded RNA, with a molecular weight of 1.9×10^6 daltons (47, 279).

Although some physical properties and the small genome of HAV are not typical for enteroviruses, it most closely resembles picornaviruses, a subgroup of the enteroviruses. The buoyant density in $CsCl_2$ gradient of most particles is 1.34 g/cm^3, similar to that of enteroviruses. In addition HAV shares with enteroviruses a cytoplasmic localization (242, 267, 275) but, in contrast to other enteroviruses, is not cytopathic in tissue culture (238).

BIOLOGY OF HA

There is a relatively uniform sequence of viral and host immune responses following HAV infection. HAV is found in the liver in the first to second week after exposure to the virus (186). The viral particles are localized within cytoplasmic vesicles of hepatocytes and Kupffer cells and can be found there several weeks after their disappearance from the feces and the normalization of the blood levels of transaminases (56). HAV can be detected in the blood about 17 days before and about 14 days after the clinical appearance of symptoms (151). The virus disappears with clinical resolution of the disease or shortly after peak serum transaminase activity in cases of anicteric hepatitis (150). Fecal excretion of the virus peaks several days to more than a week before the onset of the biochemical changes of acute hepatitis and coincides with nonspecific prodromal symptoms (46, 57, 169, 246). It is a time of peak infectivity of stools, as defined in transmission studies in humans (150). The virus disappears from the feces about 1 week after the onset of jaundice (151).

HAV has been found in bile (267), glomeruli (187), the spleen, and abdominal lymph nodes (187). It is not detected in the intestinal epithelium of experimental animals (187, 189), suggesting that the liver is the only site of viral replication. Urine collected on the first day of jaundice was shown to be infectious (91, 138).

Antibody to HAV, usually IgM, is detected in the serum during the acute illness, reaches peak levels in the convalescence period (170), and persists in the form of IgG anti-HAV indefinitely after infection (50, 60, 156, 248). The development of antibodies to HAV provides permanent immunity to this infection. IgA coproantibodies (171, 321), which can be found in stools of a few patients with acute infection, may limit the infectivity of the stools and may provide local gut immunity to reinfection. Immune serum globulin is useful for passive immunization because it contains significant titers of anti-HAV (125).

IMMUNODIAGNOSTIC MARKERS FOR HAV

The first *in vitro* test described to detect HAV and anti-HAV was immune electron microscopy. Subsequently, HAAg from the liver of infected marmosets was used for immune adherence hemagglutination to detect anti-HA (240). A modified radioimmunoassay for HAAg has now been developed (245), and the virus is now also detectable by immunofluorescence (186). The most recent test is the enzyme-linked immunosorbent assay (ELISA) (310). A reliable diagnosis of HA can be made by demonstrating rising titers of anti-HAV between acute illness and convalescence, or the presence of IgM anti-HAV in a single serum sample obtained during early infection.

NON-A, NON-B HEPATITIS

Studies of transfusion associated viral hepatitis (81, 236) and the identification of antigens and antibodies specifically related to HA and HB (77, 235) have allowed the recognition of a third major cause of human viral hepatitis, for which no agent has yet been identified. This entity, diagnosed by serologic exclusion, is known as non-A, non-B (NANB) hepatitis. Since the exclusion of HBsAg-positive donor blood transfusions, it is now apparent that NANB hepatitis is responsible for about 90% of the cases of post-transfusion hepatitis in the United States (10).

The transmission of NANB hepatitis appears to be similar to that of HBV. From 13 to 25% of reported sporadic cases of viral hepatitis are NANB (64, 216). The mode of contraction is frequently unknown in these patients, although in some cases it may be due to accidental needlesticks in health care workers (296) or to sharing of needles by drug abusers (64, 216). Spouses appear to be at somewhat higher risk, implying a sexual mode of transmission (106, 144, 306, 314).

Some observations suggest that NANB hepatitis can occur in epidemics. Recent evaluation of stored serum samples from an outbreak of hepatitis related to sewage contamination of the water supply in Dehli, India in 1955–1956 (200, 314), and studies of similar waterborn hepatitis outbreaks in Burma and Kashmir (144) revealed that there was no evidence of HA and little of HB. The clinical picture was similar to that of HA, except for an unusually high mortality rate (1%) for that malady (200), and severe cholestasis (105, 144, 280).

Studies of NANB hepatitis have been facilitated by the experimental transmission of this disorder to chimpanzees (10, 118, 295). These experiments showed that there is, indeed, an infectious agent(s) for the disease and that a chronic carrier state exists. In successfully infected chimpanzees, as well as in man, the incubation period of NANB hepatitis varies widely, ranging from 2 to 26 weeks, with a mean incubation period of 5–10 weeks after exposure (9). In general, two patterns of incubation have been noticed, one very short (2–4 weeks) and one long (8–12 weeks), suggesting that two viruses may be involved (191). The duration of the acute form of the disease is usually about 10 weeks (9).

Evidence has been presented that NANB hepatitis is more commonly associated with chronic hepatitis that HB (147, 148). Patients with transfusion-associated NANB hepatitis (25 to 50% of them) have elevated serum transaminase levels for more than 1 year after the onset of the disease (19, 79). The patients with chronic NANB hepatitis are usually asymptomatic, despite the elevations of transaminases, and in nearly 30% of patients chronic persistent hepatitis or nonspecific hepatic changes have been noted in liver biopsies (19). Chronic active hepatitis is the most common finding on liver biopsy in patients with long-standing NANB infection (19), and these patients may progress to cirrhosis (66).

Virus-like particles associated with NANB hepatitis have been described in serum and liver from infected humans and chimpanzees (29, 274, 316, 320). However, a definitive virus has not yet been identified.

In the absence of specific tests for NANB hepatitis, attention has been drawn to nonspecific tests, such as assays of the levels of liver enzymes (117), plasma carcinoembryonic antigen, and concentrations of bile acids (93), which may be raised in patients with NANB hepatitis. Most of the results are inconclusive, and little is known about the specificity of such assays for hepatitis. However, it has been estimated that 40–50% of the potential cases of transfusion hepatitis might be prevented if blood donors with an alanine aminotransferase (ALT) level greater than 45 IU/liter are excluded from donation (2). Such a standard would eliminate only 2 to 5% of healthy donors.

SUMMARY

Dramatic advances in the understanding of the pathogenesis, pathophysiology, prevention, and treatment of the major viral diseases of the liver have been made. Hepatitis B and A viruses have been identified, with specific diagnostic serologic assays commercially available for these infections. The diagnosis of non-A, non-B hepatitis is currently made by exclusion. Morphological alterations in viral hepatitis are similar, regardless of the etiologic agent. Chronic viral hepatitis may be associated with hepatitis B and non-A, non-B, but not with hepatitis A. Persistent infection with hepatitis B virus is associated with an increased incidence of primary hepatocellular carcinoma. Viruses similar to the hepatitis B virus cause the same spectrum of liver disease in certain animals. With the development of a vaccine against hepatitis B virus infection, it may be possible to prevent a large proportion of worldwide chronic liver disease, as well as primary hepatocellular carcinoma.

REFERENCES

1. Aach, R. D., and Kahn, R. A. Post-transfusion hepatitis: current perspectives. *Ann. Intern. Med.* 92: 539–546, 1980.
2. Aach, R. D., Szmuness, W., Mosley, J. W., Hallinger, F. B., Cahn, R. A., Stevens, C. E., Edwards, J. M., Wench, J. The Transfusion-transmitted Viruses Study: Serum alanine aminotransferase of donors in relation to the risk of non-A, non-B hepatitis in recipients. *N. Engl. J. Med.* 304: 989–994, 1981.
3. Acute Hepatitis Failure Study Group. Etiology and prognosis in fulminant hepatitis. *Gastroenterology* 77: 33A, 1979.
4. Agarwal, S. S., Blumberg, B. S., Gerstley, B. J. S., *et al.* Lymphocyte transformation and hepatitis. I. Impairment of thymidine incorporation and DNA polymerase activity. *Proc. Soc. Exp. Biol. Med.* 137: 1498–1502, 1971.
5. Agarwal, S. S., Lahori, U. C., Mehta, S. K., Bajpai, P. C., Warner, B., and Bradley, D. W. Hepatitis A and Indian childhood cirrhosis. *Arch. Dis. Child.* 54: 901–903, 1979.
6. Aldershvile, J., Dietrichson, O., Hardt, F., and Nielsen, J. O. Circulating T and B lymphocytes and immunoglobulin containing cells in the liver in chronic active liver disease. *Acta Pathol. Microbiol. Scand.* 85: 26–32, 1977.

7. Almeida, J. D., Rubinstein, D., and Scott, E. J. New antigen-antibody system in Australia-antigen-positive hepatitis. *Lancet 2:* 1225–1227, 1971.

8. Almeida, J. D., Zuckerman, A. J., Taylor, P. E., and Waterson, A. P. Immune electron microscopy of the Australia SH (serum hepatitis) antigen. *Microbios 2:* 117–123, 1969.

9. Alter, H. J. The dominant role of non-A, non-B in the pathogenesis of post-transfusion hepatitis: a clinical assessment. Clin. *Gastroenterol. 9:* 155–170, 1980.

10. Alter, H. J., Purcell, R. H., Holland, P. V., Feinstone, S. M., Morrow, A. G., and Moritsugu, Y. Clinical and serological analysis of transfusion-associated hepatitis. *Lancet 2:* 838–841, 1975.

11. Alter, H. J., Purcell, R. H., Holland, P. V., and Popper, H. Transmissible agent in non-A, non-B hepatitis. *Lancet 1:* 459–463, 1978.

12. Alter, H. J., Seeff, L. B., Kaplan, P. M., *et al.* Type B hepatitis. The infectivity of blood positive for antigen and DNA polymerase after accidental needlestick exposure. *N. Engl. J. Med. 295:* 909–913, 1976.

13. Balistreri, W. F., Tabor, E., and Gerety, R. J. Negative serology for hepatitis A and B viruses in 18 cases of neonatal cholestasis. *Pediatrics 66:* 269–271, 1980.

14. Bancroft, W. H., *et al.* Detection of additional antigenic determinants of hepatitis B antigen. *J. Immunol. 109:* 842–848, 1972.

15. Barker, L. F., and Murray, R. Relationship of virus dose to incubation time of clinical hepatitis and time of appearance of hepatitis-associated antigen. *Am. J. Med. Sci. 263:* 27–33, 1972.

16. Beasley, R. P., and Lin, C. C. Hepatoma risk among HBsAg carriers (abstract). *Am. J. Epidemiol. 108:* 247, 1978.

17. Beasley, R. P., Trepo, C., Stevens, C. E., *et al.* The e antigen and vertical transmission of hepatitis B surface antigen. *Am. J. Epidemiol. 105:* 94–98, 1977.

18. Beeson, P. B., *et al.* Hepatitis following injection of mumps convalescent plasma. *Lancet 1:* 814–815, 1944.

19. Berman, M. D., Alter, H. J., Ishak, K. G., *et al.* The chronic sequelae of non-A, non-B hepatitis. *Ann. Intern. Med. 91:* 1–6, 1979.

20. Bianchi, L., DeGroote, J., Desmet, V. J., Gedigh, P., Korb, G., Popper, H., Poulsen, H., Scheuer, P. J., Schmid, M., Thaler, H., and Welper, W. Acute and chronic hepatitis revisited. *Lancet 2:* 914–919, 1977.

21. Bianchi, L., and Gudat, F. Sanded nuclei in hepatitis B. Eosinophilic inclusions in liver cell nuclei due to excess in hepatitis B core antigen formation. *Lab. Invest. 35:* 1–5, 1976.

22. Bianchi, L., Simmerli-Ninng, M., and Gudat, F. Viral hepatitis. In: *Pathology of the Liver.* Edited by R. N. M. MacSween, P. P. Antony, and P. J. Scheuer, p. 164. Edinburgh, Churchill Livingstone, 1979.

23. Blumberg, B. S., Alter, H. J., and Visnich, S. A "new" antigen in leukemia sera. *J.A.M.A. 191:* 541–546, 1965.

24. Blumberg, B. S., Larouze, B., London, W. T., Werner, B., Hisser, J. E., Millman, I., Saimot, G., and Payet, M. The relation of infection with the hepatitis B agent to primary hepatic carcinoma. *Am. J. Pathol. 81:* 669–692, 1975.

25. Blumberg, B. S., and London, W. T. Hepatitis B virus and primary hepatocellular carcinoma: Relationship of "Icrons" to cancer. In: *Viruses in Naturally Occurring Cancers.* Edited by M. Essex, G. Todaro, and H. zurHausen, pp. 401–421, Cold Spring Harbor, New York, Cold Spring Harbor Laboratory, 1980.

26. Blumberg, B. S., Sutnick, A. I., London, W. T., and Melartin, L. Sex distribution of Australia antigen. *Arch. Intern. Med. 130:* 227–231, 1972.

27. Boyer, J. L. Chronic hepatitis. A perspective on classification and determinants of prognosis. *Gastroenterology 70:* 1161–1171, 1976.

28. Boyer, J. L., and Klatskin, G. Pattern of necrosis in acute viral hepatitis. Prognostic value of bridging (subacute hepatic necrosis). *N. Engl. J. Med 283:* 1063–1071, 1970.

29. Bradley, D. W., Cook, E. H., Maynard, J. E., *et al.* Experimental infection of chimpanzees with antihemophilic (Factor VIII) materials: recovery of virus-like particles associated with non-A, non-B hepatitis. *J. Med. Virol. 3:* 253–269, 1979.

30. Brechot, C., Pourcel, C., Louise, A., Rain, B., and Tiollois, P. Presence of integrated hepatitis B virus DNA sequences in cellular DNA of human hepatocellular carcinoma. *Nature 286:* 533–535, 1980.

31. Budkowska, A., Shih, J.W-K., and Gerin, J. L. Immunochemistry and polypeptide composition of hepatitis B core antigen (HBCAg). *J. Immunol. 118:* 1300–1305, 1977.

32. Bulkley, B. H., Heizer, W. D., Goldfinger, S. E., and Isselbacher, K. J. Distinctions in chronic active hepatitis based on circulating hepatitis-associated antigen. *Lancet 2:* 1323–1326, 1970.

33. Busachi, C. A., Roy, M. B., and Desmet, V. J. An immunoperoxidase technique for demonstrating membrane localized HBsAg in paraffin sections of liver biopsies. *J. Immunol. Methods 19:* 95–99, 1978.

34. Camilleri, J. P., Amat, C., Chousterman, M., Petite, J. P., Duboust, A., Boddert, A., and Parof, A. Immunohistochemical patterns of hepatitis B surface antigen (HBsAg) in patients with hepatitis, renal hemograft recipients and normal carriers. *Virchows Arch. (Pathol. Anat.). 376:* 329–341, 1977.

35. Cavalli, G., Bianchi, F. B., Bacci, G., and Casali, A. M. The histogenesis and clinical significance of acidophilic bodies in various liver diseases. *Digestion 1:* 353–369, 1968.

36. Chisari, F. V., and Edgington, T. S. Lymphocyte E rosette inhibitory factor: a regulatory serum lipoprotein. *J. Exp. Med. 142:* 1092–1107, 1975.

37. Chisari, F. V., Routenberg, J. A., and Edgington, T. S. Mechanisms responsible for defective human T-lymphocyte sheep erythrocyte rosette function associated with hepatitis B virus infections. *J. Clin. Invest. 57:* 1227–1238, 1976.

38. Chisari, F. V., Routenberg, J. A., Fiala, M., and Edgington, T. S. Extrinsic modulation of human T-lymphocyte E rosette function associated with prolonged hepatocellular injury after viral hepatitis. *J. Clin. Invest. 59:* 134–142, 1977.

39. Cochrane, A. M. G., Moussouros, A., Thomson, A. D., Eddleston, A. L. W., and Williams, R. Antibody-dependent cell-mediated (K cell) cytotoxicity against isolated hepatocytes in chronic active hepatitis. *Lancet 1:* 441–444, 1976.

40. Cockayne, E. A. Catarrhal jaundice, sporadic and epidemic and its relation to acute yellow atrophy of the liver. *Q. J. Med., 6:* 1, 1912.

40a. Colombo, M., Vernace, S. J. and Paronetto, F. T and B lymphocytes in patients with chronic active hepatitis (CAH). *Clin. Exp. Immunol. 30:* 4–9, 1977.

41. Conn, H. O. Chronic hepatitis: reducing iatrogenic enigma to a workable puzzle. *Gastroenterology 70:* 1182–1184, 1976.

42. Cook, G. C., and Scherlock, S. Jaundice and its relation to therapeutic agents. *Lancet 1:* 175–179, 1965.

43. Corey, L., and Holmes, K. K. Sexual transmission of hepatitis A in homosexual men: incidence and mechanism. *N. Engl. J. Med. 302:* 435–438, 1980.

44. Coulepis, A. G., Locarnini, S. A., Ferris, A. A., Lehmann, N. I., and Gust, I. D. The polypeptides of hepatitis A virus. *Intervirology 10:* 24–31, 1978.

45. Coulepis, A. G., Locarnini, S. A., and Gust, I. D. Iodination of hepatitis A virus reveals a fourth structural polypeptide. *J. Virol. 35:* 572–574, 1980.

46. Coulepis, A. G., Locarnini, S. A., Lehmann, N. J., and Gust, I. D. Detection of hepatitis A virus in the feces of patients with naturally acquired infections. *J. Infect. Dis. 141:* 151–156, 1980.

47. Coulepis, A. G., Tannock, G. A., Locarnini, S. A., and Gust, I. D. Evidence that the genome of hepatitis A virus consists of single-stranded RNA. *J. Virol. 37:* 473–477, 1981.

48. Dane, D. S., Cameron, C. H., and Briggs, M. Virus-like particles in serum of patients with Australia-antigen-associated hepatitis. *Lancet 1:* 659–698, 1970.

49. Daemer, R. J., Feinstone, S. M., Gust, I. D. and Purcell, R. H. Propagation of isolation and serial passage. *Infect. Immun. 32:* 388–393, 1981.

50. Decker, R. H., Overby, L. R., Ling, C-M., Frösner, G., Deinhardt, F., and Boggs, J. Serologic studies of transmission of hepatitis A in humans. *J. Infect. Dis. 139:* 74–82, 1979.

51. DeGroote, J., Desmet, V. S., Gedick, P., Korb, G., Popper, H., *et al.* A classification of chronic hepatitis. *Lancet 2:* 626–628, 1968.

52. Deinhardt, F., Holmes, A. W., Capps, R. B., and Poppert, H. Studies on the transmission of human viral hepatitis to marmoset monkeys. I. Transmission of disease, serial passages and description of liver lesions. *J. Exp. Med. 125:* 673–688, 1967.

53. Deinhardt, F. Predictive value of markers of hepatitis virus infection. *J. Infect. Dis. 141:* 299–305, 1980.

54. Desmet, V. J., and DeGroote, J. Histological diagnosis of viral hepatitis. *Clin. Gastroenterol. 3:*

337–354, 1974.

55. Dettoratius, R. J., Strickland, R. G., and Williams, R. C. T and B lymphocytes in acute and chronic hepatitis. J. Clin. Immunol. *Immunopathol. 2:* 353–360, 1974.

56. Dienstag, J. L., Feinstone, S. M., Purcell, R. H., Hoofnagle, J. H., Barker, L. F., London, W. T., Popper, H., Peterson, J. M.. and Kapikian, A. Z. Experimental infection of chimpanzees with hepatitis A virus. *J. Infect. Dis. 132:* 532–545, 1975.

57. Dienstag, J. L., Feinstone, S. M., Kapikian, A. Z., Purcell, R. H., Boggs, J. D., and Conrad, M. E. Fecal shedding of hepatitis A antigen. *Lancet 1:* 765–767, 1975.

58. Dienstag, J. L., Gust, I. D., Lucas, C. R., Wong, D. C., and Purcell, R. H. Muscle-associated viral hepatitis type A: serologic confirmation. *Lancet 1:* 561–564, 1976.

59. Dienstag, J. L., Davenport, F. M., McCollum, R. W., Hennessy, A. V., Klatskin, G., and Purcell, R. H. Non-human primate-associated viral hepatitis type A: serologic evidence of hepatitis A virus infection. *JAMA 236:* 462–464, 1976.

60. Dienstag, J. L., Alling, D. W., and Purcell, R. H. Quantitation of antibody to hepatitis A antigen by immune electron microscopy. *Infect. Immun. 13:* 1209–1213, 1976.

61. Dienstag, J. L., Popper, H., and Purcell, R. H. The pathology of viral hepatitis type A and B in chimpanzees: a comparison. *Am. J. Pathol. 85:* 131–148, 1976.

62. Dienstag, J. L., Alaama, A., Mosley, J. W., Redeker, A. G., and Purcell, R. H. Etiology of sporadic hepatitis B surface antigen-negative hepatitis. *Ann. Intern. Med. 87:* 1–6, 1977.

63. Dienstag, J. L., Feinstone, S. M., Purcell, R. H., Wong, D. C., Alter, H. J., and Holland, P. V. Non-A, non-B post-transfusion hepatitis. *Lancet 1:* 560–562, 1977.

64. Dienstag, J. L., Alaama, A., Mosley, J. W., *et al.* Etiology of sporadic hepatitis B surface antigen negative hepatitis. *Ann. Intern. Med. 87:* 1–6, 1977.

65. Dienstag, J. L., Szmuness, W., Stevens, C. E., and Purcell, R. H. Hepatitis A virus infection: New insights from seroepidemiologic studies. *J. Infect. Dis. 137:* 328–340, 1978.

66. Dienstag, J. L. Case Records of the Massachusetts General Hospital. *N. Engl. J. Med. 330:* 207, 1980.

67. Dienstag, J. L., and Ryan, D. M. Occupational exposure to hepatitis B infection or immunization. *Gastroenterology,* in press, 1981.

68. Dreesman, G. R., Chairez, R., Suarez, M., *et al.* Production of antibody to individual polypeptides derived from purified hepatitis B surface antigen. *J. Virol. 16:* 508–515, 1975.

69. Drew, J. S., London, W. T., Lustbader, E. D., and Blumberg, B. S. Cross reactivity between hepatitis B surface antigen and male-associated antigen. *Birth Defects 14:* 91–101, 1978.

70. Drew, J. S., London, W. T., Lustbader, E. D., Hesser, J. E., and Blumberg, B. S. Hepatitis B virus and sex ratio of offspring. *Science 201:* 687–692, 1978.

71. Dudley, F. J., Giustino, V., and Sherlock, S. Cell-mediated immunity in patients positive for hepatitis-associated antigen. *Br. Med. J. 4:* 754–757, 1972.

72. Edgington, T. S., and Chisari, F. V. Immunological aspects of hepatitis B virus infection. *Am. J. Med. Sci. 270:* 213–227, 1975.

73. Edmondson, H. A., and Steiner, P. E. Primary carcinoma of the liver: a study of 100 cases among 48,900 necropsies. *Cancer 7:* 462–503, 1954.

74. Edmondson, H. A., and Peters, R. L. *Liver.* In: *Pathology,* Ed. 7, p. 1412. St. Louis, C. V. Mosby, 1977.

75. Erard, P. Technical study of the leukocyte migration inhibition test in agarose. Application to PPD and to hepatitis B antigen. *Clin. Exp. Immunol. 18:* 439–448, 1974.

76. Expert Committee on Hepatitis. First report. Technical Report Series No. 62, World Health Organization, Geneva, 1953.

77. Feinstone, S. M., Kapikian, A. Z., and Purcell, R. H. Hepatitis A: detection by immune electron microscopy of a virus-like antigen associated with acute illness. *Science 182:* 1026–1028, 1973.

78. Feinstone, S. M., Kapikian, A. Z., Purcell, R. H., Alter, H. J., and Holland, P. V. Transfusion-associated hepatitis not due to viral hepatitis type A or B. *N. Engl. J. Med. 292:* 767–770, 1975.

79. Feinstone, S. M., and Purcell, R. H. Non-A, non-B hepatitis. *Annu. Rev. Med. 29:* 359–366, 1978.

80. Findlay, G. M., and MacCallum, F. O. Note on acute hepatitis and yellow fever immunization. Trans. R. Soc. Trop. *Med. Hyg. 31:* 297–308, 1937.

81. Flehmig, B., Ranke, M., Berthold, H., and Gerth, H-J. A solid-phase radioimmunoassay for

detection of IgM antibodies to hepatitis A virus. *J. Infect. Dis. 140:* 169–175, 1979.

82. Flehmig, B. Hepatitis A virus in cell culture. I. Propagation of different HAV isolates in fetal rhesus monkey kidney cell line (FRhK4). *Med. Microbiol. Immunol. 168:* 239–248, 1980.

83. Fox, J. P., *et al.* Observations on the occurrence of icterus in Brazil following vaccination against yellow fever. *Am. J. Hyg. 36:* 68–116, 1942.

84. Gazzard, B. G., Portmann, B., Murray-Lyon, I. M., and Williams, R. Cases of death in fulminant hepatic failure and relationship to quantitative histological assessment. *Q. J. Med. 45:* 615–626, 1975.

85. Geubel, A. P., Keller, R. H., Summerskill, W. H. J., Dickson, E. R., Tomasi, T. B., and Shorter, R. G. Lymphocyte cytotoxicity and inhibition studied with autologous liver cells: observations in chronic active liver disease. *Gastroenterology 71:* 450–456, 1976.

86. Gerber, M. A., Hadziyannis, S., Vissaulis, C., Shaffner, F., Paronetto, F., and Popper H. Electron microscopy and immunoelectron microscopy of cytoplasmic hepatitis B antigen in hepatocytes. *Am. J. Pathol. 75:* 489–502, 1974.

87. Gerber, M. A., Hadziyannis, S., Vernace, S., and Vissoulis, C. Incidence and nature of cytoplasmic hepatitis B antigen in hepatocytes. *Lab. Invest. 32:* 251–256, 1975.

88. Gerber, M. A., and Thung, S. N. The localization of hepatitis viruses in tissues. *Int. Rev. Exp. Pathol. 2:* 49–76, 1979.

89. Gerlish, W. H., Feitelson, M. A., Marion, P. L., and Robinson, W. S. Structural relationships between the surface antigen of ground squirrel hepatitis virus and human hepatitis B virus. *J. Virol. 36:* 787–795, 1980.

90. Gerlish, W. H., Lüer, W., Thomssen, R., *et al.* Diagnosis of acute and inapparent hepatitis B virus infections by measurement of IgM antibody to hepatitis B core antigen. *J. Infect. Dis. 142:* 95–101, 1980.

91. Giles, J. P., Liebhaber, H., Krugman, S., and Lattimer, C. Early viremia and viruria in infectious hepatitis. *Virology 24:* 107–108, 1964.

92. Giles, J. P., McCollum, R. W., Berndtson, L. W., Jr., and Krugman, S. Viral hepatitis: relation of Australia-SH antigen to the Willowbrook MS-2 strain. *N. Engl. J. Med. 281:* 119–122, 1969.

93. Gitnick, G. L., Brezina, M. L., and Mullen, R. L. Application of alanine aminotransferase, carcinoembryonic antigen and cholyglycine levels to the prevention and evaluation of acute and chronic hepatitis. In *Viral Hepatitis.* Edited by G. N. Vyas, S. N. Cohen, and R. Schmid, pp. 431–438. Philadelphia, Franklin Institute Press, 1978.

94. Giustino, V., Dudley, F. J., and Sherlock, S. Thymus dependent lymphocyte function in patients with hepatitis-associated antigen. *Lancet 2:* 850–853, 1972.

95. Goldberg, S. J., Mendenhall, C. L., Connel, A. M., and Chedid, A. "Non-alcoholic" chronic hepatitis in the alcoholic. *Gastroenterology 72:* 598–604, 1977.

96. Goldfield, M., Black, H. C., Bill, J., Srihongs, S., and Pizzuti, W. Consequences of administering blood pretested for HBsAg by 3rd generation techniques—progress report. *Am. J. Med. Sci. 270:* 335–342, 1975.

97. Good, R. A. Relations between immunity and malignancy. *Proc. Natl. Acad. Sci. USA 69:* 1026–1032, 1972.

98. Goodman, M., Wainwright, R. L., Weir, H. F., and Gall, J. C. A sex difference in the carrier state of Australia (hepatitis associated) antigen. *Pediatrics 48:* 907–913, 1971.

99. Gray, P., Edman, J. C., Valenzuela, P., Goodman, H. M., and Rutter, W. J. A human hepatoma cell line contains hepatitis B DNA and RNA sequences. *J. Supramol. Struct.* (Suppl. Y): 245, 1980.

100. Graham, G. Diabetes mellitus: a survey of changes in treatment during the last fifteen years. *Lancet 2:* 1–7, 1938.

101. Gubetta, L., Rizzetto, M., Cruielli, O., Vee, G., and Arico, S. A trichrome stain for the intrahepatic localization of the hepatitis B surface antigen (HBsAg). *Histopathology 1:* 277–288, 1977.

102. Gudat, F., Bianchi, L., Sonnabend, W., Thiel, G., Genishaenslin, W., and Stalder, G. A. Pattern of core and surface expression in liver tissue reflects state of specific immune response in hepatitis B. *Lab. Invest. 32:* 1–9, 1975.

103. Gust, I. D., Lehman, N. I., and Lucas, C. R. Relationship between prevalence of anti-HAV and age—a cohort effect? *J. Infect. Dis. 138:* 425–426, 1978.

104. Gust, I. D., Lehman, N. I., Lucas, C. R., Ferris, A. A., and Locarnini, S. A. Studies on the

epidemiology of hepatitis A in Melbourne. In *Viral Hepatitis.* Edited by G. N. Vyas, S. N. Cohen, and R. Schmid, pp. 105–112. Philadelphia, Franklin Institute Press, 1978.

105. Gupta, D. N., and Smetana, H. F. The histopathology of viral hepatitis seen in the Delhi epidemic (1955–1956). *Indian J. Med. Res. 45* (Suppl.): 101–113, 1957.

106. Guyer, B., Bradley, D. W., Bryan, J. A., *et al.* Non-A, non-B hepatitis among participants in a plasmapheresis stimulation program. *J. Infect. Dis. 139:* 634–640, 1979.

107. Gyorkey, F., Melnick, J. L., Mirkovic, R., *et al.* Experimental carcinoma of the liver in macaque monkeys exposed to diethylnitrosamine and hepatitis B virus. *J. Natl. Cancer Inst. 59:* 1451–1467, 1977.

108. Hadziyannis, S., Vissoulis, C., Moussouros, A., and Afroudakis, A. Cytoplasmic localization of Australia antigen in the liver. *Lancet 1:* 976–979, 1972.

109. Hartfall, S. J., *et al.* Gold treatment of arthritis: A review of 900 cases. *Lancet 2:* 838–842, 1937.

110. Havens, W. P. Infectious hepatitis. *J. Med. 27:* 279–326, 1948.

111. Hesser, J. E., Economidou, J., and Blumberg, B. S. Hepatitis B surface antigen in parents and sex ratio of offspring in a Greek population. *Human Biol. 47:* 415–425, 1975.

112. Hilleman, M. R., Buynak, E. B., Roehm, R. R., Tytell, A. A., Bertland, A. U., and Lampson, G. P. Purified and inactivated human hepatitis B vaccine: progress report. *Am. J. Med. Sci. 270:* 401–404, 1975.

113. Hilleman, M. R., Bertland, A. U., Buynak, E. B., Lampson, G. P., McAleer, W. J., McLean, A. A., Roehm, R. R., and Tytell, A. A. Clinical and laboratory studies of HBsAg vaccine. In *Viral Hepatitis.* Edited by G. N. Vyas, S. N. Cohen, and R. Schmid, pp. 525–537. Philadelphia, Franklin Institute Press, 1978.

114. Hirschman, S. Z. Integration enzyme hypothesis for the replication of hepatitis B virus. *Lancet 2:* 436–438, 1975.

115. Hirschman, S. Z., Gerber, M., and Garfinkel, E. Purification of naked intra nuclear particles from human liver infected by hepatitis B virus. *Proc. Natl. Acad. Sci. USA 71:* 3345–3349, 1974.

116. Hoffnagle, J. H., Gerety, R. J., and Barker, L. F. Antibody to hepatitis B core antigen. *Am. J. Med. Sci. 270:* 179–187, 1975.

117. Hollinger, F. B., Alter, H. J., Holland, P. V., *et al.* Non-A, non-B post-transfusion hepatitis in the United States. In *Non-A, Non-B Hepatitis.* Edited by R. Gerety. New York, Academic Press, in press, 1981.

118. Hollinger, F. B., Gitnick, G. L., Aach, R. D., Szmuness, W., Mosley, J. W., Stevens, C. E., Peters, R. L., Weiner, J. M., Werch, J. B., and Lander, J. J. Non-A, non-B hepatitis transmission in chimpanzees: A project of the transfusion-transmitted viruses study group. *Intervirology 10:* 60–68, 1978.

119. Holmes, A. W., Wolfe, L., Rosenblate, H., and Deinhardt, F. Hepatitis in marmosets: induction of disease with coded specimens from a human volunteer study. *Science 165:* 816–817, 1969.

120. Hoofnagle, J. H., Dusheiko, G. M., Seeff, L. B., Jones, E. A., Waggoner, J. G., and Bales, Z. B. Seroconversion from hepatitis B e antigen (HBeAg) to antibody (anti-HBe) during chronic type B hepatitis. *Ann. Intern. Med. 94:* 744–748, 1981.

121. Hoofnagle, J. H., Gerety, R. H., and Barker, L. F. Antibody to hepatitis B virus core in man. *Lancet 2:* 869–873, 1973.

122. Hoofnagle, J. H., Gerety, R. H., Ni, L. Y., and Barker, L. F. Antibody to hepatitis B core antigen, a sensitive indicator of hepatitis B virus replication. *N. Engl. J. Med. 290:* 1336–1340, 1974.

123. Hoofnagle, J. H., Gerety, R. J., Smallwood, L. A., and Barker, L. F. Subtyping of hepatitis B surface antigen and antibody by radioimmunoassay. *Gastroenterology 72:* 290–296, 1977.

124. Hoofnagle, J. H., Seeff, L. B., Bales, Z. B., Gerety, R. J., and Tabor, E. Serologic responses in hepatitis B. In *Viral Hepatitis.* Edited by G. N. Vyas, S. N. Cohen, and R. Schmid, pp. 219–242. Philadelphia, Franklin Institute Press, 1978.

125. Hoofnagle, J. H., and Waggoner, J. G. Hepatitis A and B virus workers in immune serum globulin. *Gastroenteroloy 78:* 259–263, 1980.

126. Hopf, U., Arnold, W., and Meyer Zum Büschenfeld, K. H. Studies on the pathogenesis of chronic inflammatory liver diseases. *Clin. Exp. Immunol. 22:* 1–8, 1975.

127. Hopf, U., Meyer Zum Büschenfeld, K. H., and Arnold, W. Detection of a liver-membrane autoantibody in HBsAg-negative chronic active hepatitis. *N. Engl. J. Med. 294:* 578–582, 1976.

128. Horney, J. T., and Galambos, J. T. The liver during and after fulminant hepatitis. *Gastroenter-*

ology 73: 639–645, 1977.

129. Hruska, J. F., Clayton, D. A., Rubenstein, J. L. R., and Robinson, W. S. Structure of hepatitis B particle DNA before and after the Dane particle DNA polymerase reaction. *J. Virol. 21:* 666–672, 1977.

130. Huang, S. N. Immunohistochemical demonstration of hepatitis B core and surface antigens in paraffin sections. *Lab. Invest. 33:* 88–95, 1975.

131. Huang, S. N., and Groh, V. Immunoagglutination electron microscopic study of virus-like particles and Australia antigen in liver tissue. *Lab. Invest. 29:* 353–366, 1973.

132. Huang, S. N., and Neurath, A. R. Immunohistologic demonstration of hepatitis B viral antigens in liver with reference to its significance in liver injury. *Lab. Invest. 40:* 1–17, 1979.

133. Huang, S. N., Millman, I. L., O'Connell, A., Gronoff, A., Gault, H., and Blumberg, B. S. Virus-like particles in Australia antigen associated hepatitis. An immunoelectron microscopy study of human liver. *Am. J. Pathol. 67:* 453–470, 1972.

134. Hughes, R. R. Postpenicillin jaundice. *Br. Med. J. 2:* 685–688, 1946.

135. Ibrahim, A. B., Vyas, G. N., and Perkins, H. A. Immune response to hepatitis B surface antigen. *Infect. Immun. 11:* 137–141, 1975.

136. Irwin, G. R., Jr., Hierholzer, W. J., Cimis, R., and McCollum, R. W. Delayed hypersensitivity in hepatitis B: clinical correlates of *in vitro* production of migration inhibition factor. *J. Infect. Dis. 130:* 580–584, 1974.

137. Ito, K., Nakagawa, J., Okimoto, Y., and Nakamo, H. Chronic hepatitis-migration inhibition of leukocytes in the presence of Australia antigen. *N. Engl. J. Med. 286:* 1005, 1972.

138. Joseph, P. R., Millar, J. D., and Henderson, D. A. An outbreak of hepatitis traced to food contamination. *N. Engl. J. Med. 273:* 188–194, 1965.

139. Kaff, R. S. *Viral Hepatitis.* New York, Wiley, 1978.

140. Kakumus, S., and Leevy, C. M. Lymphocyte cytotoxicity in alcoholic hepatitis. *Gastroenterology 72:* 594–597, 1977.

141. Karvountzis, G. G., Redeker, A. G., and Peters, R. L. Long-term follow-up of patients surviving fulminant viral hepatitis. *Gastroenterology 67:* 870–877, 1974.

142. Kerr, J. F. R., Wyllie, A. H., and Currie, A. R. Apoptosis: a basic biological phenomenon with wide-ranged implications in tissue kinetics. *Br. J. Cancer 26:* 239–257, 1972.

143. Kew, M. C., Ray, M. B., Desmet, V. J., *et al.* Hepatitis B surface antigen in tumor tissue and non-tumorous liver in black patients with hepatocellular carcinoma. *Br. J. Cancer 40:* 399–406, 1980.

144. Khuroo, M. S. Study of an epidemic of non-A, non-B hepatitis: possibility of another human hepatitis virus distinct from post-transfusion non-A, non-B type. *Am. J. Med. 68:* 818–824, 1980.

145. Kim, C. Y., and Bissel, D. M. Stability of the lipid and protein of hepatitis-associated (Australia) antigen. *J. Infect. Dis. 123:* 470–476, 1971.

146. Klatskin, G. Subacute hepatic necrosis and postnecrotic cirrhosis due to anicteric infections with hepatitis virus. *Am. J. Med. 25:* 333–358, 1958.

147. Knodell, R.G., Conrad, M.E., and Ishak, K.G. Development of chronic liver disease after acute non-A, non-B post-transfusion hepatitis. Role of γ-globulin prophylaxis in its prevention. *Gastroenterology 72:* 902–909, 1977.

148. Koretz, R. L., Suffin, S. C., and Gitnick, G. L. Post-transfusion chronic liver disease. *Gastroenterology 71:* 797–803, 1976.

149. Kostich, N. D., and Ingram, C. D. Detection of hepatitis B surface antigen by means of orcein staining of liver. *Am. J. Clin. Pathol. 67:* 20–30, 1977.

150. Krugman, S., Ward, R., Giles, J. P., Bodansky, O., and Jacobs, A. M. Infectious hepatitis: detection of virus during the incubation period and in clinically inapparent infection. *N. Engl. J. Med. 261:* 729–734, 1959.

151. Krugman, S., Ward, R., and Giles, J. P. The natural history of infectious hepatitis. *Am. J. Med. 32:* 717–728, 1962.

152. Krugman, S., Giles, J. P., and Hammond, J. Infectious hepatitis: evidence for distinctive clinical, epidemiological and immunological types of infection. *JAMA 200:* 365–373, 1967.

153. Krugman, S., and Giles, J. P. Viral hepatitis—new light on an old disease. *JAMA 212:* 1019–1029, 1970.

154. Krugman, S., Giles, J. P., and Hammond, J. Hepatitis virus: effect of heat on the infectivity and antigenicity of the MS-1 and MS-2 strains. *J. Infect. Dis. 122:* 432–436, 1970.

155. Krugman, S., and Giles, J. P. Viral hepatitis, type B (MS-2 strain). Further observations on natural history and prevention. *N. Engl. J. Med. 288:* 755–760, 1973.

156. Krugman, S., Friedman, H., and Lattimer, C. Viral hepatitis, type A: identification by specific complement fixation and immune adherence tests. *N. Engl. J. Med. 292:* 1141–1143, 1975.

157. Krugman, S., Hoofnagle, J. H., Gerety, R. H., Kaplan, P. M., and Gerin, J. L. Viral hepatitis, type B. (DNA polymerase activity and antibody to hepatitis B core antigen). *N. Engl. J. Med. 290:* 1331–1335, 1974.

158. Krugman, S., Overby, L. R., Mushahwar, I. K., Ling, C. M., Frösner, G. G., and Deinhardt, F. Viral hepatitis, type B. Studies on natural history and prevention re-examined. *N. Engl. J. Med. 300:* 101–106, 1979.

159. Kubo, Y., Okuda, K., Musha, H., *et al.* Detection of hepatocellular carcinoma during a clinical follow-up of chronic liver disease. *Gastroenterology 74:* 578–582, 1978.

160. Kulchar, G. V., and Reynolds, W. J. Bismuth hepatitis. *JAMA 120:* 343–346, 1942.

161. Lander, J. J., Giles, J. P., Purcell, R. H., *et al.* Viral hepatitis, type B (MS-2 strain). Detection of antibody after primary infection. *N. Engl. J. Med. 285:* 303–307, 1971.

162. Larouze, B., London, W. T., Saimot, G., Werner, B. G., Lustbader, E. D., Payet, M., and Blumberg, B. S. Host responses to hepatitis-B infection in patients with primary hepatic carcinoma and their families. A case/control study in Senegal, West Africa. *Lancet 2:* 534–538, 1976.

163. Larouze, B., Blumberg, B. S., London, W. T., Lustbader, E. D., Sankale, M., and Payet, M. Forecasting the development of primary hepatocellular carcinoma by the use of risk factors: studies in West Africa. *J. Natl. Cancer Inst. 58:* 1557–1561, 1977.

164. Lee, W. M., Reed, W. D., Mitchell, C. G., Galbraith, R. M., Eddleston, A. L. W. F., Zuckerman, A. J., and Williams, R. Cellular and humoral immunity to hepatitis B surface antigen in active chronic hepatitis. *Br. Med. J. 1:* 705–708, 1975.

165. Lee, W. M., Reed, W. D., Osman, C. G. Vahrman, J., Zuckerman, A. J., Eddleston, A. L. W. F., and Williams, R. Immune responses to the hepatitis B surface antigen and liver-specific lipoprotein in acute type B hepatitis. *Gut 18:* 250–257, 1977.

166. Lenkei, R., Babes, V. T., Dan, M. E., Mustea, A., and Dobre, I. J. Correlations between anti-albumin antibodies and HBsAg in hepatic patients. *J. Med. Virol. 1:* 29–34, 1977.

167. Lin, J. J., Liu, C., and Svoboda, D. J. Long term effect of aflatoxin B and viral hepatitis on marmoset liver. A preliminary report. *Lab. Invest. 30:* 267–278, 1974.

168. Lindberg, J., Frösner, G., Hansson, B. G., Hermodson, S., and Iwarson, S. Serologic markers of hepatitis A and B in chronic active hepatitis. *Scand. J. Gastroenterol 13:* 525–527, 1978.

169. Locarnini, S. A., Gust, I. D., Ferris, A. A., Stott, A. C., and Wong, M. L. A prospective study of acute viral hepatitis with particular reference to hepatitis A. *Bull. WHO 54:* 199–206, 1976.

170. Locarnini, S. A., Ferris, A. A., Lehmann, N. I., and Gust, I. D. The antibody response following hepatitis A infection. *Intervirology 8:* 309–318, 1977.

171. Locarnini, S. A., Coulepis, A. G., Kaldor, J., and Gust, I. D. Coproantibodies in hepatitis A: detection by enzyme-linked immunosorbent assay and immune electron microscopy. *J. Clin. Microbiol. 11:* 710–716, 1980.

172. Locarnini, S. A., Coulepis, A. G., Westaway, E. G., and Gust, I. D. Restricted replication of human hepatitis A virus in cell culture: intracellular biochemical studies. *J. Virol. 37:* 216–225, 1981.

173. London, W. T., and Blumberg, B. S. Australia antigen, hepatitis and serum protein polymorphism in nonhuman primates. In *Symposium Fourth International Congress on Primatology, Nonhuman primates and Human Diseases*, P. 30. Basel, Karger, 1973.

174. London, W. T., and Drew, J. S. Sex differences in response to hepatitis B infection among patients receiving chronic dialysis treatment. *Proc. Natl. Acad. Sci. USA 74:* 2561–2563, 1977.

175. London, W. T., Drew, J. S., Blumberg, B. S., Grossman, R. A., and Lyons, P. J. Association of graft survival with host response to hepatitis B infection in patients with kidney transplant. *N. Engl. J. Med. 296:* 241–244, 1977.

176. Lorenz, D., Barker, L., Stevens, D., Peterson, M., and Kirschstein, R. Hepatitis in the marmoset, *Saguinus mystax. Proc. Soc. Exp. Biol. Med. 135:* 348–354, 1970.

177. Lürman, A. *Berlin Klin. Wochenschr. 22:* 20, 1885 (as cited by S. Krugman. In *Viral Hepatitis.* Edited by G. N. Vyas, S. N. Cohen, and R. Schmid, pp. 3–10. Philadelphia, Franklin Institute Press, 1978.)

178. MacCallum, F. O., and Bradley, W. H. Transmission of infective hepatitis to human volunteers. *Lancet 2:* 228, 1944.

179. Macnab, G. M., Alexander, J. J., Lecatsas, G., Bey, E. M., and Urbanowicz, J. M. Hepatitis B surface antigen produced by a human hepatoma cell line. *Br. J. Cancer 34:* 509–515, 1976.

180. MacSween, N. M. R. Pathology of viral hepatitis and its sequelae. *Clin. Gastroenterol. 9:* 23–45, 1980.

181. Maddrey, W. C. Drug related acute and chronic hepatitis. *Clin. Gastroenterol. 9:* 213–224, 1980.

182. Magnius, L. O., and Espmark, J. A. New specificities in Australia antigen positive sera distinct from the LeBouvier determinants. *J. Immunol. 109:* 1117–1121, 1972.

183. Marion, P. L., Oshiro, L. S., Regnery, D. C., Scullard, G. H., and Robinson, W. S. A virus in Beechey ground squirrels that is related to hepatitis B virus of humans. *Proc. Natl. Acad. Sci. USA 77:* 2941–2945, 1980.

184. Marion, P. L., and Robinson, W. S. Hepatitis B virus and hepatocellular carcinoma. In *Viruses in Naturally Occurring Cancers.* Edited by M. Essex, G. Todaro, and H. zur Hausen, pp. 423–434. Cold Spring Harbor, NY, Cold Spring Harbor Laboratory, 1980.

185. Mason, W. S., Seal, G., and Summers, J. Virus of Pekin ducks with structural and biological relatedness to human hepatitis B virus. *J. Virol. 36:* 829–836, 1980.

186. Mathiesen, L. R., Feinstone, S. M., Purcell, R. H., and Wagner, J. Detection of hepatitis A antigen by immunofluorescence. *Infect. Immun. 18:* 524–530, 1977.

187. Mathiesen, L. R., Drucker, J., Lorenz, D., Wagner, J., Gerety, R. J., and Purcell, R. H. Localization of hepatitis A antigen in marmoset organs during acute infection with hepatitis A virus. *J. Infect. Dis. 138:* 369–377, 1978.

188. Mathiesen, L. R., Hardt, F., Dietrichson, O., Purcell, R. H., Wong, D., Skinhoj, P., Nielsen, J. O., Zoffmann, H., and Sversen, K. Copenhagen Hepatitis Acuta Programme: the role of acute hepatitis A, B, and non-A, non-B in the development of chronic active liver disease. *Scand. J. Gastroenterol. 15:* 49–54, 1980.

189. Mathiesen, L. R., Miller, A. M., Purcell, R. H., London, W. T., and Feinstone, S. M. Hepatitis A virus in the liver and intestine of marmosets after oral inoculation. *Infect. Immun. 28:* 45–48, 1980.

190. Mathiesen, L. R., Skinoj, P., Nielsen, J. O., *et al.* Hepatitis type A, B, and non-A, non-B in fulminant hepatitis. *Gut 21:* 72–77, 1980.

191. Maugh, T. H. Where is the hepatitis C virus? Non-A, non-B hepatitis is apparently caused by one or more viruses, but getting a handle on them has proved exceptionally difficult. *Science 210:* 999–1000, 1980.

192. Maupas, P., Larouze, B., London, W. T., Werner, B., Millman, I., O'Connell, A., Blumberg, B. S., Saimot, G., and Payet M. Antibody to hepatitis B core antigen in patients with primary hepatic carcinoma. *Lancet 2:* 9–11, 1975.

193. Maupas, P. H., Goudeau, A., Coursaget, P., Drucker, J., and Bargos, P. H. Immunization against hepatitis B in man. *Lancet 1:* 1367–1370, 1976.

194. Maynard, J. E. Viral hepatitis as an occupational hazard in the health care profession. In *Viral Hepatitis.* Edited by G. N. Vyas, S. N. Cohen, and R. Schmid, pp. 321–331. Philadelphia, Franklin Institute Press, 1978.

195. Maynard, J. E., Berquist, K. R., Krushak, D. H., and Purcell, R. H. Experimental infection of chimpanzees with the virus of hepatitis B. *Nature (Lond.) 237:* 514–515, 1972.

196. Maynard, J. E., Bradley, D. W., Gravelle, C. R., Ebert, J. W., and Krushak, D. H. Preliminary studies of hepatitis A in chimpanzees. *J. Infect. Dis. 131:* 194–196, 1975.

197. Mazzur, S., and Watson, T. M. Excess males among siblings of Australia antigen carriers. *Nature (Lond.) 250:* 60–61, 1974.

198. McDonald, S. *Edinb. Med. J. 15:* 208, 1908 (as cited by S. Krugman. *Perspectives on viral hepatitis infection: past, present and future.* In: *Viral Hepatitis,* Edited by G. N. Vyas, S. N. Cohen, R. Schmid, pp. 3–10. Philadelphia, Franklin Institute Press, 1978.)

199. McFarlane, E. S., Embil, J. A., Manuel, F. R., and Gorelick, M. Prevalence of antibodies to hepatitis A antigen in patients attending a clinic for treatment of sexually transmitted diseases.

Sex. Transm. Dis 7: 87–89, 1980.

200. Melnic, J. L. A water-borne urban epidemic of hepatitis. In *Hepatitis Frontiers.* Edited by F. W. Hartman, G. LoGrippo, J. G. Mateer, and J. Barron, pp. 211–225. Boston, Brown & Co., 1957.

201. Meyer Zum Büschenfeld, K. H., and Hopf, U. Studies on the pathogenesis of experimental chronic active hepatitis in rabbits. I. Induction of the disease and protective effect of allogeneic liver specific proteins. *Br. J. Exp. Pathol. 55:* 498–508, 1974.

202. Mihas, A. A., and Conrad, M. E. Hepatitis B antigen and the liver. *Medicine 57:* 129–150, 1978.

203. Miller, D. J., Dwyer, J. M., and Klatskin, G. Identification of lymphocytes in percutaneous liver biopsy cores: different T:B cells ratio in HBsAg-positive and negative hepatitis. *Gastroenterology 72:* 1199–1203, 1977.

204. Moritsugu, Y., Dienstag, J. L., Valdesuso, J., Wong, D. C., Wagner, J., Routenberg, J. A., and Purcell, R. H. Purification of hepatitis A antigen from feces and detection of antigen and antibody by immune adherence hemagglutination. *Infect. Immun. 13:* 898–908, 1976.

205. Moussouros, A., Cochrane, A. M. G., Thomson, A. D., Eddleston, A. L. W. F., and Williams, R. Transient lymphocyte-mediated hepatotoxicity in acute viral hepatitis. *Gut 16:* 835–836, 1975.

206. Mosley, J. W. Epidemiologic implications of changing trends in type A and type B hepatitis. In *Hepatitis and Blood Transfusion.* Edited by G. N. Vyas, H. A. Perkins, and R. Schmid, pp. 23–26. New York, Grune & Stratton, 1972.

207. Murata, S., Nomoto, K., Imai, M., Hattori, T., Miyakawa, Y., and Mayumi, M. Maternal transmission of hepatitis B (cont.). *N. Engl. J. Med. 296:* 692–693, 1977.

208. Murray, D. H. Acriflavine: its use by intravenous injection in the treatment of gonorrhea. *J. R. Army Med. CPS 54:* 19–27, 1930.

209. Murray, R. Viral hepatitis. *Bull NY Acad. Med. 31:* 341–358, 1955.

210. Nayak, N. C., Dhar, A., Sachdeva, R., Mittal, A., Seth, H. N., Sudarsanam, O., Reddy, B., Wagholikar, U. L., and Reddy, C. R. R. M. Association of human hepatocellular carcinoma and cirrhosis with hepatitis B virus surface and core antigens in the liver. *Int. J. Cancer 20:* 643–654, 1977.

211. Nazarewicz, T., Krawezynski, K., Sluzarczyk, J., *et al.* Cellular localization of hepatitis B virus antigens in patients with hepatocellular carcinoma coexisting with liver cirrhosis. *J. Infect. Dis. 135:* 298–302, 1977.

212. Neefe, J. R., Gellis, S. S., Stakes, J. Jr. Homologous serum hepatitis and infectious (epidemic) hepatitis: studies in volunteers bearing on immunological and other characteristics of etiological agents. *Am. J. Med. 1:* 3–22, 1946.

213. Nielson, J. O., Dietrichson, O., Elling, P., and Christoffersen, P. Incidence and meaning of persistence of Australia antigen in patients with acute viral hepatitis: development of chronic hepatitis. *N. Engl. J. Med. 285:* 1157–1160, 1971.

214. Nielson, J. O., Dietrichson, O., and Juhl, E. Incidence and meaning of the "e" determinant among hepatitis B antigen-positive patients with acute and chronic liver diseases. *Lancet 2:* 913–915, 1974.

215. Nishioka, K., Mayumi, M., Okochi, K., Okada, K., and Hirayama, T. Natural history of Australia antigen and hepatocellular carcinoma. In *Analytic and Experimental Epidemiology of Cancer,* p. 137. Baltimore, University Park Press, 1973.

216. Norkrans, G., Frosner, G., Hermodsson, S., *et al.* Clinical, epidemiological and prognostic aspects of hepatitis "non-A, non-B"; a comparison with hepatitis A and B. *Scand. J. Infect. Dis. 17:* 1–44, 1978.

217. Notkins, A. L., Mergenhagen, S. E., and Howard, R. J. Effect of virus infections on the function of the immune system. *Ann. Rev. Microbiol. 24:* 525–538, 1970.

218. Nowoslaski, A., Krawczynsky, K., Nazarewich, T., and Slusarezyk, J. Immunopathological aspects of hepatitis B. *Am. J. Med. Sci. 270:* 229–239, 1975.

219. Obada, H. *Clinician 24:* 63, 1977.

220. O'Connell, A., and London, W. T. (as cited by B. S. Blumberg). Viruses similar to hepatitis B virus (icrons). *Human Pathology,* manuscript in preparation, 1981.

221. Ohbayashi, A., Okachi, K., and Mayumi, M. Familial clustering of asymptomatic carriers of Australia antigen and patients with chronic liver disease or primary liver cancer. *Gastroenterology 62:* 618–625, 1972.

222. Okada, K., Kamiyami, I., Inomata, M., Imai, M., Miakama, Y., and Mayumi, M. E antigen and anti-e in the serum of asymptomatic carrier mothers as indicators of positive and negative

transmission of hepatitis B virus to their infants. *N. Engl. J. Med. 295:* 746–749, 1976.

223. Okochi, J., and Murakami, S. Observations on Australia antigen in Japanese. *Vox. Sang. 15:* 374–385, 1968.

224. Paronetto, F., and Vernace, S. Immunological studies in patients with chronic active hepatitis; cytotoxic activity of lymphocytes to autochthonous liver cells grown in tissue culture. *Clin. Exp. Immunol. 19:* 99–104, 1975.

225. Paul, J. R., Havens, W. P., Jr., *et al.* Transmission experiments in serum jaundice and infectious hepatitis. *JAMA 128:* 911–915, 1945.

226. Perrillo, R. P., Gelb, L., Campbell, C., *et al.* Hepatitis B e antigen DNA polymerase activity, and infection of household contacts with hepatitis B virus. *Gastroenterology 76:* 1319–1325, 1979.

227. Peters, R. K. Viral hepatitis: a pathological spectrum. *Am. J. Med. Sci. 270:* 17–31, 1975.

228. Peters, R. L., Omata, M., Ashavai, M., and Liew, C. T. Protracted viral hepatitis with impaired regeneration. In *Viral Hepatitis.* Edited by G. N. Vyas, S. N. Cohen, and R. Schmid, pp. 79–84. Philadelphia, Franklin Institute Press, 1978.

229. Phillips, M. J., and Poucell, S. Modern aspects of the morphology of viral hepatitis. *Hum. Pathol.,* manuscript in preparation, 1981.

230. Popper, H. Clinical pathologic correlation in viral hepatitis. The effect on the liver. *Am. J. Pathol. 81:* 609–628, 1975.

231. Popper, H., Dienstag, J. L., Feinstone, S. M., Alter, H. J., and Purcell, R. H. The pathology of viral hepatitis in chimpanzees. *Virchows Arch. (Pathol. Anat.) 387:* 91–106, 1980.

232. Popper, H., Paronetto, F., and Schaffner, F. Immune processes in the pathogenesis of liver disease. *Ann. NY Acad. Sci. 124:* 781–799, 1965.

233. Prates, M. D., and Torres, F. O. A cancer survey in Lourenco Marques, Portugese East Africa. *J. Natl. Cancer Inst. 35:* 729–757, 1965.

234. Prince, A. M. An antigen detected in the blood during the incubation period of serum hepatitis. *Proc. Natl. Acad. Sci. USA 60:* 814–821, 1968.

235. Prince, A. M. Immunologic distinction between I.H. and S.H. *N. Engl. J. Med. 281:* 163–164, 1969.

236. Prince, A. M., Brotman, B., Grady, G. F., *et al.* Long-incubation posttransfusion hepatitis without serological evidence of exposure to hepatitis B virus. *Lancet 2:* 241–246, 1974.

237. Propert, S. A. Hepatitis after prophylactic serum. *Br. Med. J. 2:* 677–678, 1938.

238. Provost, P. J., and Hilleman, M. R. Propagation of human hepatitis A virus in cell culture *in vitro. Proc. Soc. Exp. Biol. Med. 160:* 213–221, 1979.

239. Provost, P. J., Ittensohn, O. L., Villarejos, V. M., Arguedas, J. A., and Hilleman, M. R. Etiologic relationship of marmoset-propagated CR326 hepatitis A virus to hepatitis in man. *Proc. Soc. Exp. Biol. Med. 142:* 1257–1267, 1973.

240. Provost, P. J., Ittensohn, O. L., Villarejos, V. M., and Hilleman, M. R. A specific complement-fixation test for human hepatitis A employing CR326 virus antigen, diagnosis and epidemiology. *Proc. Soc. Exp. Biol. Med. 148:* 962–969, 1975.

241. Provost, P. J., Villarejos, V. M., and Hilleman, M. R. Suitability of the rufiventer marmoset as a host animal for human hepatitis A virus. *Proc. Soc. Exp. Biol. Med. 155:* 283–286, 1977.

242. Provost, P. J., Wolanski, B. S., Miller, W. J., Ittensohn, O. L., McAleer, W. J., and Hilleman, M. R. Physical, chemical and morphologic dimensions of human hepatitis A virus strain CR326. *Proc. Soc. Exp. Biol. Med. 148:* 532–539, 1975.

243. Purcell, R. H., Dienstag, J. L., Feinstone, S. M., and Kapikian, A. Z. Relationship of hepatitis A antigen to viral hepatitis. *Am. J. Med. Sci. 270:* 61–71, 1975.

244. Purcell, R. H., and Gerin, J. L. Hepatitis B subunit vaccine: a preliminary report of safety and efficiency tests in chimpanzees. *Am. J. Med. Sci. 270:* 395–399, 1975.

245. Purcell, R. H., Wong, D. C., Moritsugu, Y., Dienstag, J. L., Routenberg, J. A., and Boggs, J. D. A microtiter solid-phase radioimmunoassay for hepatitis A antigen and antibody. *J. Immunol. 116:* 349–356, 1976.

246. Rakela, J., and Mosley, J. W. Fecal excretion of hepatitis A virus in humans. *J. Infect. Dis. 135:* 933–938, 1977.

247. Rakela, J., Redeker, A. G., Edwards, V. M., Decker, R., Overby, L. R., and Mosley, J. W. Hepatitis and chronic active hepatitis. *Gastroenterology 74:* 879–882, 1978.

248. Rakela, J., Stevenson, D., Edwards, V. M., Gordon, I., and Mosley, J. W. Antibodies to hepatitis A virus: patterns by two procedures. *J. Clin. Microbiol. 5:* 110–111, 1977.

249. Rappaport, A. M. Anatomic considerations. In *Diseases of the Liver*, Ed. 3 edited by L. Schiff, P. I. Philadelphia, J. B. Lippincott, 1969.

250. Ray, M. B., Desmet, V. J., Bradburne, A. F., Desmyter, J., Fevery, J., and DeGroote, J. Differential distribution of hepatitis B surface antigen and hepatitis B core antigen in the liver of hepatic B patients. *Gastroenterology 71:* 462–469, 1976.

251. Redeker, A. G. Fulminant hepatitis. In *The Liver and Its Diseases*. Edited by F. Schaffner, S. Sherlock, and C. M. Levy, pp. 149–155. New York, Intercontinental Medical Book Corporation, 1974.

252. Redeker, A. G. Viral hepatitis: clinical aspects. *Am. J. Med. Sci. 270:* 9–16, 1975.

253. Rizzetto, M., Hayer, B., Canese, M. G., Shih, J. W-K., Purcell, R. H., and Gerin, J. L. Delta agent: association of Delta antigen with hepatitis B surface antigen and RNA in serum of Delta infected chimpanzees. *Proc. Natl. Acad. Sci. USA 77:* 6124–6128, 1980.

254. Robertson, J. S., and Scheared, A. V. Altered sex rates after an outbreak of hepatitis. *Lancet 1:* 532–534, 1973.

255. Robinson, W. S. Genome of hepatitis-B virus. *Ann. Microbiol. (Paris) 31:* 357–377, 1977.

256. Robinson, W. S. Hepatitis B Dane particles DNA structure and the mechanisms of the endogeneous DNA polymerase reaction. In *Viral Hepatitis*, edited by G. N. Vyas, S. N. Cohen, and R. Schmidt, pp. 139–145. Philadelphia, Franklin Institute Press, 1978.

257. Robinson, W. S., and Greenman, R. L. DNA polymerase in the core of the human hepatitis B virus candidate. *J. Virol. 13:* 1231–1236, 1974.

258. Robinson, W. S., and Lutwick, L. I. The virus of hepatitis, type B. *N. Engl. J. Med. 295:* 1168–1175, 1232–1236, 1976.

259. Routenberg, J. A., Dienstag, J. L., Harrison, W. O., Kilpatrick, M. E., Hooper, R. R., Chisari, F. V., Purcell, R. H., and Fornes, M. F. Foodborne outbreak of hepatitis A: clinical and laboratory features of acute and protracted illness. *Am. J. Med. Sci. 278:* 123–137, 1979.

260. Sanchez-Tapias, J., Thomas, H. C., and Sherlock, S. Lymphocyte populations in liver biopsy specimens from patients with chronic liver disease. *Gut 18:* 472–475, 1977.

261. Sartwell, P. E. Infectious hepatitis in relation to blood transfusion. *Bull. U. S. Army Med. Dept., 7:* 90–100, 1947.

262. Sherlock, S. Chronic hepatitis. *Gut 15:* 581–597, 1974.

263. Sherlock, S. Viral hepatitis. In *Diseases of Liver and Biliary System*, pp. 305–339. Oxford, Blackwell Scientific Publications, 1975.

264. Sherlock, S. Predicting progression of acute type B hepatitis to chronicity. *Lancet 2:* 354–356, 1976.

265. Scheuer, P. J. Acute viral hepatitis. In *Liver Biopsy Interpretation*. Ed. 3, p. 62. London, Balliere Tindall, 1980.

266. Schmid, M., and Cueni, B. Portal lesions in viral hepatitis with submassive hepatic necrosis. *Hum. Pathol. 3:* 209–216, 1972.

267. Schulman, A. N., Dienstag, J. L., Jackson, D. R., Hoofnagle, J. H., Gerety, R. J., Purcell, R. H., and Barker, L. F. Hepatitis A antigen particles in chimpanzee liver, bile and stool. *J. Infect. Dis. 134:* 80–84, 1976.

268. Schweitzer, I. L., Mosley, J. W., Aschavai, M., *et al.* Factors influencing neonatal infection by hepatitis B virus. *Gastroenterology 65:* 277–283, 1973.

269. Schweitzer, I. L., Wing, A., McPeak, C., and Spears, R. L. Hepatitis and hepatitis-associated antigen in 56 mother-infant pairs. *JAMA 220:* 1092–1095, 1972.

270. Sergiev, P. G., *et al.* Epidemic hepatitis in relation to immunizations with human sera. *Ter. Arkh. 18:* 595, 1940.

271. Shih, J. W-K., and Gerin, J. L. Immunochemistry of hepatitis B surface antigen (HBsAg): preparation and characterization of antibodies to the constituent polypeptides. *J. Immunol. 115:* 634–639, 1975.

272. Shih, J. W-K., and Gerin, J. L. Proteins of hepatitis B surface antigen. *J. Virol. 21:* 347–357, 1977.

273. Shikata, T., Karasawa, T., Abe, K., *et al.* Hepatitis B e antigen and infectivity of hepatitis B virus. *J. Infect. Dis. 136:* 571–576, 1977.

274. Shimizu, Y. K., Feinstone, S. M., Purcell, R. H., *et al.* Non-A, non-B hepatitis: ultrastructural evidence for two agents in experimental infected chimpanzees. *Science 205:* 197–200, 1979.

275. Shimizu, Y. K., Mathiesen, L. R., Lorenz, D., Drucker, J., Feinstone, S. M., Wagner, J., and Purcell, R. H. Localization of hepatitis A antigen in liver tissue by peroxidase-conjugated antibody method: light and electron microscopic studies. *J. Immunol. 121:* 1671–1679, 1978.

276. Shiraishi, H., Kohama, T., Shirachi, R., and Ishida, N. Carbohydrate composition of hepatitis B surface antigen. *J. Gen. Virol. 36:* 207–210, 1977.

277. Shouval, D., Chakraborty, P. R., Ruiz-Opazo, N., Baum, S., Spigland, I., Muchmore, E., Gerber, M. A., and Thung, S. N. Chronic hepatitis in chimpanzee carriers of hepatitis B virus: morphologic, immunologic and viral DNA studies. *Proc. Natl. Acad. Sci. USA 77:* 6147–6151, 1980.

278. Shulman, N. R. Hepatitis-associated antigen. *Am. J. Med. 49:* 669–692, 1970.

279. Siegl, G. and Frösner, G. G. Characterization and classification of virus particles associated with hepatitis A. II. Type and configuration of nucleic acid. *J. Virol. 26:* 48–53, 1978.

280. Smetana, H. F. Pathologic anatomy of early stages of viral hepatitis. In *Hepatitis Frontiers.* Edited by F. W. Hartman, G. LoGrippo, J. G. Mateer, and J. Barron, pp. 77–111. Boston, Little, Brown & Co., 1957.

281. Smith, A. L., Cochrane, A. M. G., Mowat, A. P., Eddleston, A. L. W. F., and Williams, R. Cytotoxicity to isolated rabbit hepatocytes by lymphocytes from children with liver disease. *J. Pediatr. 91:* 584–589, 1977.

282. Snyder, R. L. Longevity and disease patterns in captive and wild woodchucks. In *Proceedings,* AAZPA Regional Workshop, Indianapolis, Ind., 1977–1978.

283. Soloway, R. D. *et al.* Clinical, biochemical and histological remission of severe chronic active liver disease: a controlled study of treatments and early prognosis. *Gastroenterology 63:* 820–833, 1972.

284. Sternlieb, I., and Scheinberg, I. H. Chronic hepatitis as a first manifestation of Wilson's disease. *Ann. Intern. Med. 76:* 59–64, 1972.

285. Stevens, C. E., Silbert, J. A., Miller, D. R., Dienstag, J. L., Purcell, R. H., and Szmuness, W. Serologic evaluation of hepatitis A and B virus infections in thalassemia patients: a retrospective study. *Transfusion 18:* 356–360, 1978.

286. Storch, G., McFarland, L. M., Kelso, K., Heilman, C. J., and Caraway, C. T. Viral-hepatitis associated with day-care centers. *JAMA 242:* 1514–1518, 1979.

287. Summers, J., O'Connell, A., and Millman, I. Genome of hepatitis B virus. Restriction of enzyme cleavage and structure of DNA extracted from Dane particles. *Proc. Natl. Acad. Sci. USA 72:* 4597–4601, 1975.

288. Summers, J., Smolec, J. M., and Snyder, R. A virus similar to human hepatitis B virus associated with hepatitis and hepatoma in woodchucks. *Proc. Natl. Acad. Sci. USA 75:* 4533–4537, 1978.

289. Summers, J., Smolec, J. M., Werner, B. G., Kelly, T. J., Tyler, G. V., and Snyder, R. L. Hepatitis B virus and woodchuck hepatitis virus are members of a novel class of DNA viruses. In *Viruses in Naturally Occuring Cancers,* Cold Spring Harbor Conferences on Cell Proliferation, Vol. 7, p. 459. Cold Spring Harbor, NY, Cold Spring Harbor Laboratory, 1980.

290. Swift, W. E., Jr., *et al.* Clinical course of viral hepatitis and the effect of exercise during convalescence. *Am. J. Med. 8:* 614–622, 1950.

291. Szmuness, W., Dienstag, J. L., Purcell, R. H., Prince, A. M., Stevens, C. E., and Levine, R. W. Hepatitis type A and hemodialysis: a seroepidemiologic study in 15 U.S. centers. *Ann. Intern. Med. 87:* 8–12, 1977.

292. Szmuness, W., Dienstag, J. L., Purcell, R. H., Harley, E. J., Stevens, C. E., and Wong, D.C. Distribution of antibody to hepatitis A antigen in urban adult populations. *N. Engl. J. Med. 295:* 755–759, 1976.

293. Szmuness, W., Harley, E. J., Ikram, H., and Stevens, C. E. Sociodemographic aspects of the epidemiology of hepatitis B. In *Viral Hepatitis.* Edited by G. N. Byas, S. N. Cohen, and R. Schmid, pp. 297–320. Philadelphia, Franklin Institute Press, 1978.

294. Tabor, E., Gerety, R. J., Vogel, C. L., Bayley, A. C., Anthony, P. P., Chan, C. H., and Barker, L. F. Hepatitis B virus infection and primary hepatocellular carcinoma. *J. Natl. Cancer Inst. 58:* 1197–1200, 1977.

295. Tabor, E. R., Gerety, R. J., Drucker, J. A., Seef, L. B., Hoofnagle, J. H., Jackson, D. R., April, M., Barker, L. F., and Dineda-Tamondong, G. Transmission of non-A, non-B hepatitis from man to chimpanzee. *Lancet 1:* 463–465, 1978.

296. Tabor, E. R., Seef, L. B., and Gerety, R. J. Chronic non-A, non-B hepatitis carrier state: transmissible agent documented in one patient over a six-year period. *N. Engl. J. Med. 303:* 140–143, 1980.

297. Tapp, E., and Jones, D. M. HBsAg and HBcAg in the livers of asymptomatic hepatitis B antigen carrier. *J. Clin. Pathol. 30:* 671–677, 1977.

298. Tong, M. J., Sun, S-G., Schaeffer, T., Chang, N-K., and Lo, K-J. Hepatitis-associated antigen and hepatocellular carcinoma in Taiwan. *Ann. Intern. Med. 75:* 687–691, 1971.

299. Tong, M. J., Wallace, A. M., Peters, R. L., and Reynolds, T. V. Lymphocyte stimulation in hepatitis B infection. *N. Engl. J. Med. 293:* 318–322, 1975.

300. Tong, M. J., Stevenson, D., and Gordon, I. Correlation of e antigen, DNA polymerase activity and Dane particles in chronic benign and chronic active type B hepatitis infections. *J. Infect. Dis. 135:* 980–984, 1977.

301. Tong, M. J., Rakela, J., McPeak, C. M., Thursby, M. W., Edwards, V. M., and Mosley, J. W. Studies in infants born to mothers with type A hepatitis and acute non-A, non-B hepatitis during pregnancy (abstract). *Gastroenterology 75:* 991, 1978.

302. Trepo, G., Vitvitski, L., Neurath, R., Hashimoto, N., Schafer, R., Nemoz, G., and Prince, A. M. Detection of e antigen in immunofluorescence in cytoplasm of hepatocytes of HBsAg carriers. *Lancet 1:* 486, 1976.

303. Trevisian, A., Realdi, G., Losi, C., *et al.* Hepatitis B virus antigens in primary hepatic carcinoma: immunofluorescent techniques on fixed liver tissue. *J. Clin. Pathol. 31:* 1133–1139, 1978.

304. Turbitt, M. L., Patrick, R. S., Gouldie, R. B., *et al.* Incidence in South-West Scotland of hepatitis B surface antigen in the liver of patients with hepatocellular carcinoma. *J. Clin. Pathol. 30:* 1124–1128, 1977.

305. Vannfalt, K. A. On the combination of diabetes mellitus and acute hepatitis. *Acta Med. Scand. 117:* 462–473, 1944.

306. Villarejos, V. M., Visona, K. A., Eduarte, A., *et al.* Evidence for viral hepatitis other than type A or type B among persons in Costa Rica. *N. Engl. J. Med. 293:* 1350–1352, 1975.

307. Virchow, R. Ueber das Vorkommen und den Nachweis des hepatogenen, insbesondere des katarrhabischen icterus. *Virchows Arch.* (*Pathol Anat.*) *32:* 117, 1865, (as cited by J. W. Mosley and J. Galambos. Viral hepatitis. In *Diseases of the Liver.* Edited by L. Schiff. Philadelphia, J. B. Lippincott.)

308. Vogel, C. L., Anthony, P. P., Sadikali, F., Barker, L. F., and Peterson, M. R. Hepatitis-associated antigen and antibody in hepatocellular carcinoma: results of a continuing study. *J. Natl. Cancer Inst. 48:* 1583–1588, 1972.

309. Vyas, G. N., Peterson, D. L., Townsend, R. M., Danle, S. R., and Magnius, L. O. Hepatitis B "e" antigen: an apparent association with lactate dehydrogenase isozyme-5. *Science 198:* 1068–1070, 1977.

310. Walters, G., Kuijpers, L., Kacaki, J., and Schuurs, A. Solid phase enzyme-immunoassay for detection of hepatitis B surface antigen. *J. Clin. Pathol. 29:* 873–879, 1976.

311. Wands, J. R., and Isselbacher, F. J. Lymphocyte cytotoxicity to autologous liver cells in chronic active hepatitis. *Proc. Natl. Acad. Sci. USA 72:* 1301–1303, 1975.

312. Williams, A., and LeBouvier, G. L. Heterogeneity and thermolability of "e." *Bibl. Haematol. 42:* 71–75, 1976.

313. Williams, S. V., Huff, J. C., and Bryan, J. A. Hepatitis A and facilities for preschool children. *J. Infect. Dis. 131:* 491–495, 1975.

314. Wong, D. C., Purcell, R. H., Sreennivasan, M. A., *et al.* Epidemic and endemic hepatitis in India: evidence for a non-A, non-B hepatitis virus etiology. *Lancet 2:* 876–879, 1980.

315. Wright, R. Type B hepatitis: progression to chronic hepatitis. *Clin. Gastroenterol. 9:* 97–115, 1980.

316. Wyke, R. J., Tsiquaye, K. N., Thorton, A. *et al.* Transmission of non-A, non-B hepatitis to chimpanzees by factor-IX concentrates after fatal complications in patients with chronic liver disease. *Lancet 1:* 520–524, 1979.

317. Yamada, G., and Nakane, P. K. Hepatitis B core and surface antigens in liver tissue. *Lab. Invest. 36:* 649–659, 1977.

318. Yeung Laiwah, A. A. C., Chaudhuri, A. K. R., and Anderson, J. R. Lymphocyte transformation and leucocyte migration—Inhibition by Australia antigen. *Clin. Exp. Immunol. 15:* 27–34, 1973.

319. Yoshizawa, H., Itoh, Y., Simonetti, J. P. *et al.* Demonstration of hepatitis B e antigen in hepatitis core particles obtained from the nucleus of hepatocytes infected with hepatitis B virus. *J. Gen. Virol. 42:* 513–519, 1979.

320. Yoshizawa, H., Akahane, Y., Itoh, Y. *et al.* Virus-like particles in a plasma fraction (fibrinogen) and in the circulation of apparently healthy blood donors capable of inducing non-A, non-B hepatitis in humans and chimpanzees. *Gastroenterology 79:* 512–520, 1980.

321. Yoshizawa, H., Itoh, Y., Iwakiri, S., Tsuda, F., Nakano, S., Miyakawa, Y., and Mayumi, M. Diagnosis of type A hepatitis by fecal IgA antibody against hepatitis A antigen. *Gastroenterology 78:* 114–118, 1980.

Chapter 12

Rickettsial Diseases: An Update

DAVID H. WALKER

A clear, meaningful definition for the term rickettsia is now possible, although there is still a strong tendency to include miscellaneous microorganisms of uncertain taxonomic status in this category. The genus *Rickettsia* may be defined as small, obligate intracellular, coccobacillary gram-negative bacteria (Fig. 12.1) which spend all or a portion of their life in an arthropod host and which contain antigens of spotted fever group, typhus group, or scrub typhus group. Recent studies of DNA homology have confirmed that representative members of the genus share 40–70% of genetic information, a proportion consistent with genus level of relatedness (23). Of the other bacterial species considered fairly closely related to genus *Rickettsia*, *Coxiella burnetii* has considerable biologic and pathologic differences, and *Rochalimaea quintana* has been cultivated on cell-free medium (53).

In addition to the recognized agents of human rickettsial diseases in North America, numerous spotted fever group rickettsiae (7, 29) of undefined pathogenic significance have been identified in tick reservoirs (Table 12.1). These rickettsiae are not rare; in fact, they outnumber *Rickettsia rickettsii* in natural tick populations. Two new ecologic situations have been observed involving typhus group organisms: *R. canada* (2, 22), another rickettsia of unknown pathogenic importance, and *R. prowazeki*, the etiologic agent of classic typhus fever originating in a zoonotic cycle involving flying squirrels (3). This latter problem has resulted in human disease resembling Rocky Mountain spotted fever (RMSF) except for its seasonal occurrence between November and March.

The principal rickettsiosis in the United States is Rocky Mountain spotted fever. Over the last two decades its incidence has risen sharply from 0.11 cases per 100,000 population in 1959 to 0.50 cases per 100,000 population in 1977 (8). The disease occurs more often in the Southeastern states, in children, in males, and between mid-April and mid-September (14). These epidemiologic factors are determined by the distribution of infected ticks and their opportunity to feed on humans. The central role of the tick as reservoir and vector for *R. rickettsii* is emphasized by the mechanism of maintenance of the organism in nature, highly efficient transovarial transmission (Fig. 12.2), and the mechanism of transmission to man, regurgitation of infected salivary secretions during feeding (6) (Fig. 12.3).

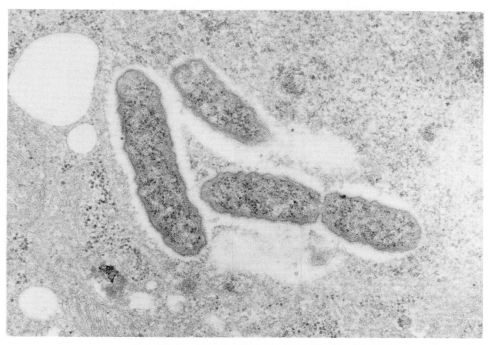

FIG. 12.1. Electron micrograph of *Rickettsia rickettsii* in cytosol of primary chick embryo cell culture. Rickettsiae have ultrastructural morphology characteristic of gram-negative bacteria. A rickettsia is undergoing binary fission. Uranyl acetate-lead citrate stain. ×40,040.

TABLE 12.1. RICKETTSIAE OF NORTH AMERICA

Group	Organism	Disease	Vector
Spotted fever	*R. rickettsii*	Rocky Mountain spotted fever	Dermacentor variabilis Dermacentor andersoni Rhipicephalus sanguineus
	R. akari	Rickettsialpox	Allodermanyssus sanguineus
	R. parkeri	NK[a]	Amblyomma maculatum
	R. montana	NK	Dermacentor variabilis Dermacentor andersoni
	R. rhipicephali	NK	Rhipicephalus sanguineus Dermacentor variabilis Dermacentor andersoni
	Unnamed species	NK	Amblyomma americanum
	Unnamed species	NK	Dermacentor occidentalis
	Unnamed species	NK	Ixodes pacificus
	Unnamed species	NK	Dermacentor parumapertus
Typhus	*R. mooseri*	Murine typhus	Xenopsylla cheopis
	R. prowazeki	Typhus	Ectoparasite of flying squirrels
		Recrudescent ty-phus	None
	R. canada	NK	Haemophysalis leporispalustris
Scrub typhus	None		

[a] None known.

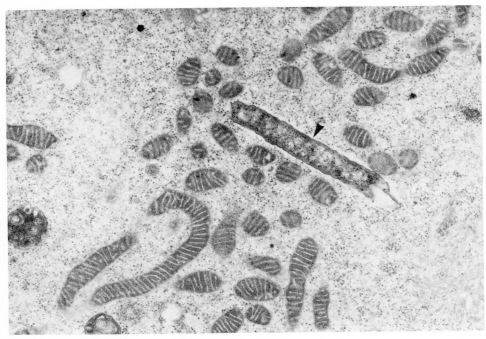

FIG. 12.2. Electron micrograph of a spotted fever rickettsia (*arrow*) in the cytoplasm of a cell in the ovary of *Dermacentor variabilis*, the common dog tick. Highly efficient transovarial transmission maintains the rickettsia in the environment. Uranyl acetate-lead citrate stain. ×23,970.

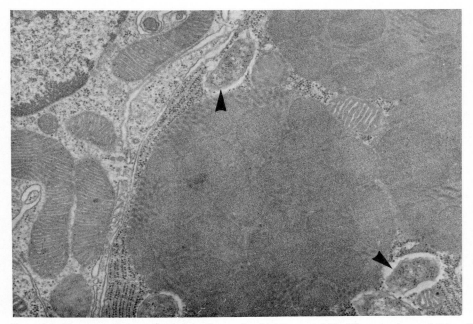

FIG. 12.3. Electron micrograph of the salivary gland of *D. variabilis*. The cytoplasm of this cell, which contains secretory granules and spotted fever rickettsiae (*arrowheads*), is released into the blood meal during feeding. Uranyl acetate-lead citrate stain. ×24,000.

CLINICAL AND PATHOLOGIC FEATURES OF ROCKY MOUNTAIN SPOTTED FEVER (RMSF)

The sequence of pathogenic events in RMSF appears to consist of intradermal inoculation of regurgitated rickettsiae by a feeding tick, lymphatic and hematogenous spread of the organisms, invasion of vascular endothelium (Fig. 12.4), intracellular replication by binary fission, local spread to involve many contiguous endothelial cells, and injury to parasitized endothelial cells. The results of endothelial injury are increased vascular permeability (13) and vasculitis in many organs (19, 56). Recent clinicopathologic studies have yielded new information on several pathologic lesions and the associated clinical complications.

A complication of major clinical importance is noncardiogenic pulmonary edema. Rickettsiae infect the pulmonary microcirculation (Fig. 12.5), and this is the likely mechanism of endothelial injury and increased vascular permeability (51). Investigation of the pulmonary pathology of RMSF has demonstrated the consequences of vascular permeability and vasculitis in this site: increased lung weight due to edema and congestion; interstitial pneumonia and edema (Fig. 12.6); and alveolar edema, fibrin, and hemorrhages (51). Clinical involvement of the lower respiratory tract includes rales, abnormal chest radiographs, and abnormal gas exchange (9). That pulmonary edema is noncardiogenic has been documented by measurement of pulmonary capillary wedge pressure, chest radiography, and postmortem cardiac examination (18, 40, 49). The recognition of this complication should lead to judicious fluid management to attempt to maintain perfusion of vital organs without raising the likelihood of pulmonary edema. Documentation of the presence or absence of pulmonary edema by the pathologist at necropsy should provide important feedback to the clinicians in charge of managing such cases.

In contrast, studies of cardiac pathology in fatal RMSF have shown little evidence to support significant loss of function (5, 50). Although there is usually moderate interstitial mononuclear myocarditis (Fig. 12.7) and rarely involvement

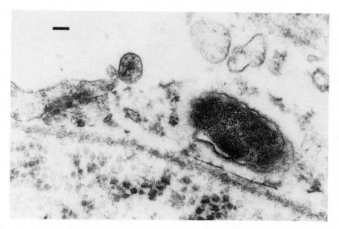

FIG. 12.4. Electron micrograph of endothelium of a patient with fatal Rocky Mountain spotted fever. *R. rickettsii* is present in the cytoplasm of an endothelial cell. Uranyl acetate-lead citrate stain. ×40,000. *Bar*, 0.1 µm.

FIG. 12.5. Photomicrograph of lung from a patient with RMSF. Immunofluorescent *R. rickettsii* are demonstrated in alveolar septa. FITC-rabbit anti-*R. rickettsii* globulin. ×350.

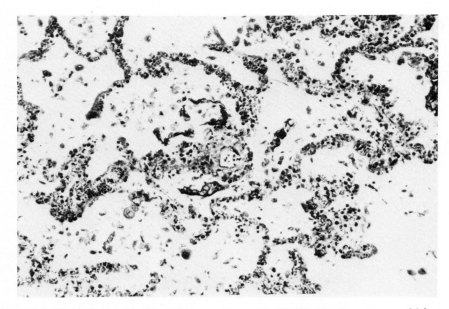

FIG. 12.6. Photomicrograph of lung from a patient with RMSF. Alveolar septa are thickened by interstitial pneumonia. Darkly stained fibrinous exudate is present in alveoli adjacent to an inflamed septal blood vessel. Phosphotungstic acid-hematoxylin stain. ×150.

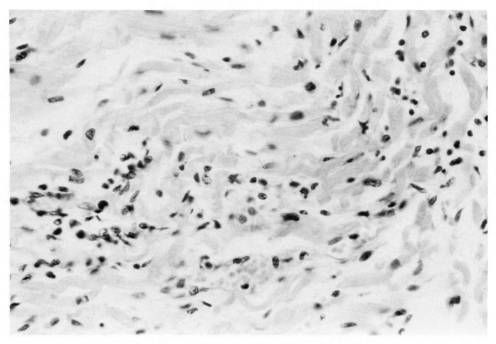

FIG. 12.7. Photomicrograph of heart from a patient with RMSF demonstrates mononuclear interstitial myocarditis with no myocardial cell necrosis. Hematoxylin-eosin stain. ×375.

FIG. 12.8. Photomicrograph of brain from a patient with RMSF. Immunofluorescent *R. rickettsii* infect a small cerebral blood vessel. FITC-rabbit-anti-*R. rickettsii* globulin. ×800.

of the conduction system, the left ventricle is not grossly dilated, and myocardial cell necrosis occurs extremely rarely and even then only focally.

Clinically, the cause of death is usually related to manifestations of rickettsial encephalitis such as seizures, multiple focal neurologic signs, cardiorespiratory arrest, and coma. Rickettsiae infect cerebral blood vessels (Fig. 12.8), and the associated pathologic lesion is quite characteristic of rickettsial disease. This classic lesion consists of accumulation of lymphocytes and macrophages around a small blood vessel with infiltration of the adjacent neuropil by macrophages (Figs. 12.9 and 12.10). In cases of RMSF which have survived for 11 or more days from onset of symptoms, identification of this lesion by the pathologist is a reliable observation suggesting a rickettsial etiology to the disease process (19).

The liver is not usually an important target organ in RMSF. However, occasionally a patient has severe hyperbilirubinemia with or without modest elevations of serum hepatic enzymes (1, 17, 33). Rickettsiae infect mainly arteries and veins of the portal triads, and the consequent pathologic lesions are portal vasculitis and portal triaditis with large mononuclear cells and polymorphonuclear leukocytes (1) (Fig. 12.11). Hepatomegaly may reflect hepatic edema. Erythrophagocytosis is a prominent observation. Hyperbilirubinemia presumably results from a combination of biliary obstruction at the level of the inflamed portal triad and increased bilirubin production due to hemolysis. Hepatocytes are not infected, hepatic necrosis is minimal to mild, and hepatic metabolic function appears to be intact.

Acute renal failure usually accompanies fatal RMSF and complicates many severe cases in which the patients ultimately survive (45). The renal pathophysiology has been shown to be either prerenal azotemia secondary to hypovolemia or oliguric acute renal failure (acute tubular necrosis) secondary to shock. The most frequent lesion, multifocal perivascular interstitial nephritis occurring at the corticomedullary junction and in the outer medulla, does not seem to produce a

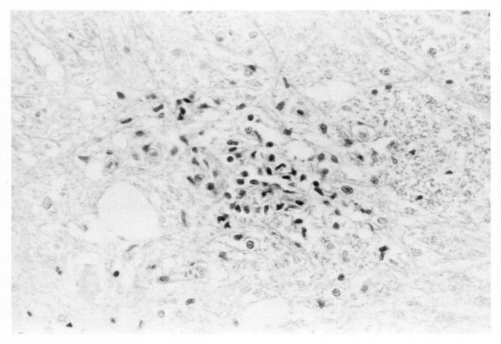

FIG. 12.9. Photomicrograph of brain from a patient with RMSF demonstrates a typical lesion. Perivascular neuropil is infiltrated by mononuclear cells. Hematoxylin-eosin stain. ×370.

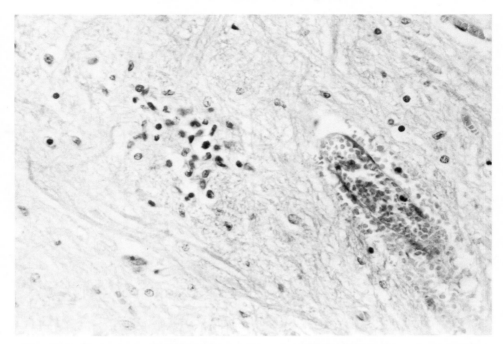

FIG. 12.10. Photomicrograph of brain from a patient with RMSF demonstrates two types of CNS vascular lesions observed in rickettsial diseases. The "typhus nodule" with perivascular mononuclear cellular infiltration (*left*) is seen uniformly in patients dying 11 or more days after onset of symptoms. In patients dying of fulminant RMSF less than 5 days after onset, perivascular ring hemorrhage without leukocytic reaction (*right*) is the manifestation of vascular injury. Hematoxylin-eosin stain. ×370.

discernible effect on renal function (4, 45). This lesion is the major site of rickettsial infection in the kidney (45). Thrombosis of glomerular capillaries is rarely observed, except in cases of fulminant RMSF (5, 25, 40, 45), which by definition causes death within 3–5 days of onset of symptoms (28).

The coagulopathy of RMSF is quite variable, yet tends to reflect the severity of the disease in the individual patient (17) (Table 12.2). Patients may maintain normal platelet counts and coagulation times, may develop thrombocytopenia with normal coagulation times, or may have thrombocytopenia with prolonged prothrombin and partial thromboplastin times. Fibrinogen levels are usually within the normal range, although in the severest cases they too may be depressed. Although these laboratory data have been used to diagnose disseminated intra-vascular coagulation (DIC) and a few have even advocated heparin therapy, thrombi are observed only in foci of the microcirculation which are infected and injured by *R. rickettsii* (45) (Fig. 12.12). Normal uninfected, uninjured microcirculation does not manifest DIC. The thrombi are usually nonocclusive and appear located to achieve hemostasis appropriately (Fig. 12.13).

Hallmarks of RMSF are fluid and electrolyte imbalance secondary to increased vascular permeability (13). This disease is regularly accompanied by edema and hypovolemia and is at times complicated by acute renal failure. Hyponatremia is

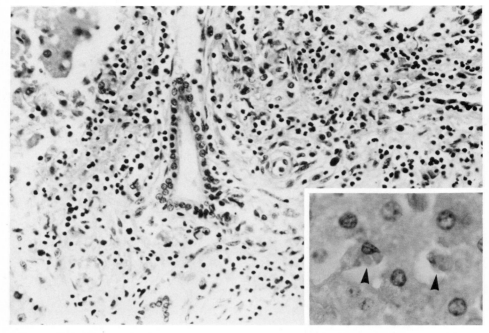

FIG. 12.11. Photomicrograph of liver from a patient with RMSF. Portal triaditis is characterized by presence of polymorphonuclear leukocytes and large mononuclear cells. Hematoxylin-eosin stain. ×300. *Inset*, erythrophagocytosis by Kupffer cells (*arrowheads*). Hematoxylin-eosin stain. ×600.

TABLE 12.2. COAGULATION LABORATORY VALUES IN ROCKY MOUNTAIN SPOTTED FEVER

Clinical Severity	Platelets	PT[a] and PTT	Fibrinogen
Mild	Normal	Normal	Normal
Moderate	Normal or decreased	Normal or prolonged	Normal
Severe	Decreased	Prolonged	Normal or decreased

[a] PT, prothrombin time; PTT, partial thromboplastin time.

so frequently observed that it is often considered as supporting evidence for the diagnosis of RMSF. In severe RMSF, hypocalcemia and hypoalbuminemia are often noted. The pathophysiologic mechanisms underlying hyponatremia, hypoalbuminemia, and hypocalcemia have not been elucidated completely, although it is probable that albumin passes into the extravascular interstitial fluid as a result of capillary leakage (10, 13). Whether the calcium ion levels are low or whether only the calcium bound to albumin is depressed has not been determined. Moreover, although the syndrome of inappropriate secretion of antidiuretic hormone has been suggested as the mechanism of hyponatremia (36), it would seem that in the face of a hypovolemic state, secretion of antidiuretic hormone would be, in fact, appropriate. Clearly, research on fluid management could provide valuable information for clinical care.

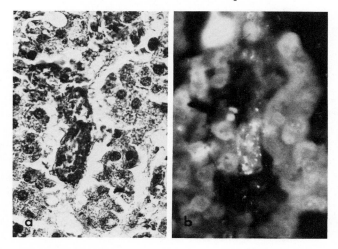

FIG. 12.12. Photomicrographs of serial sections from adrenal of patient with fulminant RMSF. (*A*) Histochemical demonstration of an isolated focus of sinusoidal fibrin thrombus. Phosphotungstic acid-hematoxylin stain. ×400. (*B*) The same sinusoidal focus is the site of intense rickettsial infection. FITC-rabbit anti-*R. rickettsii* globulin. ×400.

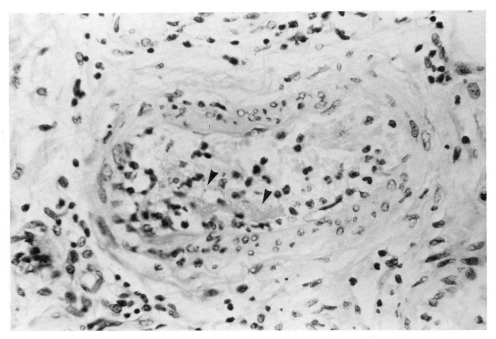

FIG. 12.13. Photomicrograph of skin from a patient with RMSF. A dermal artery shows evidence of rickettsial vasculitis, mural and perivascular infiltration composed principally of mononuclear cells, and a nonocclusive thrombus (*arrowheads*). Hematoxylin-eosin stain. ×368.

Pathogenesis

Consideration of current data on factors associated with virulence in RMSF reveals several host factors and suggestions of rickettsial factors (Table 12.3). Fatality-to-case ratios are higher for males, for persons over 30 years of age, and for blacks (14). Black males with glucose-6-phosphate dehydrogenase (G-6-PD) deficiency appear to be predisposed to a more severe course of RMSF (41, 47). This problem is the subject of ongoing research in our laboratory using blood submitted from any severe or fatal case of RMSF in a black male. Data suggesting that there may be rickettsial strain differences for virulence in RMSF are historical observations of marked geographic variation in mortality rates (20, 21) and strain differences in virulence for guinea pigs (32). Other rickettsial factors are dose of inoculum (26) and the state of reversible activation of rickettsiae in the tick at the time of inoculation (39).

The weight of experimental evidence at present indicates that host-mediated pathogenic mechanisms such as immunopathology (24, 26, 44), Schwartzman-like blood coagulation (24, 40), and the inflammatory process are not the primary mechanisms of injury in infection by *R. rickettsii* (Table 12.4). However, a recent clinical investigation of RMSF has demonstrated activation of the kallikrein-kinin system with elevated serum kallikrein and depressed serum prekallikrein and kininogen (58). Because kallikrein inhibitor levels were only reduced to half of normal levels, it is not likely that the elevated kallikrein would have had a systemic effect in the patients who were studied. On the other hand, it is conceivable that the blanchable, erythematous maculopapule surrounding the focus of rickettsial vasculitis in the dermis might represent vasodilatation due to local effects of kallikrein or another inflammatory mediator. Moreover, there may

TABLE 12.3. FACTORS ASSOCIATED WITH VIRULENCE IN RMSF

1. Host factors
   a. Sex
   b. Age
   c. Race
   d. G-6-PD deficiency
2. Rickettsial factors
   a. Geographic
   b. Strain differences in virulence for guinea pigs
   c. Dose of inoculum
   d. State of reversible activation

TABLE 12.4. HYPOTHETICAL MECHANISMS OF INJURY IN ROCKY MOUNTAIN SPOTTED FEVER

A. Host-mediated
   1. Immunopathology
   2. Coagulation
   3. Inflammation
B. Rickettsia-mediated
   1. Toxin
   2. Metabolic competition
   3. Cell membrane lysis
   4. ATP parasitism

be patients with severe RMSF in whom the kallikrein inhibitor mechanism is overwhelmed, resulting in systemic effects. Even under these circumstances, however, the inflammatory events would be secondary to the primary mechanism of injury.

Furthermore, *R. rickettsii* is directly cytopathic in cell culture systems devoid of any complex host-mediated mechanism such as the immune system, coagulation mechanism, or inflammatory reaction (Fig. 12.14). The most heavily parasitized host cells are most likely to manifest cytopathology or to undergo necrosis (46). Association of cell injury with rickettsial parasitism has been shown not only for plaque assay systems such as primary chick embryo cells and VERO cells (African green monkey kidney) but also for human umbilical vein endothelial cell cultures (52).

The pathogenic mechanism for injury to the infected cell is not known. However, certain hypotheses seem more likely based on our current state of knowledge. No toxin has ever been isolated and identified from *R. rickettsii*. Lipopolysaccharides from other rickettsiae have been shown to be relatively nontoxic (12, 34, 35), and conclusive evidence has not been demonstrated that endotoxin is an important pathogenic mechanism in any rickettsial disease. The cell culture plaque model indicates that a diffusible exotoxin is unlikely, for uninfected cells adjacent to even heavily infected cells exhibited no cytopathology (46). On the other hand, production of an intracellular toxin which is active within the infected cell is a possibility that cannot be excluded.

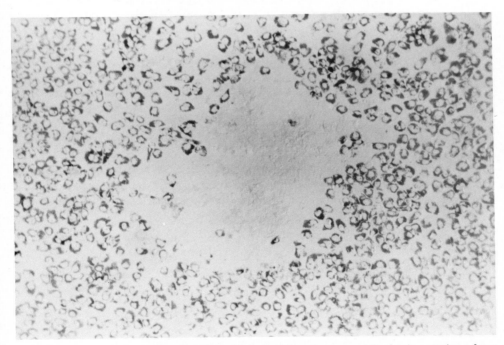

FIG. 12.14. A monolayer of endothelial cells derived from human umbilical vein contains a focus of cellular necrosis due to infection by *R. rickettsii*. Phase contrast microscopy of cell culture with viable cells containing cytoplasmic neutral red, a supravital stain. ×149.

In contrast, evidence is accumulating that injury occurs to the cell membrane on penetration into and release from the host cell by rickettsiae. Massive penetration of a cell by typhus group rickettsiae can cause cytolysis. Release of typhus group rickettsiae from the host cell occurs as a burst associated with cytolysis (55). The mechanism of penetration has been shown to involve action of phospholipase A on the host cell membrane with concomitant production of lysophosphatides and cytolysis (54). Thus, phospholipase enzymatic host cell membrane injury on penetration and possibly release seems a likely pathogenic mechanism. Moreover, the cytopathologic lesion, dilated rough endoplasmic reticulum, suggests increased cellular permeability to water (38, 46). Other hypothetical mechanisms of injury by rickettsiae to the infected cell include competition for crucial metabolic substrates and ATP parasitism (53). Although rickettsiae have been shown to utilize host cell metabolites and ATP, neither substrate nor energy parasitism has been demonstrated to cause pathologic effects in rickettsial infections. Further investigation is needed in order to ascertain the roles of the various hypothetical rickettsial pathogenic mechanisms and their relative importance.

DIAGNOSTIC TESTS

Until recently, the diagnosis of RMSF at the clinically relevant time of presentation was based on examination for rash and fever and history of severe headache and tick exposure. Laboratory confirmation was performed for completion of the individual's medical record, epidemiologic reports, and the physician's desire to evaluate his diagnostic accuracy. A fourfold rise in titer of serum agglutination of *Proteus* OX-19 or OX-2 provided sensitive evidence for recent rickettsial infection. However, the Weil-Felix test has been demonstrated to yield many false-positive results (16, 48). The complement fixation test was recognized as having greater specificity.

Currently, several sensitive and specific newer tests have been developed for detecting antibodies to *R. rickettsii* Table 12.5). These are indirect fluorescent antibody (31), latex agglutination (15), passive hemagglutination (37), and microagglutination (11). Recent comparisons of serologic methods for diagnosis of RMSF suggest that indirect fluorescent antibody, passive hemagglutination, and latex agglutination are quite sensitive and specific (27, 30). The complement fixation text varies in its sensitivity from laboratory to laboratory, depending apparently on the source of reagents (27, 30). In some laboratories the complement

TABLE 12.5. RELATIVE SENSITIVITY AND SPECIFICITY OF SEROLOGIC TESTS FOR ROCKY MOUNTAIN SPOTTED FEVER

Test	Sensitivity	Specificity	Availability
Weil-Felix Proteus OX-19	+++	+	++++
Weil-Felix Proteus OX-2	++	++	++++
Indirect fluorescent antibody	+++	++++	++
Latex agglutination	+++	++++	++
Passive hemagglutination	++++	+++	+
Microagglutination	++	++++	+
Complement fixation	+	++++	++

+, poor; ++, fair; +++, good; ++++, excellent.

fixation test missed half of the cases of RMSF, which were documented by other specific methods. The indirect fluorescent antibody test seems to be replacing the complement fixation test in many public health laboratories, although lack of availability of reagents has limited its use in hospital laboratories. The technical simplicity of the latex agglutination test makes it likely to become available commercially in the future. It will probably prove to be approximately equal to indirect fluorescent antibody in sensitivity and specificity in the immediate convalescent period. However, none of these tests may be relied upon for the acute diagnosis of RMSF. Few patients have detectible antibodies at the time of presentation for medical care (48).

A new approach, demonstration of *R. rickettsii* in punch biopsies of skin lesions by direct immunofluorescence, has been shown to offer a rapid method for diagnosis of RMSF (43, 57). Frozen sections of foci of dermal vasculitis reacted with a specific conjugate for spotted fever rickettsiae yield diagnostic results within 3 hours from the time of biopsy in 70% of patients with RMSF (43, 48). These laboratory results have proved useful in distinguishing RMSF from meningococcemia, enteroviral exanthems, secondary syphilis, immune-complex vasculitides, thrombotic thrombocytopenic purpura, idiopathic thrombocytopenic purpura, and other febrile exanthems. Although most histochemical stains described for rickettsiae, such as Wolbach's Giemsa stain, usually fail to demonstrate rickettsiae, a newly rediscovered modification of the Brown-Hopps stain does stain rickettsiae distinctly. Its sensitivity relative to specific direct immunofluorescence on formalin fixed, paraffin-embedded tissue (42) or on frozen sections remains to be determined. The greatest challenges to pathologists by rickettsial diseases during the next decade will lie in development and application of better diagnostic tools and assistance to research laboratories in unraveling the host and rickettsial factors in severity of illness. In particular, isolation and speciation of rickettsiae for an etiologic diagnosis and the study of rickettsial virulence factors for furthering our understanding of rickettsial pathogenesis require that pathologists send samples of blood and tissues such as spleen collected at necropsy to national reference and research laboratories such as the Rocky Mountain Laboratory in Hamilton, Montana. Ultimately, the goals of rapid diagnosis, prediction, management, and possibly prevention of particular complications such as noncardiogenic pulmonary edema, elucidation of pathogenic mechanisms, and prevention by an effective, long-lasting vaccine may be achieved.

REFERENCES

1. Adams, J. S., and Walker, D. H. The liver in Rocky Mountain spotted fever, *Am. J. Clin. Pathol.*, 75: 156–161, 1981.
2. Bozeman, F. M., Elisberg, B. L., Humphries, J. W., Runcik, K., and Palmer, D. B., Jr. Serologic evidence of *Rickettsia canada* infection of man. *J. Infect. Dis. 121:* 367–371, 1970.
3. Bozeman, F. M., Masiello, S. A., Williams, M. S., and Elisberg, B. L. Epidemic typhus rickettsiae isolated from flying squirrels. *Nature 255:* 545–547, 1975.
4. Bradford, W. D., Croker, B. P., and Tisher, C. C. Kidney lesions in Rocky Mountain spotted fever. A light-, immunofluorescence-, and electron-microscopic study. *Am. J. Pathol. 97:* 381–390, 1979.
5. Bradford, W. D., and Hackel, D. B. Myocardial involvement in Rocky Mountain spotted fever. *Arch. Path. Lab Med. 102:* 357–359, 1978.
6. Burgdorfer, W. Tick-borne diseases in the United States: Rocky Mountain spotted fever and Colorado tick fever. *Acta Tropica 34:* 103–126, 1977.

7. Burgdorfer, W., Sexton, D. J., Gerloff, R. K., Anacker, R. L., Philip, R. N., and Thomas, L. A. *Rhipicephalus sanguineus*: Vector of a new spotted fever group rickettsiae in the United States. *Infect. Immun. 12:* 205–210, 1975.

8. D'Angelo, L. J., Winkler, W. G., and Bregman, D. J. Rocky Mountain spotted fever in the United States, 1975–1977. *J. Infect. Dis. 138:* 273–276, 1978.

9. Donohue, J. F. Lower respiratory tract involvement in Rocky Mountain spotted fever. *Arch. Intern. Med. 140:* 223–227, 1980.

10. Fegin, R. D., Kissane, J. M., Eisenberg, C. S., and Kahn, L. I. Rocky Mountain spotted fever. Successful application of new insights into physiologic changes during acute infections to successful management of a severely ill patient. *Clin. Pediatr. 8:* 331–343, 1969.

11. Fiset, P., Ormsbee, R. A., Silberman, R., Peacock, M., and Spielman, S. H. A microagglutination technique for detection and measurement of rickettsial antibodies. *Acta Virol. 13:* 60–66, 1969.

12. Fumarola, D., Munno, I., Monno, R., and Miragliotta, G. Lipopolysaccharides from *Rickettsiaceae*: *Limulus* endotoxin assay and pathogenetic mediators in rickettsiosis (letter to the editor). *Acta Virol. 24:* 155, 1980.

13. Harrell, G. T., and Aikawa, J. K. Pathogenesis of circulatory failure in Rocky Mountain spotted fever. *Arch. Intern. Med. 83:* 331–347, 1949.

14. Hattwick, M. A. W., O'Brien, R. J., and Hanson, B. F. Rocky Mountain spotted fever: epidemiology of an increasing problem. *Ann. Intern. Med. 84:* 732–739, 1976.

15. Hechemy, K., Anacker, R., Philip, R., Kleeman, K., MacCormack, J. N., Sasowski, S., and Michaelson, E. Detection of Rocky Mountain spotted fever antibodies by a latex agglutination test. *J. Clin. Microbiol. 12:* 144–150, 1980.

16. Hechemy, K. E., Stevens, R. W., Sasowski, S., Michaelson, E. E., Casper, E. A., and Philip, R. N. Discrepancies in Weil-Felix and microimmunofluorescence test results for Rocky Mountain spotted fever. *J. Clin. Microbiol. 9:* 292–293, 1979.

17. Kaplowitz, L. G., Fischer, J. J., and Sparling, P. F. In *Current Clinical Topics in Infectious Disease.* Edited by J. S. Remington and M. N. Swartz, Vol. 2, pp. 89–108. New York, McGraw-Hill, 1980.

18. Lankford, H. V., and Glauser, F. L. Cardiopulmonary dynamics in a severe case of Rocky Mountain spotted fever. *Arch. Intern. Med. 140:* 1357–1360, 1980.

19. Lillie, R. D. The pathology of Rocky Mountain spotted fever. *Natl. Inst. Health Bull. 177:* 1–46, 1941.

20. Maxey, E. E. Some observations on the so-called spotted fever of Idaho. *Med. Sentinel 7:* 433–438, 1899.

21. McCullough, G. T. Spotted fever. *Med. Sentinel 10:* 225–228, 1902.

22. McKiel, J. A., Bell, E. J., and Lackman, D. B. *Rickettsia canada*: a new member of the typhus group of rickettsiae isolated from *Haemaphysalis leporispalustris* ticks in Canada. *Can. J. Microbiol. 13:* 503–510, 1967.

23. Meyers, W. F., and Wisseman, C. L., Jr. Genetic relatedness among the typhus group of rickettsiae. *Int. J. Syst. Bacteriol. 30:* 3–150, 1980.

24. Moe, J. B., Mosher, D. F., Kenyon, R. H., White, J. D., Stookey, J. L., Bagley, L. R., and Fine, D. P. Functional and morphologic changes during experimental Rocky Mountain spotted fever in guinea pigs. *Lab. Invest. 35:* 235–245, 1976.

25. Moon, J. H., and Silverberg, S. G. Febrile exanthem in 14-year-old boy with subsequent development of coagulopathy. *Va. Med. Monthly 98:* 271–278, 1971.

26. Mosher, D. F., Fine, D. P., Moe, J. B., Kenyon, R. H., and Ruch, G. L. Studies of the coagulation and complement system during experimental Rocky Mountain spotted fever in rhesus monkeys. *J. Infect. Dis. 135:* 985–989, 1977.

27. Newhouse, V. F., Shepard, C. C., Redus, M. D., Tzianabos, T., and McDade, J. E. A comparison of the complement fixation, indirect fluorescent antibody, and microagglutination tests for the serological diagnosis of rickettsial diseases. *Am. J. Trop. Med. Hyg. 28:* 387–395, 1979.

28. Parker, R. R. Rocky Mountain spotted fever. *J.A.M.A. 110:* 1185–1188, 1273–1278, 1938.

29. Philip, R. N., Casper, E. A., Burgdorfer, W., Gerloff, R. K., Hughes, L. E., and Bell, E. J. Serologic typing of rickettsiae of the spotted fever group by microimmunofluorescence. *J. Immun. 121:* 1961–1968, 1978.

30. Philip, R. N., Casper, E. A., MacCormack, J. N., Sexton, D. J., Thomas, L. A., Anacker, R. L., Burgdorfer, W., and Vick, S. A comparison of serologic methods for diagnosis of Rocky Mountain spotted fever. *Am. J. Epidemiol. 105:* 56–67, 1977.

31. Philip, R. N., Caspter, E. A., Ormsbee, R. A., Peacock, M. G., and Burgdorfer, W. Microimmunofluorescence test for the serological study of Rocky Mountain spotted fever and thyphus. *J. Clin. Microbiol. 3:* 51–61, 1976.

32. Price, W. H. The epidemiology of Rocky Mountain spotted fever. I. The characterization of strain virulence of *Rickettsia rickettsii. Am. Hyg. 58:* 248–268, 1953.

33. Ramphal, R., Kluge, R., Cohen, V., and Feldman, R. Rocky Mountain spotted fever and jaundice. Two consecutive cases acquired in Florida and a review of the literature on this complication. *Arch. Intern. Med. 138:* 260–263, 1978.

34. Schramek, S., Brezina, R., and Kazar, J. Some biological properties of an endotoxic lipopolysaccharide from the thyphus group rickettsiae. *Acta Virol. 21:* 439–441, 1977.

35. Schramek, S., Brezina, R., and Tarasevich, I. V. Isolation of a lipopolysaccharide antigen from *Rickettsia* species. *Acta Virol. 20:* 270, 1976.

36. Sexton, D. J., and Clapp, J. Inappropriate antidiuretic hormone secretion. Occurrence in a patient with Rocky Mountain spotted fever. *Arch. Intern. Med. 137:* 362–363, 1977.

37. Shirai, A., Dietel, J. W., and Osterman, J. V. Indirect hemagglution test for human antibody to typhus and spotted fever group rickettsiae. *J. Clin. Microbiol. 2:* 430–437, 1975.

38. Silverman, D. J., and Wisseman, C. L. *In vitro* studies of rickettsia-host cell interactions: ultrastructural changes induced by *Rickettsia rickettsii* infection of chicken embryo fibroblasts. *Infect. Immun. 26:* 714–727, 1979.

39. Spencer, R. R., and Parker, R. R. Studies on Rocky Mountain spotted fever. U. S. Public Health Service. *Hyg. Lab. Bull. 154:* 1–116, 1930.

40. Walker, D. H. Unpublished observations.

41. Walker, D. H., Kirkman, H. N., and Wittenberg, P. H. Genetic states possibly associated with enhanced severity of Rocky Mountain spotted fever. Proceedings of the Conference on Rickettsia and Rickettsial Diseases. New York, Academic Press, in press, 1982.

42. Walker, D. H., and Cain, B. G. A method for specific diagnosis of Rocky Mountain spotted fever on fixed, paraffin-embedded tissue by immunofluorescence. *J. Infect. Dis. 137:* 206–209, 1978.

43. Walker, D. H., Cain, B. G., and Olmstead, P. M. Laboratory diagnosis of Rocky Mountain spotted fever by immunofluorescent demonstration of *Rickettsia rickettsii* in cutaneous lesions. *Am. J. Clin. Pathol. 69:* 619–623, 1978.

44. Walker, D. H., and Henderson, F. W. Effect of immunosuppression on *Rickettsia rickettsii* infection in guinea pigs. *Infect. Immun. 20:* 221–227, 1978.

45. Walker, D. H., and Mattern, W. D. Acute renal failure in Rocky Mountain spotted fever. *Arch. Intern. Med. 139:* 443–8, 1979.

46. Walker, D. H., and Cain, B. G. The rickettsial plaque. Evidence for direct cytopathic effect of *Rickettsia rickettsii. Lab. Invest. 43:* 388–396, 1980.

47. Walker, D. H., and Kirkman, H. W. Rocky Mountain spotted fever and deficiency in glucose-6-phosphate dehydrogenase. *J. Infect. Dis. 142:* 771, 1980.

48. Walker, D. H., Burday, M. S., and Folds, J. D. Laboratory diagnosis of Rocky Mountain spotted fever. *Southern Med. J. 73:* 1443–1446, 1980.

49. Walker, D. H., and Mattern, W. D. Rickettsial vasculitis. *Am. Heart. J. 100:* 896–906, 1980.

50. Walker, D. H., Paletta, C. E., and Cain, B. G. Pathogenesis of myocarditis in Rocky Mountain spotted fever. *Arch. Pathol. Lab. Med. 104:* 171–174, 1980.

51. Walker, D. H., Crawford, C. G., and Cain, B. G. Rickettsial infection of the pulmonary microcirculation, the basis of interstitial pneumonitis of Rocky Mountain spotted fever. *Hum. Pathol. 11:* 263–272, 1980.

52. Walker, D. H., Firth, W. T., and Edgell, C. J. Plaques in human endothelial cell cultures caused by *Rickettsia rickettsii* (abstract). FASEB Meeting, Atlanta, Georgia, April 14, 1981.

53. Weiss, E. Growth and physiology of rickettsiae. *Bacteriol. Rev. 37:* 259–283, 1973.

54. Winkler, H. H., and Miller, E. T. Phospholipase A activity in the hemolysis of sheep and human erythrocytes by *Rickettsia prowazeki. Infect. Immun. 29:* 316–321, 1980.

55. Wisseman, C. L., Jr., and Waddell, A. D. *In vitro* studies on rickettsia-host cell interactions:

intracellular growth cycle of virulent and attenuated *Rickettsia prowazeki* in chicken embryo cells in slide chamber cultures. *Infect. Immun. 11:* 1391–1401, 1975.

56. Wolbach, S. B. Studies on Rocky Mountain spotted fever. *J. Med. Res. 41:* 2–197, 1919.
57. Woodward, T. E., Pedersen, C. E., Jr., Oster, C. N., Bagley, L. R., Romberger, J., and Snyder, M. J. Prompt confirmation of Rocky Mountain spotted fever. Identification of rickettsiae in skin tissues. *J. Infect. Dis. 134:* 297–301, 1976.
58. Yamada, T., Harber, P., Pettit, G. W., Wing, D. A., and Oster, C. N. Activation of the kallikrein-kinin system in Rocky Mountain spotted fever. *Ann. Intern. Med. 88:* 764–768, 1978.

Chapter 13

Diagnostic Features of Three Unusual Infections: Micronemiasis, Pheomycotic Cyst, and Protothecosis

DANIEL H. CONNOR, DEAN W. GIBSON, AND ANNEMARIE ZIEFER

Viruses, chlamydia, rickettsiae, spirochetes, bacteria, mycobacteria, fungi, protozoans, and metazoans all infect man. The relatively few species of these that cause disease are the traditional pathogens. In the past two decades, however, the widespread use of immunosuppressive therapy has paved the way for two new patterns of infectious disease. First, there are some traditional pathogens that infect immunosuppressed patients with increased frequency and with increased virulence. Herpesvirus infections and tuberculosis are examples. Second, immunosuppression has opened the doors to new infectious agents. These have been called "opportunists" or "opportunistic infections." In one sense, all infections are opportunistic, but the concept of opportunism is valid, for usually benign organisms may cause progressive infections in patients with suppressed immunity. Three new opportunistic infections—*micronemiasis, pheomycotic cyst*, and *protothecosis*—will be discussed in detail in this chapter.

MICRONEMIASIS

INTRODUCTION

Micronemiasis is infection by free-living nematodes of the genus *Micronema* (3, 6, 7). *Micronema* spp. are saprophytes that live in soil, manure, and decaying humus. Although normally not pathogenic, *Micronema delextrix* has caused lesions in horses (1, 2, 4, 9–11, 13, 16) and rarely in man.

CLINICAL FEATURES

There are three known fatal infections of man (Table 13.1).

Patient 1 was a 5-year-old boy who lived on a farm in Manitoba (7, 8). He fell into a manure spreader, passed through its mechanism, and sustained multiple

* This work was supported in part by the World Health Organization (WHO), Geneva. Specimens from a patient with pheomycotic cyst associated with an onchocercal nodule are from the WHO Reference Laboratory for Filarial Infections of Man at the Armed Forces Institute of Pathology (AFIP). The opinions or assertions contained herein are the private views of the authors and are not to be construed as official or as reflections of the views of the Department of the Army or the Department of Defense (USA), or WHO.

TABLE 13.1. MICRONEMIASIS IN THREE PATIENTS

Patient	Age/Sex	Yr	Location	Predisposition or Antecedent	Onset	CSF	Duration (days)	References
1	5/M	1968	Manitoba	Lacerations contaminated with manure	Lethargy	100–300 Lymphocytes & macrophages	6	7, 8
2	47/M	1978	Texas	Unknown (from horses on ranch?)	Painful legs and confusion		19	15
3	54/M	1977	Washington, D.C.	Indigent, alcoholic, diabetic, decubitus ulcers	Disorientation	Xanthochromic; WBC, 50–110; 90% lymphocytes; protein, 214 mg$^+$; sugar, 50 mg%	11	5

lacerations and fractures. Originally his wounds were heavily contaminated with horse manure, but they healed satisfactorily. Eighteen days after his injury, however, he became lethargic. Two lumbar punctures revealed about 300 cells/ ml, with approximately equal numbers of lymphocytes and macrophages. No organisms were recovered. In the ensuing hours the lethargy progressed to coma; he died 24 days after the accident and 6 days after the onset of encephalitis. Microscopic examination revealed many nematodes, *Micronema* spp., in all portions of brain, cord, and meninges and fewer in the pituitary and alveolar walls of the lung. The nematodes probably entered his body from the equine manure that heavily contaminated his wounds at the time of his accident.

Patient 2 was a 47-year-old man who owned a small ranch near Dallas, Texas (15). Although a few horses were stabled on his ranch, he had little to do with the animals and had no unusual accidents or incidents on the ranch or elsewhere. Ten days before coming to the hospital, the patient noticed pain in the right middiaphragmatic area and intermittent pain and paresthesias in his legs. On admission he had acute pains in his legs and had progressive mental confusion. The patient's condition progressively deteriorated to coma 4 days after admission and to death 19 days after admission. His brain contained many nematodes identified as *Micronema* spp.

Patient 3 was a 54-year-old male resident of Washington, D.C. (5). During the 6 months before admission he lost 35 pounds and had many episodes of diarrhea. He had no known antecedent trauma, no known association with horses, but had a large decubitus ulcer on each buttock. On admission he was febrile (100.1°F), cachetic, disoriented, and had general wasting of muscles, and bilateral conjunctivitis. His temperature rose to 106°F on the 2nd hospital day, and he became semicomatose. On the 3rd day he developed shallow respirations and hypotension. A neurologist identified bilateral internuclear ophthalmoplegia. Three spinal punctures revealed xanthochromic fluid with WBC, 50–110, 90% lymphocytes, protein 214 mg%, and sugar, 50 mg%. Although a culture of cerebrospinal fluid yielded no growth, he was treated with gentamycin, isoniazid (INH), ethambutol, and chloramphenicol, but his coma deepened. The patient died on the 11th hospital day. At autopsy, microscopic examination revealed many nematodes, *Micronema* spp., in the brain and rare micronemas in the liver and heart. We suspect that the worms entered his body through the decubitus ulcers.

Gross Findings

The brain of patient 1 had hyperemic white matter. Cut surfaces had white foci of inflammation in all portions of the brain (Fig. 13.1). The brain of patient 2 was soft and had numerous focal necrotic areas (15). The brain of patient 3 was soft, fragmenting, and autolyzed (5).

Microscopic Features

Microscopically, the three brains had extensive meningoencephalitis. Throughout the parenchyma and especially around vessels, there was an inflammatory cell infiltrate comprised of lymphocytes, plasma cells, giant cells, neutrophils, and

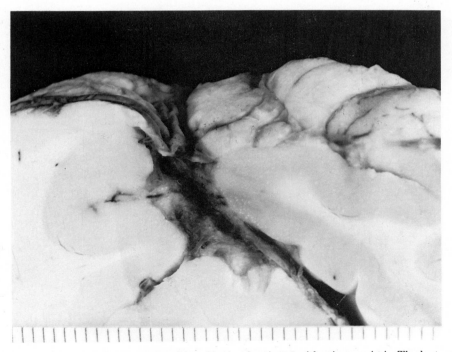

FIG. 13.1. Gross appearance, cut surface of brain of patient 1 with micronemiasis. The leptomeninges are thickened, and foci of inflammation are seen in the gray matter as minute white spots. (×3, AFIP Neg. 75-14475).

swollen microglial cells. In the brain of patient 3, there were eosinophils as well. Worms (*Micronema* spp.) were in the inflamed areas (Figs. 13.2–13.6), in vessel walls, and in portions of brain without inflammatory cells. Worms have also been seen in capillaries of the brain, in the spinal cord, in the walls and lumen of ventricles, in the central canal, and within the pituitary. Occasionally, worms have been identified in microabscesses in the liver, in the heart, and within capillaries of alveolar walls of lung. Micronemas were also in formalin in which the brain of patient 1 had been fixed (7, 8). Whole worms were recovered by trypsin digestion of the brain from patient 2 (15), and other whole worms were teased from formalin-fixed brain of patient 3.

MORPHOLOGIC FEATURES OF MICRONEMA SPECIES

The worms are small rhabdoid nematodes. The mature female worms measure between 250 and 450 μm long by 15–25 μm across (Fig. 13.4). There is a thin cuticle with fine transverse striations. One of the most characteristic features of *Micronema* spp. is the rhabditiform esophagus, which is about 85 μm long and consists of a corpus, isthmus, and bulb (Fig. 13.5). Another characteristic feature is the single ovary which shows dorsal reflection (Fig. 13.6). There is usually only one egg present measuring 4 to 6 μm by 9 to 11 μm.

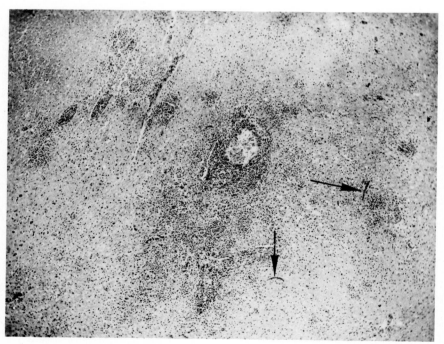

FIG. 13.2. Microscopic appearance of the brain of patient 1. There is edema, congestion, and meningoencephalomyelitis with inflammatory cells throughout the parenchyma and around vessels. There are several sections of *Micronema* sp. (*arrows*). (H&E, ×45; AFIP Neg. 70-1487).

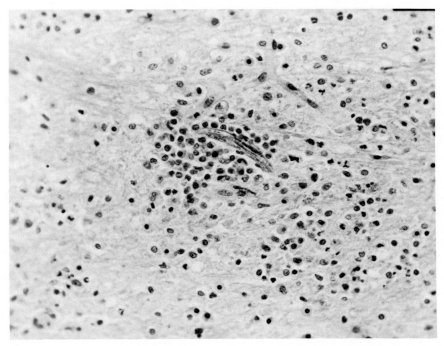

FIG. 13.3. Fragment of *Micronema* sp. in the parenchyma of the brain of patient 1. The worm is surrounded by lymphocytes, plasma cells, histiocytes, and neutrophils. (H&E, ×275; AFIP Neg. 70-1488).

DISCUSSION

Severe generalized trauma and heavy contamination of deep wounds with horse manure were apparently predisposing to micronemiasis in patient 1. Patient 2 owned a ranch in Texas with horses, but there was no known accident which would contribute to his micronemiasis. Patient 3 had a history of alcoholism, malnutrition, diabetes, and decubitus ulcers, all of which may have predisposed to infection of *Micronema* spp. It is not known what contact he may have had with horse manure.

Micronemiasis was suspected in none of these patients before death, so antihelminthics have not been tried. If in the future a clinical suspicion can be confirmed by identification of micronemas in the cerebral spinal fluid, then drugs such as thiabendazole or mebendazole can be tried—as used in treatment of strongyloidiasis (12, 14).

The contrast of micronemiasis with other helminthic infections of man is striking. Infections with cestodes, trematodes, filarial worms, and other nematodes are generally chronic or subacute and often subclinical, persisting for months and years in man. These worms are generally well adapted to man's tissues, causing little inflammation or damage other than by the gradual accumulation of scar tissue around eggs, degenerating larva, or adult worms. Micro-

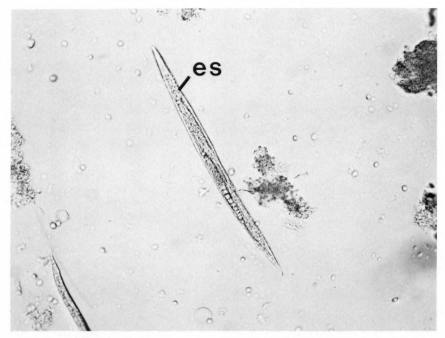

Fig. 13.4. Mature female *Micronema* sp. teased from formalin-fixed brain of patient 3. The worm is about 450 μm long and 25 μm across. The most characteristic feature is the rhabditiform esophagus (*es*). There is a single genital tube usually containing one mature egg. The pointed tail is about 70 μm long. (×160; AFIP Neg. 77-9965).

nemiasis, on the other hand, causes a rapidly progressive and fatal meningoencephalitis. Tissue and blood eosinophilia are conspicuous in most helminthic infections of man, but in micronemiasis, eosinophils are inconspicuous.

PHAEOMYCOTIC CYST (PHEOMYCOSIS)

Introduction

Pheomycotic cyst consists of infection of the deep dermis and subcutaneous tissue by brown fungi. The name is derived from the Greek *phaios*, meaning "dusky" or "gray," and refers to the brown color of these fungi both *in vivo* and *in vitro*. *Phialophora* spp. are worldwide saprophytes and grow naturally in soil, especially in humus. They may darken new lumber and eventually decay it (38).

Man becomes infected when the fungus is carried into the deep dermis or subcutaneous tissue with a foreign body—usually a sliver. Accordingly, the lesion develops on an exposed part of the limb. Early infections are small stellate pyogranulomatous foci which grow and coalesce to form abscesses with central cavities. When pus is removed, a thick-walled cavity remains. Pheomycotic cysts remain localized. None has spread locally, by lymphatics to lymph nodes, or to deep organs. The circumscribed abscess, localized in the subcutis beneath normal skin, and the pigmented polymorphous fungus are the characteristic features of pheomycotic cyst. Recent reviews include refs. 22, 30, 32, and 48.

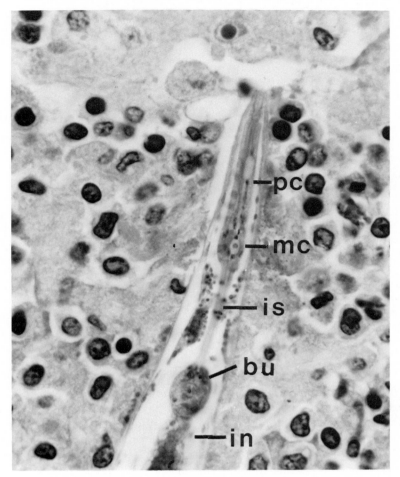

FIG. 13.5. The anterior end of a mature female *Micronema* sp. in the brain of patient 1. The rhabditiform esophagus includes the procorpus (*pc*), metacorpus (*mc*), isthmus (*is*), bulb (*bu*), and intestine (*in*). (H&E, ×1040; AFIP Neg. 74-11156.) (Fig. 6 in ref. 8.) (Reproduced with permission from J. Hoogstraten and W. G. Young (8).)

This condition was first described in 1907 by de Beurmann and Gougerot (21), who interpreted the lesion as a variant of sporotrichosis. The fungus and lesions were subsequently known by a number of different names (22, 25, 27–32, 34, 35, 39–42, 44, 48).

In 1977, the fungus was renamed *Exophiala jeanselmei*, which is considered a synonym of *Phialophora gougerotii* and *Phialophora jeanselmei* (36, 37). Nevertheless, we prefer the name *Phialophora* and accept *P. gougerotii* and *P. jeanselmei* as two distinct species (22, 48).

Ajello *et al.* (17–19) proposed "pheohyphomycosis" as an inclusive term for all cutaneous, subcutaneous, and systemic infections by dark-walled hyphomycetes. Thus "pheohyphomycosis" is a broader term than "pheomycotic cyst," which is restricted to circumscribed, subcutaneous abscesses beneath normal skin. The

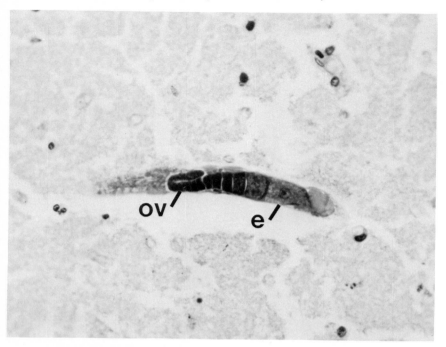

FIG. 13.6. Adult female *Micronema* sp., in the brain of patient 3. The single ovary (*ov*) shows the characteristic dorsal reflection and contains a uninucleate egg (*e*). (H&E, ×485; AFIP Neg. 77-8830).

term "pheomycotic cyst" was suggested by Binford and Dooley (22, 28) because it "defines a clinical and pathological entity that should not be confused with human sporotrichosis or equine hyphomycosis." We stress that pheomycotic cyst does not provoke hyperplasia of the epidermis, does not ulcerate, does not cause infiltrative growth, does not form sinus tracts, or contain grains. For example, the ulcerating cutaneous macule caused by *Drechslera specifera* (31), termed "pheo-hyphomycosis," does not meet the criteria for "pheomycotic cysts." For a more detailed discussion of these matters, see ref. 48.

CLINICOPATHOLOGIC STUDIES AT THE AFIP

Between 1959 and 1981, specimens from 33 patients with pheomycotic cysts have been studied at the AFIP (Table 13.2). Patients 1 through 25 were included in our recent review (48). Patients 5, 8, 9, and 14 were also in previous publications (28, 39, 42, and 47, respectively). Pheomycotic cysts from patients 26 to 33 were received between 1979 and 1981. Ten patients had an associated chronic debilitating disease (Table 13.2). The patients each had a single pheomycotic cyst, on a variety of exposed anatomic locations (Table 13.2 and Fig. 13.7). Seven patients remembered trauma at the site. Sixteen patients estimated the duration of the lesions at between 2 weeks and 10 years, with a peak at 6–12 months.

The pheomycotic cysts varied from firm to fluctuant. The cyst on the scalp of patient 8 progressed from firm to fluctuant over a period of 3 months (39). None of the lesions were tender or painful. The overlying skin was smooth, not red, swollen, or hyperplastic (Fig. 13.8).

TABLE 13.2. PHEOMYCOTIC CYST IN 33 PATIENTS

Patient	Age/Sex	Location	Associated Disease	Site of Lesion	Size (cm)	Configuration
1	38/M	Zaire		Wrist	5.0	Cyst
2	39/M	Zaire	Polyfilariasis[a]	Foot	7.0	Cyst
3	4.5/M	Hawaii		Eyelid	0.7	Solid
4	26/M	Germany		Foot	1.6	Stellate
5	33/M	Tennessee	Tuberculosis	Wrist	3.2	Stellate
6	78/F	U.S. (?)		Thumb	1.3	Cyst
7	28/F	Washington, D. C.		Knee	1.6	Cyst
8	38/M	Zaire	Leprosy[b] Diabetes	Scalp	4.0	Stellate
9	80/M	New York		Finger	1.5	Cyst
10	35/M	Malawi		Foot	Large	Cyst
11	50/F	Malawi		Ankle	4.3	Cyst
12	45/M	Haiti		Knee	3.0	Cyst
13	35/F	North Carolina	Uterine dysplasia	Foot	4.0	Cyst
14	47/F	Maryland	Cardiovascular disease[c]	Foot	3.0	Cyst
15	77/F	Missouri		Thumb	2.0	Cyst
16	60/M	Zaire		Leg	1.5	Cyst
17	59/M	Australia		Forearm	Large	Cyst
18	83/M	North Carolina	Leukemia[d]	Finger	Unknown	Stellate
19	31/F	Georgia		Leg	0.5	Stellate
20	69/F	Florida		Foot	1.5	Stellate
21	70/F	North Carolina		Foot	2.5	Cyst
22	Unknown	Oklahoma		Finger	0.8	Cyst
23	42/M	Nebraska		Hand	Unknown	Stellate
24	61/F	Florida	Lymphoma[d]	Hand	0.9	Cyst
25	75/M	West Virginia		Finger	2.0	Stellate
26	56/M	Nigeria	Lepromatous leprosy	Shin	2.5	Cyst
27	59/M	Illinois & Wisconsin	Renal failure (10 yr) with hemodialysis	Elbow (Ølecranon bursa)	6.0	Cyst
28	85/M	Oregon		Finger	1.0	Solid
29	86/M	Tennessee		Hand	4.0	Cyst
30	70/F	Maryland		Hallux	3.0	Cyst
31	60/F	Maryland		Hand	2.5	Stellate
32	15/F	Washington, D. C.		Forearm	2.0	Cyst
33	48/F	California	Diabetes	Forearm	2.5	Cyst

[a] Onchocerciasis, loiasis, dipetalonemiasis, and bancroftian filariasis.
[b] Erythema nodosum leprosum, with corticosteroid therapy.
[c] Hypertension with intraventricular block.
[d] Immunosuppressive therapy.

Incisions and aspirations were performed on seven patients, and patient 5 developed a sinus tract after repeated aspirations. All of the cysts were eventually excised (Fig. 13.9). For 32 patients the cysts were described as lying in the subcutaneous tissue beneath uninvolved skin, and attachment to muscle, bone, and deep fascia were not mentioned.

The size of 29 cysts was recorded as varying between 0.5 and 7.0 cm, with a mean of 3.25 cm (Table 13.2). All but two cysts had a distinct capsule. Contents

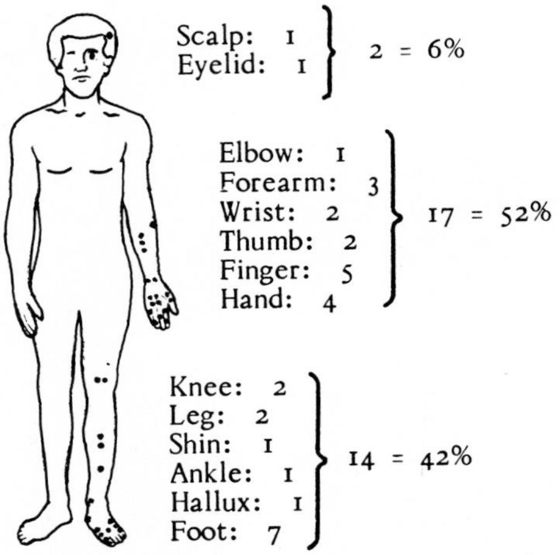

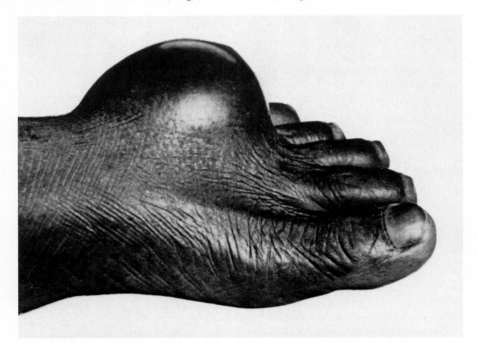

FIG. 13.7. Anatomic locations of 33 pheomycotic cysts. All but two were on the limbs and concentrated on the hands and feet, fingers and toes (AFIP Neg. 81-13877).

FIG. 13.8. The 7-cm pheomycotic cyst on the foot of patient 2 was nontender, tense, and fluctuant. (×0.7; AFIP Neg. 68-100645).

of the cysts were described variously as solid or friable, creamy or viscid, and yellow-tan, brown, or grey-green (Fig. 13.9).

MICROSCOPIC FEATURES OF PHEOMYCOTIC CYSTS

Except for the lesion in the olecranon bursa (patient 27), all cysts were in the deep dermis or the subcutaneous tissue and did not involve the fascia, muscle, or

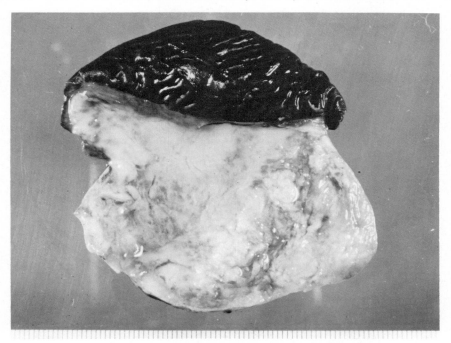

Fig. 13.9. The 7-cm cyst with attached skin (patient 2) has been opened and the pus washed away, to reveal a shaggy lining. (×1.2; AFIP Neg. 68-10064-4).

bone (Figs. 13.9–13.12). None showed any epidermal changes such as ulceration, hyperkeratosis, acanthosis, or epidermal hyperplasia (in contrast to sporotrichosis and chromomycosis).

The walls of the cysts showed three distinct layers: an outer layer of hyalinized scar tissue; a middle layer of more vascularized scar tissue; and an inner layer of mixed suppurative and granulomatous inflammation (predominantly epithelioid cells, histiocytes, foreign body and Langhans' giant cells, and neutrophils). In 26 cysts there were also numerous eosinophils.

Patients 3 and 28 showed solid granulomas, without cavities. Nine lesions were partially solid with stellate abscesses (Fig. 13.13). Twenty-two lesions showed a dominant cystic cavity with varying degrees of infolding and papillary change (Fig. 13.10). In the latter category the infolds of the cavity were reminiscent of the earlier stellate pattern and are thought to represent a later stage of development of the lesion. The exudate in the cavities was comprised mainly of fibrin and neutrophils. Portions of vegetable fiber were seen in or beside the cysts of eight patients. During excision of two other cysts, the surgeons noted a foreign body discarded with the pus.

Cysts that were firm clinically revealed an essentially uniform granulomatous reaction, with scattered small stellate abscesses intermixed. Clinically soft cysts had cavities formed by coalesced stellate abscesses, and fluctuant cysts each had a single dominant cavity. The more solid lesions in patients 3 and 5 had been present for a shorter time (2–8 weeks). In contrast, the large 5-cm and 7-cm cysts in patients 1 and 2 each had a single large central cavity (Figs. 13.8 and 13.9). We

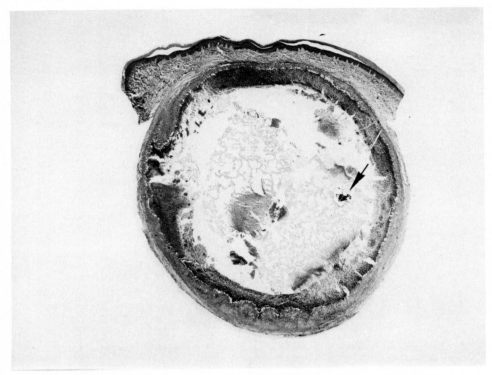

FIG. 13.10. The 0.9-cm pheomycotic cyst from the finger of patient 24. The cyst lies within and has expanded the dermis, but the overlying skin is not involved. The cyst has a papillomatous lining, central liquefaction, and contains a sliver (*arrow*). (H&E, ×6.0; AFIP Neg. 79-685).

believe these are among the oldest lesions—in malnourished Africans who delayed seeking treatment—although we could not establish a consistent relationship between size and stated duration of the cysts.

The large, 6-cm lesion in the olecranon bursa of patient 27 also had a long and unusual history (Dr. J. E. Williams, personal communication, Mount Sinai Medical Center, Milwaukee, Wisc.). Over a 10-year period the patient had renal insufficiency and recurrent swellings of the right elbow. Whenever he bumped it (five or six times a year), the olecranon bursa would swell from its usual 1-cm diameter to about 4 cm. The swelling would resolve without treatment in a few days. While hunting in October 1977, he hit his elbow—which swelled over 2 days to about 6 cm. The olecranon bursa was aspirated in December 1977, and again in January, 1978—with 50 ml of grossly bloody aspirate obtained on the second occasion. *E. jeanselmei* was cultured from both aspirates. The olecranon bursa was excised in February 1978, and light microscopy revealed pigmented fungi consistent with *Exophiala* sp.

Lesions from these 33 patients contained brown fungi with morphologic features characteristic of *Phialophora* spp. They were in the exudate but most numerous in histiocytes and giant cells lining the abscesses (Figs. 13.14–13.16). They were also present within the silver in one lesion. Fungi were not found in the scar

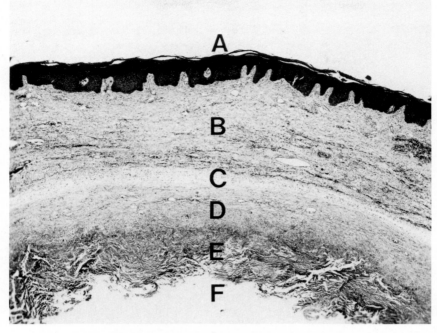

FIG. 13.11. The wall of the cyst from patient 1 shows several layers: (*A*) uninvolved epidermis; (*B*) uninvolved dermis; (*C*) loose connective tissue between dermis and cyst wall; (*D*) scar tissue; (*E*) organizing exudate lining the cyst; and (*F*) cavity of the cyst. (Russel-Movat, ×20; AFIP Neg. 79-623).

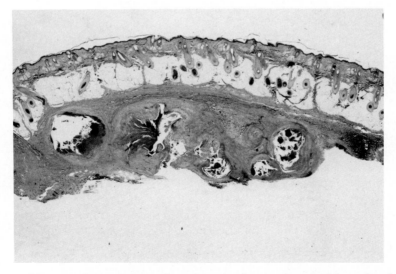

FIG. 13.12. The 4-cm pheomycotic cyst from the scalp of patient 8, excised 2 months after needle aspiration and wall curettage (39). Note abscesses with coalescence and surrounding granuloma. (H&E, ×4; AFIP Neg. 79-12312).

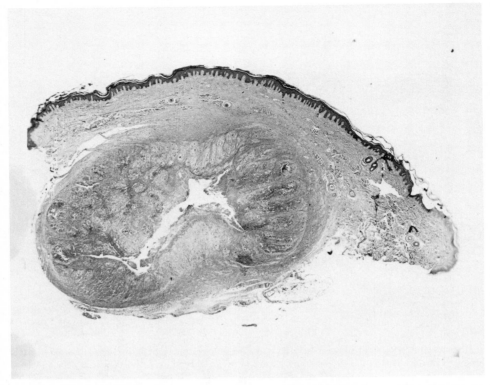

Fig. 13.13. In the cyst from patient 5, some of the stellate abscesses have coalesced to form a clearly defined central abscess which appears as a cavity after the pus has run out. (H&E, ×10; AFIP Neg. 78-8606).

tissue or outside the cyst wall. The fungi were polymorphous, with single cells in 32 lesions and hyphae in 20 lesions (Figs. 13.14 to 13.16). In 32 cysts there were budding cells (yeasts); in 8 cysts, yeast-like cells with single septa; and in 25 cysts, chain formation. The number of fungi did not appear to be related to the duration, size, or pattern of the cyst. The width of the yeasts varied between 2 and 12 μm, but averaged 5 to 6 μm. All forms of the fungus were intensely slivered with the GMS stain and showed PAS-positive walls and cytoplasm. Hematoxylin stained the fungi strongly in only one lesion. Examination of H&E sections and unstained sections revealed varying patterns of pigmentation of the fungi.

Occasionally, rounded aggregates of hyphae, in addition to numerous single hyphae, were found in the biopsy specimen and aspirated material from the cyst in patient 8. These microcolonies were comparable to grains in eumycetoma, and measured 20–110 μm. The pigmented fungus *Phialophora repens* was repeatedly cultured from that cyst (39).

INVOLVEMENT OF VEGETABLE FIBERS IN PHEOMYCOTIC CYSTS

In 10 of the 33 lesions there were fragments of sliver (wood) in or beside the cyst of eight and in the aspirated pus of two. Within the substance of one sliver there were fungi having morphologic characteristics of *Phialophora* spp. Thus

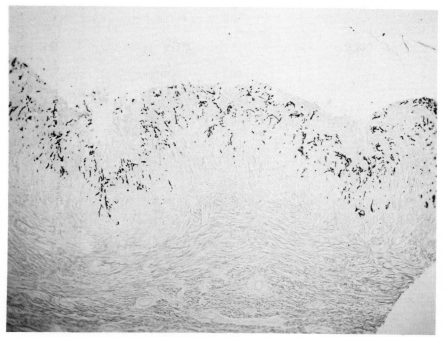

FIG. 13.14. The exudate lining the cyst from patient 17 contains numerous fungi. (GMS, ×42; AFIP Neg. 78-8970).

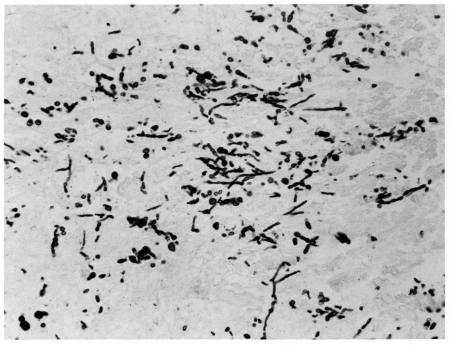

FIG. 13.15. Higher magnification of Fig. 14.14, showing pleomorphism of the fungi: yeasts, single and in chain formation, and hyphae. (GMS, ×250; AFIP Neg. 79-688-4).

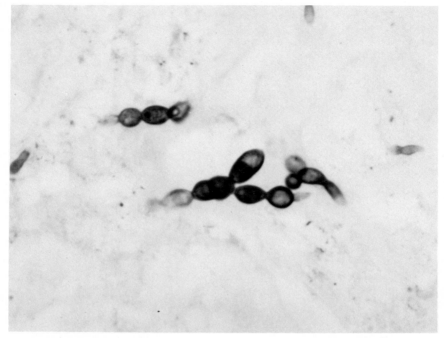

FIG. 13.16. Budding yeasts and chain formation, in the exudate of the cyst from patient 20. (GMS, ×675; AFIP Neg. 78-6533).

slivers were identified in 30% of the lesions in our series. Although slivers are common, pheomycotic cysts are rare. We suspect that only retained, deeply penetrating slivers cause pheomycotic cysts. The sliver acts as both foreign body and source of the infecting fungus. When experimental animals were inoculated with *P. gougerotii* without foreign material, no infection was produced, but infection resulted when foreign material was included (A. Ziefer, unpublished results).

The proposed involvement of vegetable fibers (slivers) is supported by the facts that all lesions in our series were in the deep dermis or subcutis (except the olecranon bursa of patient 27), and the cysts were all on exposed surfaces of the body—predominantly on distal parts of the limbs.

Other Predisposing Factors for Pheomycotic Cyst

Immunodeficiency of the host appears to be a predisposing factor for some patients in our series. Four of the 33 patients were receiving immunosuppressive therapy when their lesions developed. Of these, two were being treated for tumors of the reticuloendothelial system (leukemia and lymphoma); one, for leprosy in reaction, and one, in conjunction with chronic renal insufficiency (10 years) with hemodialysis (5 years) (see Table 13.2). Other patients had infections which are associated with depressed or altered immune mechanisms: polyfilariasis, tuberculosis, lepromatous leprosy, and diabetes mellitus. Malnutrition may have suppressed immunity in five patients from rural Africa (Zaire, 2; Malawi, 2; Nigeria, 1) where starvation is common and adequate dietary protein is the exception. Nine patients (27%) were over 70 years old—suggesting immunodeficiency from old age. Thus twenty patients (61%) may have had at least some degree of immunodeficiency for one reason or another. Pheomycotic cysts may become more common as use of immunosuppressive therapy increases.

PROTOTHECOSIS

INTRODUCTION

Protothecosis is a rare infection caused by achloric algae of the genus *Prototheca*. The first infection of man was recognized in 1964 in a West African rice farmer from Sierra Leone (59–61). Since then, at least 30 cases have been reported (Table 13.3). These can be generally divided into two groups, those who are immunosuppressed and those with competent immunity. In immunosuppressed patients, protothecosis involves skin and tends to persist in spite of treatment. In patients with competent immunity, however, the olecranon bursa is usually infected and simple excision is curative. There are several reviews of protothecosis (57–59, 63, 65, 73, 76, 79, 83, 109, 114).

The index human case was studied by Dr. P. O. Wakelin, while working in the town of Segbwema in Sierra Leone. The patient presented himself in August 1961 with a small lesion on the right foot which he claimed had been present for 7 years. By 1963, the lesion had encircled the foot (Fig. 13.17). Microscopic examination revealed organisms that were at first thought to be a peculiar fungus (Figs. 13.19 and 13.20). Later, culture of skin scrapings showed the organisms to be *Prototheca* spp., which was named *Prototheca segbwema* (64). Dr. Wakelin saw the patient again in 1965 when the lesion had begun to spread up the leg (Fig. 13.18). Biopsy specimens of skin and femoral lymph node were cultured, and *P. segbwema* was cultured from both (65). *P. segbwema* subsequently was shown to be identical to *Prototheca zopfi* by carbohydrate and alcohol assimilation tests (50, 68, 76, 99) and by immunofluorescent staining (83, 115). Since that first study, human protothecosis has been identified in China, South Africa, Vietnam, New Zealand, Iran, Panama, France, and the United States (Table 13.3). In all other lesions where culture or immunofluorescence has identified the species, it has been *Prototheca wickerhamii* (Table 13.3; ref. 83).

ETIOLOGIC AGENT

The *Prototheca* spp. are achloric algae that were originally isolated from the mucus flux of trees. They have subsequently been isolated from potato skin, stools of patients with tropical sprue, grass, cow's milk, waste-stabilizing ponds, dogs, a cat, and a fruit bat (51, 52, 83, 84, 92). They are distinguished from the *Chlorella* spp. (green algae) by a number of features (56). In particular, the *Prototheca* spp. do not have chloroplasts, whereas *Chlorella* spp. have chloroplasts that are readily seen with the GMS, PAS, and Gridley fungus stains.

In tissue sections, *Prototheca* spp. are ovoid or spherical and range from 3 to 15 μm (*P. wickerhamii*) or from about 7 to 30 μm (*P. zopfii*) (Figs. 13.21–13.23). They stain with fungal stains such as GMS, PAS, and Gridley fungus, but are distinguished from fungi, especially by the form of division. The *Prototheca* cell divides asexually by septation to form internal spores—first 2, then 8 or more—before the theca or wall of the parent cell ruptures, discharging the spores.

As mentioned, there is great variation in size and shape for organisms in any

TABLE 13.3. HUMAN PROTOTHECOSIS IN 30 PATIENTS

Patient	Age/Sex	Year	Location	Occupation	Predisposition or Antecedent	Site*	Outcome/Comment	Etiologic Agent*					References†
								Spec.	Cult.	FA	LM	EM	
1	30/M	1961	Sierra Leone	Rice farmer	Malnutrition, barefoot in rice patties	Foot, leg, femoral lymph node	Spread to leg and femoral node by 1965; lost to follow-up	P. zop.	+	+	+	+	63–65 (56, 57, 76, 83, 97, 114, 118)
2	63/M	1964	Florida	Businessman		Olecranon bursa	Bursectomy	P. sp.			+		118 (49, 76, 83, 86)
3	45/F	1967	N. Carolina	Housewife	Diabetes, breast cancer, shaved leg (a)	Leg	(a)‡	P. wic.	+	+	+	+	86, 118 (76, 83, 114)
4	43/M	1968	Mississippi	Physician	Cleaned aquarium after surgery (b)	Wrist	Excised ganglion on wrist (b)	P. sp.			+		118
5	36/F	1968	Virginia	Nurse		Olecranon bursa	Bursectomy	P. sp.			+		AFIP (49, 83, 98)
6	62/M	1969	Florida	Meat dealer	Injured elbow (c)	Olecranon bursa	Bursectomy	P. sp.			+		118 (49, 83, 98)
7	58/M	1970	S. Vietnam	Solider	Injured elbow (d)	Olecranon bursa	Bursectomy	P. wic.		+	+		98 (49, 83)
8	60/M	1971	Washington, D.C.	Veteran		Olecranon bursa		P. sp.			+		AFIP (49, 83, 98)
9	40/M	1971	Transvaal, South Africa	Ditch digger	Alcoholic, malnutrition (e)	Forehead & scalp	Regression and recurrence	P. wic	+	+	+	+	71, 90, 112, (83)
10	?/F	1972	Hong Kong			Cheek, conjunctival mucosa	Nodule excised	P. wic.	+	+	+		124, 125 (83, 114)
11	30/M	1973	Maryland	Oyster handler, Seafood market (f)	Diabetes with renal transplant, immunosuppressive drug(s)	Forearm	Died of renal failure	P. wic.	+		+		62, 123 (83)

No.	Age/Sex	Year	Location	Occupation	Clinical features	Site	Treatment/Outcome	Organism				Reference
12	29/M	1974	New Zealand	Truck driver	Viral hepatitis, with depressed cellular immunity	Forehead, nose, peritoneal cavity	Regressed after IV amphotericin B & transfer factor	*P. wic*	+	+	+	61 (83)
13	17/F	1974	Iran	Student	Insect bite on leg, by seashore (g)	Leg	No response to topical & systemic antibiotics	*P. sp*		+		95 (79)
14	30/F	1973	California		Diabetes, chronic vaginal candidiasis, surgery on palm (h)	Palm	Wound infection, 1 month after palm surgery	*P. wic.*	+	+	+ +	87 (49, 83)
15	20/F	1972	Missouri	Housewife	Not known	Cheek	Regressed after 5 wk of IV amphotericin B	*P. wic.*	+	+	+	91 (83)
16	48/M	1977	Illinois			Olecranon bursa	Bursectomy	*P. wic.*		+		*AFIP, (unpublished)* (i)
17	72/M	1978	Minnesota & California	Law professor	Steroid injection of olecranon bursa (j)	Olecranon bursa	Bursectomy	*P. sp.*		+		49
18	39/M	1974	Panama	Sanitation worker	Injured elbow, cleaned septic tank (k)	Olecranon bursa	Bursectomy	*P. wic.*	+	+		79 (49, 83)
19	70/M	1979	Washington state		Arthritis; steroids; Felty's syndrome; leukopenia; splenectomy	Olecranon bursa	Bird bath is possible source of algae infection	*P. wic.*	+	+		(l)
20	44/M	1979	Massachusetts		Diabetes, bilateral vascular disease, renal failure	Finger thumb		*P. sp.*		+		*AFIP,* unpublished (m)

TABLE 13.3. HUMAN PROTOTHECOSIS IN 30 PATIENTS—*continued*

No.	Age/Sex	Year	Location	Occupation	Predisposing factor	Site	Clinical course	Organism				Reference
21	61/F	1980	Washington, D. C.	Housewife	Uterine cancer, immunosuppressed (X-ray, chemotherapy) (n)	Finger thumb	Died of acute cardiopulmonary arrest	*P. wic.*	+		+	*AFIP*, 80
22	65/M	1966	New York		Not known	Thumb		*P. wic.*	+		+	(45)
23	12/M	1971	France			Inguinal skin		*P. sp.*	+			108, (95)
24	42/M	1976	North Carolina		Injured elbow	Olecranon bursa	Bursectomy	*P. wic.*		+	+	CDC, 83
25	65/M	1976	North Carolina		Injured elbow	Olecranon bursa	Bursectomy	*P. wic.*		+	+	CDC, 83
26	18/F	1977	Virginia		Excision of ganglion; steroid injection; cleaned aquarium	Hand	Lesion developed at site of previous surgery	*P. wic.*		+	+	122, (83)
27	?/?	1977	Venezuela			Foot		*P. wic.*	+		+	117
28	73/F	1979	Texas		Diabetes, breast cancer (mastectomy, X-ray, drugs), heart & renal failure, lymphocytic leukemia	Skin/??	Progressive skin rash	*P. wic.*	+		+	*AFIP*, unpublished (o)
29	34/F	1979	Illinois	Housekeeper & governess	Defective neutrophils; topical corticosteroids	Shoulder back, neck, chest, proximal extremities	Regressed after IV amphotericin B & tetracycline	*P. wic.*	+	+	+	*AFIP*; in press (p)

| 30 | 48/F | 1980 | Michigan | Renal transplant, immunosuppressive drug therapy | Forearm | *P. wic.* | + | + | 93 |

* *Etiologic agent: P. wic, Prototheca wickerhamii; P. zop., Prototheca zopfii, (P. segbuema); Spec., species; Cult., grown in culture on routine laboratory media without cycloheximide; soft, white-tan "yeast-like" colonies within 48 hr; FA, fluorescent antibody staining (83); LM, light microscopic demonstration in tissue sections; EM, electron microscopy.

† *References: principal references,* by original authors; *secondary references,* citation in reviews and by other secondary authors, including further characterization of organisms at Communicable Disease Center (CDC) by FA (83). *AFIP,* diagnostic report from Armed Forces Institute of Pathology.

‡ Additional comments about individual patients: (a) Patient 3 had diabetes and breast cancer, treated by radical mastectomy, X-irradiation, and steroid chemotherapy; source of infection suspected to be scummy water drawn from a cistern, with which she shaved her legs; she died of breast cancer (86, 118). (b) After ganglionectomy on wrist, patient 4 cleaned a fish tank that was apparently contaminated with *Prototheca* sp. (118). (c) Patient 6 fell in bathtub, causing nonpenetrating injury to elbow; swollen elbow, cured by excision of olecranon bursa (118). (d) Patient 7 suffered nonpenetrating injury to elbow in South Vietnam; swollen elbow; olecranon bursa excised (98). (e) Patient 9 dug ditches for electric cables; contact with soil is suspected source of infection (71, 90, 112). (f) Patient 11 had contact with contaminated water while working as oyster handler at seafood market in Maryland (62, 123). (g) Patient 13 related lesion to insect bite on leg while walking barefoot on shore of Caspian Sea in Iran (95). (h) Patient 14, a diabetic, had surgery for swelling in palm—diagnosed as early nodular Dupuytren's contracture; surgical wound became infected with *P. wickerhamii* within 1 month (87). (i) Patient 16—unpublished AFIP case submitted by Dr. J. Costa, St. Clair Med. Lab, Belleville, Ill. (j) Patient 17 noted draining mass over olecranon process, and bursa was injected with steroids, stopping drainage; patient moved from Minn. to Calif.; swelling recurred several months later; bursa aspirated and again injected with steroids; drained clear fluid 1 month after second injection; olecranon bursa excised (49). (k) Patient 18 fell during a drunken brawl in Panama and lacerated elbow; 2 days later, while cleaning a septic tank, "he accidentally splashed dirty waste water over his injured elbow, thoroughly wetting the dressing. Within 10 days he noted swelling" (79). (l) Patient 19—case reported by Dr. J. W. Young, St. Peter Hospital, Olympia, Washington; see brief Case Report by F. Boyce, D. L. Longerier, J. W. Young, and K. Partlow, *Prototheca* as a Pathogen. *Clin. Microbiol. Newsletter 1* (23): 4–5, 1979. (m) Patient 20—unpublished AFIP case submitted by Dr. F. Von Lichtenberg, Harvard Medical School and Peter Bent Brigham Hospital. (n) Patient 21 received chemotherapeutic injection of blood; nodules developed on fingers and thumbs, 3 days later (80). (o) Patient 28—unpublished AFIP case submitted by Dr. J. L. Smith, Jr., M. D. Anderson Hospital and Tumor Institute, Houston, Texas. (p) Patient 29—AFIP case submitted by Dr. J. E. Williams, Northwestern University School of Medicine (now Mt. Sinai Hosp., Milwaukee, Wisc.). F. R. Venezio, E. Laboo, J. E. Williams, C. R. Zeiss, W. A. Caro, F. E. Dunlop. M. Mangkornkanok-Mark, and J. P. Phair. Progressive cutaneous protothecosis, manuscript in preparation.

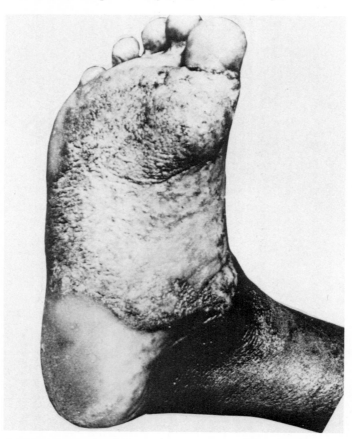

FIG. 13.17. Foot of the index human case of protothecosis (patient 1) in March 1963, 9 years after the infection began as a small papule on the instep. The lesion is raised, crusted and weeping and at this stage has encircled the foot (AFIP Neg. 75-12872-1). (Reproduced with permission from P. O. Wakelin *et al.* (64).)

given lesion caused by *P. zopfii* or *P. wickerhamii*. For example, some of the *P. wickerhamii* organisms have a characteristic morula form or "daisy" (Fig. 13.23). This form was not seen in the single human case caused by *P. zopfii*. In the earlier literature, several "different" *Prototheca* species were described in culture or in animals, based on morphologic criteria (reviewed in ref. 83). As a result of carbohydrate and alcohol assimilation tests and immunofluorescent staining, however, only three distinct species are now accepted: *Prototheca stagnora*, *P. wickerhamii*, and *P. zopfii* (50, 67, 68, 72, 76, 83, 99, 115). The earlier literature includes another species termed *Prototheca filamenta* that is no longer considered a *Prototheca* species, but rather *Fissuricella filamenta* (50, 83, 85, 96, 102).

CLINICOPATHOLOGIC FEATURES

We know of 30 cases of human protothecosis, including several unpublished cases from the files of the AFIP (Table 13.3). There are in general two forms of

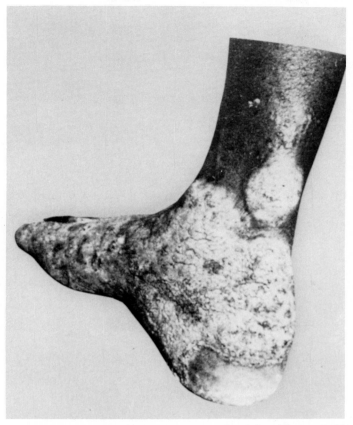

Fig. 13.18. Foot of patient 1 in October 1965 (2½ years later than Fig. 14.17). The lesion has a coarse, granular surface that involves most of the foot (excepting toes and heel) and has formed a satellite lesion that spreads up the posterior aspect of the leg (AFIP Neg. 75-12872-2). (Reproduced with permission from P. O. Wakelin *et al.* (67).)

the disease. Patients with suppressed immunity have a papular or eczematoid dermatitis, often over an extremity (foot, hand, finger, thumb, etc.), and disseminated in a few patients. Patients with apparently normal immunity have a localized infection of the subcutaneous tissues, usually over the elbow and involving the olecranon bursa.

The rice farmer (patient 1) had a chronic scaling dermatitis which began as a papule on the instep and gradually spread over an 11-year period to involve most of the foot and part of the leg ("*Introduction*"; Figs. 13.17 and 13.18). Microscopically, a biopsy specimen from the foot taken in the 9th year revealed hyperkeratosis, parakeratosis, and acanthosis with marked elongation of the rete ridges. There were *P. zopfii* organisms in the keratin layer, the germinal layer, and the upper dermis (Figs. 13.19–13.22). The dermis was hyperemic and had an inflammatory cell infiltrate comprised of lymphocytes, histiocytes, neutrophils, and eosinophils. The infection subsequently spread to the femoral lymph nodes by the 11th year. The patient was malnourished, but apparently had a normal

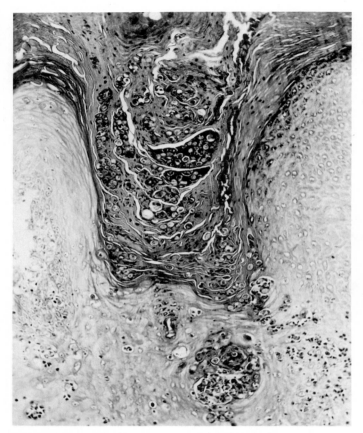

FIG. 13.19. Biopsy specimen from margin of lesion on foot of patient 1 (Figs. 14.17 and 14.18). There is acanthosis and hyperkeratosis. *P. zopfii* organisms are in the dermis and in all levels of the epidermis. Here they are crowded into the hyperkeratotic layer forming clusters of organisms. (H&E, ×115; AFIP Neg. 67-4737).

immune system. He was lost to follow-up after 1965 (("Introduction"; refs. 63–65).

Some of the patients had suppressed immunity associated with cancer and its chemotherapy or radiation therapy. Two patients had disseminated protothecosis associated with suppressed immunity or defective leukocytes.

Patients 4 and 26 developed lesions on the wrist or hand after cleaning aquariums that were apparently contaminated by algae (83, 118, 122). Each had previously had a ganglion excised from the site, and steroid injection had followed the surgery for patient 26. Identification of *P. wickerhamii* was confirmed by culture for patient 26.

Eleven (37%) of the 30 patients had protothecosis on the elbow—involving the olecranon bursa (Table 13.3; patients 2, 5–8, 16–19, 24, and 25). Their lesions had developed within several days to several weeks after injuries to the elbow. Surgical specimens showed soft caseating centers surrounded by granulation tissue and fibrous tissue that contained foreign body and Langhans' giant cells (Fig. 13.24).

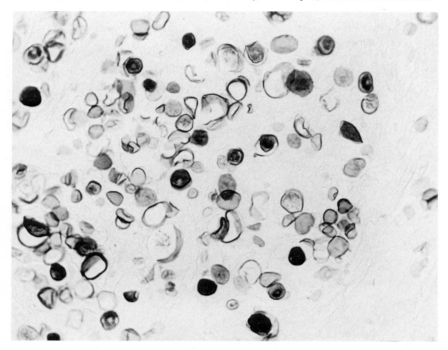

FIG. 13.20. The walls of *P. zopfii* are stained well with the Girdley fungus stain (patient 1). Characteristic features include the great variation in size from 2 to 16 μm. Note the presence of collapsed forms, crescent-shaped organisms, and some which appear as hollow spheres. Some organisms have a well-stained central body. (Gridley fungus, ×400; AFIP Neg. 67-3943).

The *Prototothecae* were located in the caseating centers and were scattered (Fig. 13.25), in contrast to the solid or clustered configurations in the cutaneous lesions. Attempts to culture organisms from lesions in the olecranon bursae were unsuccessful for most patients—except that *P. wickerhamii* was cultured from patients 16 and 19 (Table 13.3). Greater success was obtained by immunofluorescent staining, which identified *P. wickerhamii*, in the bursae of patients 7, 18, 14, and 15 (83).

TREATMENT

Lesions involving the olecranon bursa have generally been cured by simple bursectomy. Some cutaneous lesions in immunosuppressed patients, however, have resisted treatment and persisted over several years and spread to other sites (*e.g.*, patients 1, 10, and 29). Several topical treatments were tried. Systemic treatments have generally had no demonstrable effect—including treatment with griseofulvin, penicillin, emetine hydrochloride, and pentamidine isothionate (61, 83, 110, 114, 123). Cutaneous lesions of patient 9 regressed after oral treatment with potassium iodide (90). The lesions, however, became active again a year later and healed spontaneously (71). The systemic lesions of patient 12 regressed after combined treatment with intravenous amphotericin B and transfer factor (61). He simultaneously recovered from his immune deficiency, however, so the

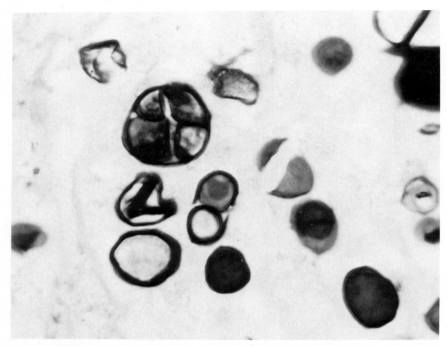

Fɪɢ. 13.21. Higher magnification of *P. zopfii* (patient 1) reveals a distinct outer wall or theca with internal spores separated by septa. (GMS, ×1080; AFIP Neg. 67-5798).

therapeutic effects of such combined treatment are difficult to assess. The cutaneous lesion on the cheek of patient 15 was successfully treated with intravenous amphotericin B over a 5-week period (91). The lesion appeared less indurated after 4 weeks of treatment. Repeated skin biopsies after 2, 4, and 7 months showed progressively fewer *Prototheca*, and cultures failed to grow the *P. wickerhamii* that was found in pretreatment cultures. The disseminated lesions of patient 29 were likewise successfully treated with intravenous amphotericin B over a 4-month period—accompanied by tetracycline during the first 5 weeks. After treatment, her skin lesions resolved, and repeated skin biopsies showed degenerating *Prototheca* but no growth in culture—in contrast to *P. wickerhamii* cultured from pretreatment specimens.

Pʀᴏᴛᴏᴛʜᴇᴄᴏsɪs ɪɴ Aɴɪᴍᴀʟs

Prototheca spp. infect many animals, as well as man. *P. zopfii* and *P. wicker-hamii* both cause disseminated infections in dogs, with *P. zopfii* reported more frequently (54, 55, 81–83, 114, 116, 119–121). Infection of the eye of dogs is especially common, but infections have also been reported in the brain, kidney, liver, heart, colon, lymph nodes, lung, arteries, ear, nares, and para-adrenal connective tissue. *P. zopfii* likewise more frequently than *P. wickerhamii* causes mastitis in cows (53, 70, 77, 83, 88, 94, 103, 107, 114, 118). Green lesions in lymph nodes of three cows and an ox were originally diagnosed as protothecosis, but

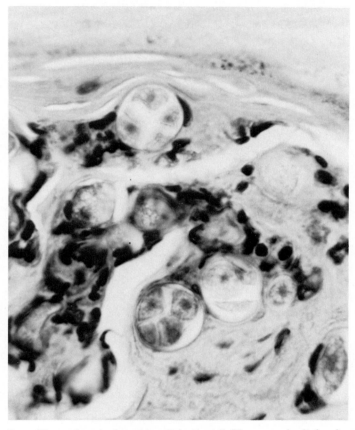

FIG. 13.22. *P. zopfii* organisms in the epidermis (patient 1). They are spherical and contain distinct internal spores. (H&E, ×1080; AFIP Neg. 67-5797).

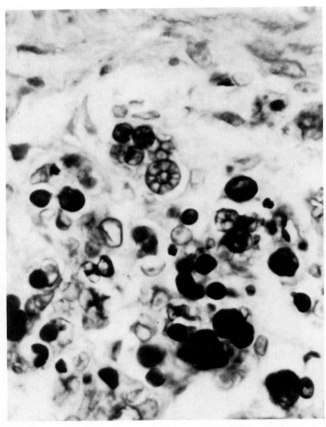

Fig. 13.23. A concentration of *Prototheca* organisms in the skin of the leg of patient 3. There is considerable variation in size and polymorphism of the organisms but a distinct morula form ("daisy") is present in the center of the field. The morula form characteristic of *P. wickerhamii* and has daughter cells surrounding a central daughter cell. (PAS, ×1000; AFIP Neg. 75-10327). (Reproduced with permission from Dr. G. K. Klintworth *et al.* (86).

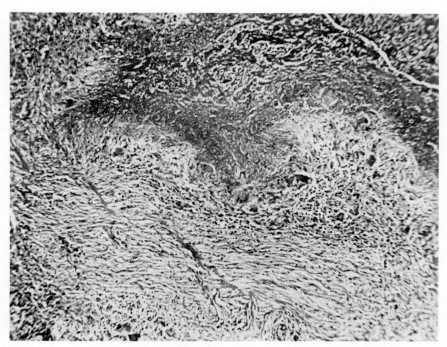

FIG. 13.24. Wall of necrotic area, olecranon bursa of Patient 7. The stellate configuration to the necrosis is shown. There are epithelioid cells, Langhans' giant cells, lymphocytes, and plasma cells. The surrounding tissue is hyperemic (H&E, ×90; AFIP Neg. 74-2693).

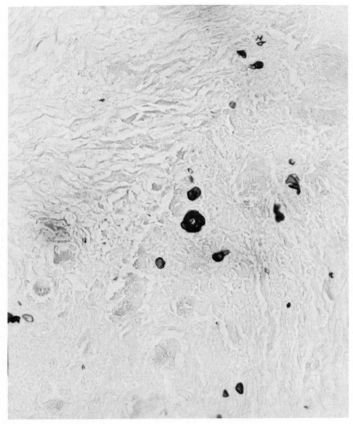

Fɪɢ. 13.25. Organisms in patient 7 (Fig. 14.24). They are located in the necrotic tissue and lining the wall of the necrotic area. The *P. wickerhamii* organisms vary in size, and there are morula forms present. (GMS, ×440; AFIP Neg. 74-2694).

were subsequently shown to be caused by *Chlorella* (56, 94, 106). Green lesions in lymph nodes, liver, and lung of sheep are likewise caused by *Chlorella* (56, 60, 83). Green nodules in the dermis of a beaver pelt, originally diagnosed as protothecosis, are also caused by *Chlorella* (56, 83, 111). Infection of a deer, originally diagnosed as *P. zopfii*, was shown by immunofluorescent staining to be caused by *P. wickerhamii* (78, 83). *P. wickerhamii* also caused disseminated infection of the lymph node, spleen, heart, muscle, and kidney of a fruit bat (83, 92) and infected the subcutaneous tissue in the tarsus region of a cat (83, 84).

REFERENCES ON MICRONEMIASIS

1. Alstad, A. D., Berg, I. E., and Samuel, C. Disseminated *Micronema deletrix* infection in the horse. *J. Am. Vet. Med. Assoc. 174:* 264–266, 1979.
2. Anderson, R. V., and Bemrick, W. J. *Micronema deletrix* n. sp., a saprophagous nematode inhabiting a nasal tumor of a horse. *Proc. Helminthol. Soc. Wash. 32:* 74–75, 1965.
3. Chitwood, M., and Lichtenfels, J. R. Other rhabditida (*Micronema deletrix*); In *Parasitological Review—Identification of a Parasitic Metazoa in Tissue Sections. Exp. Parasitol. 32:* 407–519, 1972.

4. Ferris, D. H., Levine, N. D., and Beamer, P. D. *Micronema deletrix* in equine brain. *Am. J. Vet. Res. 33:* 33–38, 1972.

5. Gardiner, C. H., Koh, D. S., and Cardella, T. A. *Micronema* in man: Third fatal infection. *Am. J. Trop. Med. Hyg., 30:* 586–589, 1981.

6. Goodey, T., and Goodey, J. B. *Soil and Freshwater Nematodes.* London, Methuen & Co., 1963.

7. Hoogstraten, J., Connor, D. H., and Neafie, R. C. Micronemiasis. In *Pathology of Tropical and Extraordinary Diseases.* Vol. 2, edited by C. H. Binford and D. H. Connor, pp. 468–470. Washington, D. C., Armed Forces Institute of Pathology, 1976.

8. Hoogstraten, J., and Young, W. G. Meningo-encephalomyelitis due to the saprophagous nematode, *Micronema deletrix. Can. J. Neurol. Sci. 2:* 121–126, 1975.

9. Johnson, K. H., and Johnson, D. W. Granulomas associated with *Micronema deletrix* in the maxillae of the horse. *J. Am. Vet. Med. Assoc. 49:* 155–159, 1966.

10. Pletcher, J. M., and Howerth, E. *Micronema deletrix* infection in horses. *J. Am. Vet. Med. Assoc. 177:* 1090, 1980.

11. Powers, R. D., and Benz, G. W. *Micronema deletrix* in the central nervous system of a horse. *J. Am. Vet. Med. Assoc. 170:* 170–177, 1977.

12. Purtilo, D. T., Meyers, W. M., and Connor, D. H. Fatal strongyloidiasis in immunosuppressed patients. *Am. J. Med. 56:* 488–493, 1974.

13. Rubin, H. L., and Woodard, J. C. Equine infection with *Micronema deletrix. J. Am. Vet. Med. Assoc. 165:* 256–258, 1974.

14. Scowden, E. B., Schaffner, W., and Stone, W. J. Overwhelming strongyloidiasis: an unappreciated opportunistic infection. *Medicine 57:* 527–544, 1978.

15. Shadduck, J. A., Ubelaker, J., and Telford, V. Q. *Micronema deletrix* meningoencephalitis in an adult man. *Am. J. Clin. Pathol. 72:* 640–643, 1979.

16. Stone, W. M., Steward, R. B., and Peckham, J. C. *Micronema deletrix* Anderson and Bemrick, 1965, in the central nervous system of a pony. *J. Parasitol. 56:* 986–987, 1970.

PHAEOMYCOTIC CYST

17. Ajello, L. Phaeohyphomycosis: Definition and etiology. In *Mycoses, Scientifique Publication. Pan American Health Organization 304:* 126–133, 1975.

18. Ajello, L. Chromoblastomycosis, chromomycosis and phaeohyphomycosis: a confusion of terms. *Hum. Animal Mycol. Int. Cong. Ser. 480:* 187–189, 1980.

19. Ajello, L., George, L. K., Steigbigel, R. T., and Wang, C. J. K. A case of phaeohyphomycosis caused by a rare species *Phialophora. Mycologia 66:* 490–498, 1974.

20. Amma, S. M., Paniker, C. K. J., Iype, P. T., and Rangaswamy, S. Phaeohyphomycosis caused by *Cladosporium bantianum* in Kerala (India). *Sabouraudia 17:* 419–423, 1979.

21. Beurmann, L. de, and Gougerot, H. Association morbides dan les sporotrichoses. *Bull. Mém. Soc. Méd. Hôp. Paris, Ser. 3, 24:* 591–596, 1907.

22. Binford, C. H., and Dooley, J. R. Phaeomycotic cysts. In *Pathology of Tropical and Extraordinary Diseases,* Vol. 2, edited by C. H. Binford, and D. H. Connor, pp. 591–592, 1976.

23. Borelli, D. *Sporotrichum gougerotii, Hominiscium dermatitidis, Phialophora jeanselmei: Phialophora gougerotii* (Matruchot 1910) comb. n. *Mem. VI Conf. Venezolano Ci. Med. 5:* 2945–2971, 1955.

24. Carrión, A. L., and Silva, M. Sporotrichosis: special reference; a revision of so-called *Sporotrichum gougerotii. Arch. Dermatol. 72:* 523–534, 1955.

25. Cooke, W. B. A taxonomic study in the "black yeasts." *Mycopathologia 17:* 1–43, 1962.

26. Corrado, M. L., Weitzman, I., Stanek, A., Goetz, R., and Agyare, E. Subcutaneous infection with *Phialophora richardsiae* and its susceptibility to 5-fluorocytosine, amphotericin B and miconazole. *Sabouraudia 18:* 97–104, 1980.

27. Di Salvo, A. F., and Chew, W. H. *Phialophora gougerotii:* an opportunistic fungus in a patient treated with steroids. *Sabouraudia 6:* 241–245, 1968.

28. Dooley, J. R. Case for diagnosis (phaeomycotic cyst). *Milit. Med. 138:* 807, 827, 1973.

29. Emmons, C. W. Pathogenic dematiaceous fungi. *Jap. J. Med. Mycol. 7:* 233–245, 1966.

30. Emmons, C. W., Binford, C. H., Utz, J. P., and Kwon-Chung, K. J. Phaeomycotic cyst. In *Medical Mycology,* edited by C. W. Emmons, C. H. Binford, J. P. Utz, and K. J. Kwon-Chung, pp. 425–536. Philadelphia, Lea & Febiger, 1977.

31. Estes, S. A., Merz, W. G., and Maxwell, L. G. Primary cutaneous phaeohyphomycosis caused by *Drechslera spicifera*. *Arch. Derm. 113:* 813–815, 1977.

32. Ichinose, H. Subcutaneous abscesses due to brown fungi. In *Human Infection with Fungi, Actinomycetes and Algae.* Edited by R. D. Baker, pp. 719–730. New York, Springer-Verlag, 1971.

33. Kempson, R. L., and Sternberg, W. H. Chronic subcutaneous abscesses caused by pigmented fungi, a lesion distinguishable from chronic chromoblastomycosis. *Am. J. Clin. Pathol. 39:* 598–606, 1963.

34. Mariat, F., Ségrétain, G., Destombes, P., and Darasse, H. Kyste sous cutané mycosique (phaeosporotrichose) à *Phialophora gougerotii* (Matruchot 1910) Borelli 1955. *Sabouraudia 5:* 209–219, 1967.

35. Matruchot, L. Sur un nouveau groupe de champignons pathogènes, agents des sporotrichoses. *C. R. Acad. Sci. Paris 150:* 67–84, 1910.

36. McGinnis, M. Human pathogenic species of *Exophiala, Phialophora* and *Wangiella*. In *The Black and White Yeasts*, Sci. Publ. No. 356, pp. 37–59. Washington, D. C., Pan Am. Health Organization, 1978.

37. McGinnis, M. R., and Pathye, A. A. *Exophiala jeanselmei*, a new combination for *Phialophora jeanselmei*. *Mycotaxon 5:* 341–352, 1977.

38. Melin, E., and Nannfeldt, J. A. Researches into the bluing of ground wood pulp. *Svenska Skogsvards. Tidskr. 32:* 307–585, 1934.

39. Meyers, W. M., Dooley, J. R., and Kwon-Chung, K. J. Mycotic granuloma caused by *Phialophora repens*. *Am. J. Clin. Pathol. 64:* 549–555, 1975.

40. Nielson, H. S., and Conant, N. F. A new human pathogenic *Phialophora*. *Sabouraudia 6:* 228–231, 1968.

41. Schol-Schwarz, M. B. *Rhinocladiella*, its synonym *Fonsecaea* and its relations to *Phialophora*. *Antonie van Leeuwenhoek 34:* 119–152, 1968.

42. Schwartz, I. S., and Emmons, C. W. Subcutaneous cystic granuloma cuased by fungus of wood pulp (*Phialophora richardsiae*). *Am. J. Clin. Pathol. 49:* 500–505, 1968.

43. Sussman, A. S., Lingappa, Y., and Bernstein, J. A. Effect of light media upon growth and melanin formation in *Cladosporium mansoni*. *Mycologia 49:* 307–314, 1963.

44. Thasnakorn, P., and Bhadrakom, S. Isolation of *Phialophora gougerotii* from a Thai patient. *J. Med. Assoc. Thai. 54:* 449–452, 1971.

45. Weidman, F. D., and Rosenthal, L. H. Chromoblastomycosis: a new and important blastomycosis in North America: report of a case in Philadelphia. *Arch. Dermatol. Syphil. 43:* 62–84, 1941.

46. Young, N. A., Kwon-Chung, K. J., and Freeman, J. Subcutaneous abscess caused by *Phoma* sp. resembling *Pyrenochaeta romeroi*. *Am. J. Clin. Pathol. 59:* 810–816, 1973.

47. Young, J. M., and Ulrich, E. Sporotrichosis produced by *Sporotrichum gougerotii*. *Arch. Dermatol. 67:* 44–52, 1953.

48. Ziefer, A., and Connor, D. P. Phaeomycotic cyst: a clinicopathologic study of twenty-five patients. *Am. J. Trop. Med. Hyg. 29:* 901–911, 1980.

PROTOTHECOSIS

49. Ahbel, D. E., Alexander, A. H., Kleine, L. L., and Lichtman, D. M. Protothecal olecranon bursitis: a case report and review of the literature. *J. Bone Joing Surg. (Am.) 62:* 835–836, 1980.

50. Arnold, P., and Ahearn, D. G. The systematics of the genus *Prototheca* with a description of a new species *P. filamenta*. *Mycologia 64:* 265–275, 1972.

51. Ashford, B. K., Ciferri, R., and Dalmau, L. M. A new species of *Prototheca* and a variety of the same isolated from the human intestine. *Arch. Protistenk. 70:* 619–638, 1930.

52. Bernstein, L. H., Lepow, H., Wagle, A., Doran, T., and Brand, B. Is tropical sprue an algal disease of man? *Gastroenterology 64:* 697, 1973.

53. Bodenhoff, J., and Madsen, P. S. Bovine protothecosis: a brief report of ten cases. *Acta Pathol. Microbiol. Scand. (B) 86:* 51–52, 1978.

54. Buyukmihci, N., Rubin, L. F., and Deapoli, A. Protothecosis with ocular involvement in a dog. *J. Am. Vet. Med. Assoc. 167:* 158–161, 1975.

55. Carlton, W. W., and Austin, L. Ocular protothecosis in a dog. *Vet. Pathol. 10:* 274–280, 1973.

56. Chandler, F. W., Kaplan, W., and Callaway, C. S. Differentiation between *Prototheca* and morphologically similar green algae in tissue. *Arch. Pathol. Lab. Med. 102:* 353–356, 1978.

57. Connor, D. H., and Neafie, R. C. Protothecosis. In *Pathology of Tropical and Extraordinary Diseases*, Vol. 2, edited by C. H. Binford, and D. H. Connor, pp. 684–689, 1976.
58. Cooke, W. B. Studies in the genus *Prototheca*. I. Literature review. *J. Elisha Mitchell Sci. Soc. 84:* 213–216, 1968.
59. Cooke, W. B. Studies in the genus *Prototheca*. II. Taxonomy. *J. Elisha Mitchell Sci. Soc. 84:* 217–222, 1968.
60. Cordy, D. R. Chlorellosis in a lamb. *Vet. Pathol. 10:* 171–176, 1973.
61. Cox, G. E., Wilson, J. D., and Brown, P. Protothecosis: a case of disseminated algal infection. *Lancet 2:* 379–382, 1974.
62. Dagher, F. J., Smith, A. G., Pankoski, D., and Ollodart, R. M. Skin protothecosis in a patient with renal allograft. *South. Med. J. 71:* 222–224, 1978.
63. Davies, R. R. Protothecosis and opportunist fungal infections. *Trans. St. John's Hosp. Dermatol. Soc. 58:* 38–42, 1972.
64. Davies, R. R., Spencer, H., and Wakelin, P. O. A case of human protothecosis. *Trans. R. Soc. Trop. Med. Hyg. 58:* 448–451, 1964.
65. Davies, R. R., and Wilkinson, J. L. Human protothecosis: supplementary studies. *Ann. Trop. Med. Parasitol. 61:* 112–115, 1967.
66. De Almeida, F., Lacaz, C. A., and Forattini, O. Consideracoes sobre tres casos de micoses humanas, de cujas lesoes foram isoladas ao lado dos cogulmelos responsaveis, Algas provavelmente do genero *Chlorella*. *Ann. Fac. Med. Sao Paulo 22:* 295–299, 1946.
67. De Camargo, Z. P., and Fischman, O. *Prototheca stagnora*, an encapsulated organism. *Sabouraudia 17:* 197–200, 1979.
68. De Camargo, Z. P., and Fischman, O. Use of morphophysiological characteristics for differentiation of the species of *Prototheca*. *Sabouraudia 17:* 275–278, 1979.
69. De Camargo, Z. P., Fischman, O., and Silva, M. R. R. Experimental protothecosis in laboratory animals. *Sabouraudia 18:* 237–240, 1980.
70. Dion, W. M. Bovine mastitis due to *Prototheca zopfii*. *Can. Vet. J. 20:* 221–222, 1979.
71. Dogliotti, M., Mars, P. W., Rabson, A. R., and Rippey, J. J. Cutaneous protothecosis. *Br. J. Dermatol. 93:* 473–474, 1975.
72. El-Ani, A. S. Life cycle and variation of *Prototheca wickerhamii*. *Science 156:* 1501–1503, 1967.
73. Emmons, C. W., Binford, C. H., Utz, J. P., and Kwon-Chung, K. J. Protothecosis. In *Medical Mycology*, Ed. 3, edited by C. W. Emmons, C. H. Binford, J. P. Utz, and K. J. Kwon-Chung, pp. 511–517. Philadelphia, Lea & Febiger, 1977.
74. Feo, M. 262 Levaduras del hombre aisladas en Caracas, Venezuela. *Mycopathol. Mycol. 39:* 299–303, 1969.
75. Feo, M. Cinco cepas de *Prototheca* de origen humano. *Mycopathol. Mycol. 46:* 53–59, 1972.
76. Fetter, B. F., Klintworth, G. K., and Nielsen, H. S., Jr. Protothecosis—Algal infection. In *Human Infection with Fungi, Actinomycetes and Algae*. Edited by R. D. Baker, pp. 1081–1093. New York, Springer-Verlag, 1971.
77. Frank, N., Ferguson, L. C., Cross, R. F., and Redman, D. R. *Prototheca*, a cause of bovine mastitis. *Am. J. Vet. Res. 30:* 1785–1794, 1969.
78. Frese, K., and Gedek, B. Ein Fall von Protothecosis beim Reh. *Berl. Muench. Tieraerztl. Wochenschr. 9:* 174–178, 1968.
79. Grocott, R. G., Huffaker, A. K., and White, C. B. Protothecal bursitis: a case from Panama. *Lab. Med. 10:* 89–96, 1979.
80. Hadfield, T. L., and Albert, M. Personal communication.
81. Holscher, M. A., Shasteen, W. J., Powell, H. S., and Burka, N. R. Disseminated canine protothecosis: a case report. *J. Am. Anim. Hosp. Assoc. 12:* 49–52, 1976.
82. Imes, G. D., Jr., Lloyd, J. C., and Brightman, M. P. Disseminated protothecosis in a dog. *Onderstepoort J. Vet. Res. 44:* 1–6, 1977.
83. Kaplan, W. Protothecosis and infections caused by morphologically similar green algae. In *The Black and White Yeasts*, Pan Amer. Hlth. Org., Sci. Publ. No. 356: 218–232, 1978.
84. Kaplan, W., Chandler, F. W., Holzinger, E. A., Plue, R. E., and Dickinson, R. O., III. Protothecosis in a cat: first recorded case. *Sabouraudia 14:* 186–281, 1976.
85. King, D. S., and Jong, S. C. *Sarcinosporon*: A new genus to accommodate *Trichosporon inkin* and *Prototheca filamenta*. *Mycotaxon 3:* 84–94, 1975.

238   *Current Topics in Inflammation and Infection*

86. Klintworth, G. K., Fetter, B. F., and Nielsen, H. S., Jr. Protothecosis, an algal infection: report of a case in man. *J. Med. Microbiol. 1:* 211–216, 1968.
87. Lee, W. S., Lagios, M. D., and Leonards, R. Wound infection by *Prototheca wickerhamii*, saprophytic alga pathogenic for man. *J. Clin. Microbiol. 2:* 62–66, 1975.
88. Lerche, M. Einen durch Algen (*Prototheca*) hervorgerufene Mastitis der Kuh. *Berl. Muench. Tieraerztl. Wochenschr. 65:* 64–69, 1952.
89. Mariana, P. L. Ricerche sperimentali intorno ad alcune alghe parassite dell' uonomo. *Boll. Soc. Ital. Microbiol. 14:* 113–115, 1942.
90. Mars, P. W., Rabson, A. R., Rippey, J. J., and Ajello, L. Cutaneous protothecosis. *Br. J. Dermatol. 85 (Suppl. 7):* 76–84, 1971.
91. Mayhall, C. G., Miller, C. W., Eisen, A. Z., Kobayashi, G. S., and Medoff, G. Cutaneous protothecosis: successful treatment with amphotericin B. *Arch. Dermatol. 112:* 1749–1752, 1976.
92. Mettler, F. Generalisierte Protothecose bei einem Flughund (*Pteropus lylei*). *Vet. Pathol. 12:* 118–124, 1975.
93. Mezger, E., Eisses, J. F., and Smith, M. J. Protothecal cellulitis in a renal transplant patient. *Lab. Invest. 44:* 81A, 1981.
94. Migaki, G., Garner, F. M., and Imes, G. D., Jr. Bovine protothecosis: a report of three cases. *Pathol. Vet. 6:* 444–453, 1969.
95. Nabai, H., and Mehregan, A. H. Cutaneous protothecosis: report of a case from Iran. *J. Cutan. Pathol. 1:* 180–185, 1974.
96. Nadakavukaren, M. J., and McCrecken, D. A. *Prototheca*: an alga or a fungus? *J. Phycol. 9:* 113–116, 1973.
97. Neafie, R. C., Connor, D. H., and Binford, C. H. Case for diagnosis (protothecosis). *Milit. Med. 133:* 925, 928, 1968.
98. Nosanchuk, J. S., and Greenberg, R. D. Protothecosis of the olecranon bursa caused by achloric algae. *Am. J. Clin. Pathol. 59:* 567–573, 1973.
99. Padhye, A. A., Baker, J. G., and D'Amato, R. F. Rapid identification of *Prototheca* species by the API20C system. *J. Clin. Microbiol. 10:* 579–582, 1979.
100. Pore, R. S. Nutritional basis for relating *Prototheca* and *Chlorella. Can. J. Microbiol. 18:* 1175–1177, 1972.
101. Pore, R. S. Selective medium for the isolation of *Prototheca. Appl. Microbiol. 26:* 648–649, 1973.
102. Pore, R. S., D'Amato, R. F., and Ajello, L. *Fissuricella* gen. Nov.: a new taxon for *Prototheca filamenta. Sabouraudia 15:* 69–78, 1977.
103. Povey, R. C., Austwick, P. K. C., Pearson, H., and Smith K. C. A case of protothecosis in a dog. *Pathol. Vet. 6:* 396–402, 1969.
104. Pringsheim, E. C. *Farblose Algen: Ein Beitrag zur Evolutionsforschung.* Stuttgart, Gustav Fischer Verlag, 1963.
105. Redaelli, P., and Ciferri, R. La patogenicita per animali di alghe acloriche coprofite del genera *Prototheca. Boll. Soc. Ital. Biol. Sper. 10:* 809–811, 1935.
106. Rodger, R. J. Protothecal lymphadenitis in an ox. *Anat. Vet. J. 50:* 281–283, 1974.
107. Schiefer, B., and Gedek, B. Zum Verhalten von *Prototheca*-Species im Gewebe von Saugetieren. *Berl. Muench. Tieraerztl. Wochenschr. 24:* 485–490, 1968.
108. Schnitzler, L., Belperron, P., and Hocquet, P. Dermatose inguinale chez un enfant. Peut-on incriminer le rôle pathogene d'une algue du genre *Prototheca. Bull. Soc. Fr. Dermatol. Syphiligr. 79:* 126–130, 1972.
109. Schwimmer, M., and Schwimmer, D. Medical aspects of phycology. In *Algae, Man, and the Environment.* Edited by D. F. Jackson, pp. 279–358. Syracuse, Syracuse University Press, 1968.
110. Segal, E., Padhye, A. A., and Ajello, L. Susceptibility of *Prototheca* species to antifungal agents. *Antimicrob. Agents Chemother. 10:* 75–79, 1976.
111. Sileo, L., and Palmer, N. C. Probable cutaneous protothecosis in a beaver. *J. Wildlife. Dis. 9:* 320–322, 1973.
112. Silk, M. H. Human cutaneous protothecosis—an ultrastructural study. *S. Afr. J. Med. Sci. 38:* 1–11, 1973.
113. Stropnik, Z. Alge rodu *Prototheca*, patogene za človeka in živali (Czech). [Algae of the genus *Prototheca*, pathogenic for man and animals.] *Zdrav. Vestn. 43:* 267–270, 1974.

114. Sudman, M. S. Protothecosis: a critical review. *Am. J. Clin. Pathol. 61:* 10–19, 1974.

115. Sudman, M. S., and Kaplan, W. Identification of the *Prototheca* species by immunofluorescence. *Appl. Microbiol. 25:* 981–990, 1973.

116. Sudman, M. S., Majka, J. A., and Kaplan, W. Primary mucocutaneous protothecosis in a dog. *J. Am. Vet. Med. Assoc. 163:* 1372–1374, 1973.

117. Tejera, G. E. Dermatose d'un pied produite par une *Protothèque. Bordeaux Médical 10:* 707–710, 1977.

118. Tindall, J. P., and Fetter, B. F. Infections caused by achloric algae (protothecosis). *Arch. Dermatol. 104:* 490–500, 1971.

119. Tyler, D. E., Lorenz, M. D., Blue, J. L., Munnell, J. F., and Chandler, F. W. Disseminated protothecosis with central nervous system involvement in a dog. *J. Am. Vet. Med. Assoc. 176:* 987–993, 1980.

120. Van Kruiningen, H. J. Protothecal entercolitis in a dog. *J. Am. Vet. Med. Assoc. 157:* 56–63, 1970.

121. Van Kruiningen, H. J., Garner, F. M., and Schiefer, B. Protothecosis in a dog. *Pathol. Vet. 6:* 348–354, 1969.

122. Walker, A. N., and Fechner, R. E. The evolution of the inflammatory response to *Prototheca wickerhamii. Lab. Invest. 44:* 71A, 1981.

123. Wolfe, I. D., Sacks, H. G., Samorodin, C. S., and Robinson, H. M. Cutaneous protothecosis in a patient receiving immunosuppressive therapy. *Arch. Dermatol. 112:* 829–832, 1976.

124. Yip, S. Y., Huang, C. T., and Clark, W. H. Protothecosis, an infection by algae. Report of a case from Hong Kong. *J. Dermatol. (Tokyo) 3:* 309–315, 1976.

125. Yip, S. Y., Huang, C. T., and Clark, W. H. Protothecosis, an infection by algae. Report of a case from Hong Kong. *Jap. J. Dermatol. 86:* 105, 708, 1976.

Index